VOICE AND ARTICULATION

Dr. **KENNETH C. CRANNELL**
Emerson College

WADSWORTH PUBLISHING COMPANY
Belmont, California
A Division of Wadsworth, Inc.

Communication Editor: Kristine M. Clerkin
Editorial Associate: Naomi S. Brown
Production Editor: Jerilyn Emori
Managing Designers: Andrew H. Ogus, Paula Shuhert
Print Buyer: Ruth Cole
Design: Vargas/Williams/Design
Copy Editor: Paul Monsour
Technical Illustrator: Joan Carol
Cover: Vargas/Williams/Design

Printed in the United States of America   **34**

1 2 3 4 5 6 7 8 9 10—91 90 89 88 87

Library of Congress Cataloging-in-Publication Data
Crannell, Kenneth C.
   Voice and articulation.
   Includes index.
   1. Voice culture. I. Title.
PN4162.C73 1987   808.5   86-18918
ISBN 0-534-07164-3

ACKNOWLEDGMENTS:
Chapter 5: "Lay of the Deserted Influenzaed," reprinted from *An Almanac of Words at Play* by Willard R. Espy. Copyright © 1975 by Willard R. Espy. Used by permission of Clarkson N. Potter, Inc.
Chapter 10: "The Wild Duck," reprinted from *Eleven Plays* by Henrik Ibsen. Originally published by The Scribner Book Companies, Inc.
Chapter 12: Excerpt from *Miss Julie: Masters of Modern Drama* by August Strindberg; translated by Elizabeth Sprigge; reprinted by permission of A. P. Watt Ltd.
Chapter 13: "Ode to a Toad Who Died on the Road" and "Tigers and Stew and Young Krishna Panju" by Eugene Lyttle; reprinted by permission of the author.

DEDICATED TO

"Pop-Pop" and Ma Ed and Louise

Jack and Bill

Pat

Chuck and Tracy

Speech is a mirror of the soul:
as a man speaks, so is he.

PUBILIUS SYRUS, *Maxim* 1073

C O N T E N T S

P R E F A C E

THE STUDENT

This text is designed for beginning and advanced students in voice and speech classes. It is intended for, but not limited to, students who wish to have a career in which strong verbal skills are important. Because of its content and suggested techniques, this text would also be a helpful guide for persons studying English as a second language. The material is presented in a clear and concise manner yet is sufficiently detailed to be used by advanced as well as beginning students. Most voice and speech teachers acknowledge the fact that changes take place very slowly. A teacher is successful if he or she has been able to motivate a student to the point where, with concerted effort, the student is able to control the speech/voice during specific drills or exercises. It will take many months (even years!) before the positive changes have become a permanent part of the speaker's verbal patterns.

THE BASICS

This book makes no attempt to force the student to rid himself of regional speech or sound production. It is a recognized fact that some communication experts wish to retain these cultural aspects of speech. I wish to see them preserved as well—but not necessarily for careers in the communication arts and sciences. The emphasis in this text is on *flexibility* of voice and speech. Although an individual will never totally *lose* regional speech characteristics, a good communicator wants to be able to minimize them if they are a career disadvantage.

Each chapter in the book begins with a glossary that contains terms introduced or discussed in that chapter. If the material is to be meaningful and remain with the reader, it must be understood. The text presents those terms and functions necessary for basic understanding.

In addition, appropriate anatomical and physiological discussions are introduced as needed for the students' basic understanding. Students must understand a concept if they are to retain it.

I wish to emphasize that as students and teacher progress through this text, they will need mechanical aids if significant progress is to be made. It is imperative, for example, that the student possess a cassette recorder with tapes. The availability of VCR equipment is also profitable, especially for speech occasions that will occur in the last half of the semester or term.

APPROACH AND APPLICATION

This text is different from other texts in a number of important ways. First, the student is encouraged to develop professional speech through the exercise of a technique called negative practice, in which the student not only becomes aware of the professional manner of speech and voice but also is capable of reproducing either old habits or just plain incorrect speech and voice.

Second, a basic principle governing this text is that both teacher and student can learn by experiencing vocal and articulatory extremes. When these extremes or exaggerations are achieved, we are more likely to make the discovery that the voice and speech we are presently using are, perhaps, inadequate and inappropriate. For we may not know what is out of proportion until we have experienced it. Often the student is in no position to determine what is overdone and feels self-conscious with any modification that is different from habit. It sometimes takes feedback from an objective or semiobjective observer (the teacher or peers), coupled with the student's willingness to experiment, before the right *feeling* is achieved. Being able to hear and reproduce vocal and articulatory extremes is an aid to flexibility.

Third, the text is interested in the application of improved voice and speech skills to various communication occasions, as well as personal development. Personal vocal changes are often easier and more effectively made when attention is given to communication situations and experiences intended for an audience.

Career or professional standards of speech are applied to oral performance and include oral reading of various kinds from literature to oral reports. Because of the book's focus on the application concept of voice and speech, many selections from various speech occasions are included.

In addition, the text discusses the acquisition as well as the elimination of common vocal and verbal habits such as glottal shock and vocal fry. Stage or British/London speech and selected American/foreign dialects that might be important to student career goals are detailed.

Finally, this text is different from other texts in its concern with the role played by kinesics in the communication process. There is a very strong interaction between voice/speech and the use of the body in creating a *whole* experience for the communicator. The speaker must appeal to both the ear (voice/speech) and the eye (kinesics) of the audience.

IN CONCLUSION

No attempt has been made to provide detailed information of an anatomical, physiological, or acoustical nature. The material included should clarify the purpose of specific exercises or drills.

Some of the drills and exercises are the "Old Faithfuls." They are used because they are effective and they work! A note about the use of newscasts: These have been included not because of their content, which often becomes outdated before they are broadcast, but for their style of delivery.

Many of the philosophical tenets of this text have their foundation in the teachings of Charles Wesley Emerson, the founder of Emerson College. Other concepts and drills have been included to give this text additional substance.

I want to emphasize my appreciation to a number of individuals without whose help and direction this text would still be in my lowest bureau drawer. To:

my students, present and past, who have contributed their vocal strengths (and weaknesses) and encouragement to this project;

to my colleagues at Emerson College—Professor Frances La Shoto, my dear friend, who taught and continues to teach me; Cynthia Alcorn, Robert Amelio, the Delucas (Tony and Michele), Arthur Roidoulis, Vicki Nelson, Timothy Thompson, and Jean Gibson—all of whom encouraged and gave me invaluable input;

John Zacharis and Judith and Allen Koenig for their personal and administrative support;

Marsha Della-Guistina of Emerson College for the news and commercial materials;

Inga Karetnikova of Emerson College, Jürgen Hoffmann of the University of Stuttgart, and Consuela Roberto for their help with the Russian, German, and Spanish pronunciations, respectively;

Wilma and Joseph Messina for their technical knowledge and treasured friendship;

Rett Rich of Monmouth College;

Vito Silvestri, my "boss" and friend who persuaded me that I had something to say and made sure that I said it succinctly;

Lea Queener of Memphis State University who continues to make significant contributions to my personal and professional growth in spite of overpowering odds;

Carl W. Eastman, Northeastern University; Dwight Freshley, The University of Georgia; Thomas L. Isbell, Ithaca College; and Willie B. Morgan, Eastern Michigan University, who reviewed the original draft of the manuscript;

my children Ken and Tracy who are a constant source of encouragement, insight, and inspiration;

and finally, Patricia, my wife and special friend, who not only drew the sketches for this text but is also my sounding board to whom I owe—oh so very much!

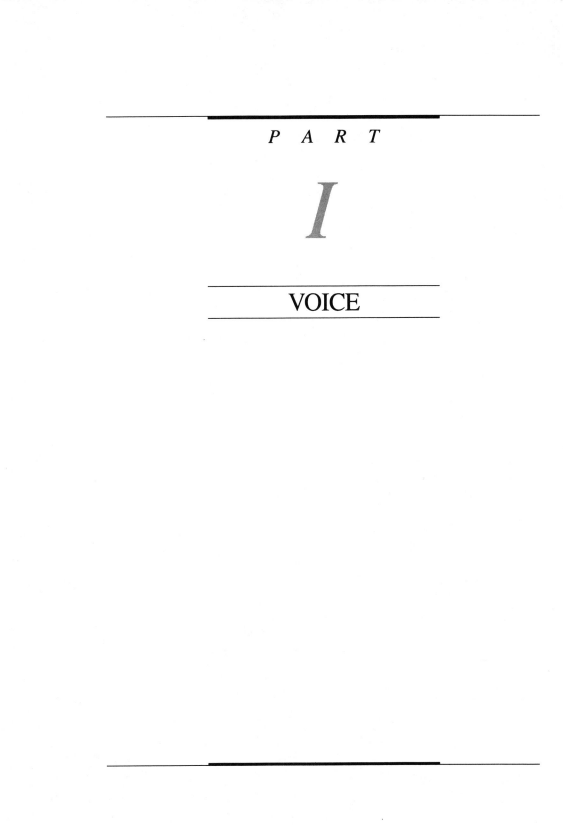

P A R T

I

VOICE

1

MOTIVATION
AND
EXPECTATION

GLOSSARY

Affected Speech/Voice   Spoken or vocal characteristics that are not habitual. Any deviation or change in present speech and voice habits will seem affected. When such changes are developed, they seem natural.

Articulatory Mold   The place where the sound is made.

Career Speech   Voice and speech that are of professional quality.

Cartilage   Soft bone.

Consonant   A speech sound in which the flow of breath is stopped either partially or totally. The consonants give spoken language clarity.

Diphthong   A speech sound composed of two vowel sounds but perceived as one. Any two vowels coming together within the same syllable constitute a diphthong.

Flexibility   Ability to make changes in voice and speech to underscore changes of meaning in connected or dynamic speech.

Habitual   Pertaining to that which is customary or usual. In describing voice and speech, it refers to your present verbal characteristics.

Inflection   A vocal technique that brings attention to thoughts and ideas through variations of pitch.

International Phonetic Alphabet (IPA)   An alphabet of symbols that represent sounds.

Mimesis   Imitation. *Mimetic* is the adjective form.

Muscle   A fibrous tissue capable of being contracted and relaxed.

Natural   Pertaining to that which is not artificial. The only truly natural characteristics are those with which you were born. In regards to voice and speech, the anatomical, physiological, and muscular systems are natural. These are, however, capable of being developed. Since speech is a learned process, it is artificial.

Negative Practice   The learning technique of *consciously* practicing an error.

Nonverbal   Pertaining to everything in communication that is not spoken, such as gestures, facial expressions, and so on.

Phoneme   A sound family.

Pitch   The perception of the highs and lows of sound.

Projection   The action achieved through the carrying power of the voice.

Quality   The subjective interpretation of sound determined by the complexity of the vibration.

Resonance Cavities   The important cavities in which sound can resonate. For voice production the mouth, nose, and throat cavities are the most important.

Speech   How the individual components of vocal sound are produced, combined, and presented.

Speech Environment   The circumstances surrounding a speaking occasion, including the audience and occasion. The speech environment determines the style of speech to be used.

Tempo   Rate at which words are spoken; affects rhythm.

Verbal   Pertaining to words.

Vocal Individuality   A voice response that reflects the most positive qualities of your personality.

Voice   The quality and condition of the sound produced at the larynx by the exhaled breath passing between the vocal folds and causing them to vibrate. The vocal sound is magnified and made resonant by the resonance cavities.

Volume   The amount of force or energy applied to the production of the vocal sound.

Vowel   A free, unobstructed flow of vibrating breath through the articulatory mold. The vowels give the language beauty and carrying power.

The purpose of **speech** is to communicate effectively. Everyone would agree that voice and articulation constitute an important part of that effectiveness. Not everyone would agree, however, on the importance of **voice** and articulation in the total communication process. This textbook maintains that voice and articulation play significant roles in communication. Because of its importance, we will use the term **career speech** (or *professional speech*) to indicate the quality of speech to be achieved in this course. Career speech is defined as the type of speech expected in a career where communication is important. It is not necessarily the speech of the educated, because one can be highly educated and yet have poor speech. It is speech that reflects the best vocal characteristics, with a control of regional speech patterns.

A career in which **verbal** communication plays an integral part demands a different standard of speech and language from a career that is not people oriented. Some of the careers that should encourage professional speech are teaching, theater, the media (radio, television, etc.), business (sales, executive training), law, and the clergy.

HABIT AND NATURE

A student often asks, "Why do we speak as we do?" The answer is somewhat complex. Speech (and often voice) is a learned process that becomes habitual if the speaker's intelligence and physical structure are relatively normal. **Habit** is a pattern of behavior acquired by repetition. When you have a habit, you are addicted to a certain type of behavior. **Natural,** on the other hand, could be defined as not artificial. In all probability, your present speech and voice are a result of habit. It will be difficult for you at first to distinguish habit from nature. You will be frequently reminded not to confuse the two terms.

Much habitual speech is determined and molded by factors that are environmental as well as physiological. The local regionalisms that most of us have developed result from an idiosyncratic manner of speaking that we heard as infants. If you are from Massachusetts and repeatedly heard during your childhood something like "*Lindar* had a great time in *Asiar,*" it would sound quite affected when Aunt Matilda and Uncle Ned from Chicago said, "So Linda had a great time in Asia."

The best time for learning a foreign language is in the early, formative years of life. At that time you are a sand dune just waiting for a footprint! What you hear and mimic while learning to talk seems natural. Now, however, any and all attempts by you, and especially your teacher, to modify or change your speech or voice will feel unnatural or **affected.** This class will be like a war between your habitual and professional speech habits.

In addition to environment, heredity plays an important part in determining **pitch, quality,** and **tempo.** You were given at birth **resonance cavities** and **muscles** that resemble those of your parents. This is a natural phenomenon caused by genes. So the die has been cast. If your anatomical and physiological structure is very similar to that of one of your parents, how much easier it will be for you to sound like that parent. Thus, we have the great similarity between

Liza Minnelli and her mother, Judy Garland. Ms. Minnelli has a Garlandesque quality of voice that she acquired through heredity. In addition, her phrasing, pronunciation, and **inflection** in both singing and speech are very reminiscent of her mother and were in all probability made habitual through imitation, or **mimesis.**

Your voice is not necessarily *you* at present. Although it is the momentary *habitual you,* it may not be the *natural you.* The sound you produce now is created by muscles and **cartilage** manipulated by habit. As you progress in this class, you will experiment with new vocal techniques. Try them all before you choose those that work, and eliminate those that do not. However, before you reject a suggestion, make certain that you do not do so because you are self-conscious. Unless you have perfect speech at the moment, which is unlikely, you are going to be self-conscious about making changes in your voice and speech until such modifications become habitual. Being self-conscious is a good sign because it shows that you are trying something new. You will be trying new speech and voice techniques in exercises. Any self-consciousness is a healthy feeling and should be encouraged in the early stages of change.

Just for fun and to establish a goal or model for yourself, make a list of the positive aspects of voice in speakers you admire. What do you like about them? Surely one thing is their **vocal individuality,** expressed by their voice and speech. But a distinctive voice is not necessarily a positive factor. There are some distinctive voices and speech that you remember because they are produced with a great deal of tension or have such a whining inflection that they are irritating. The fact that we can identify an individual by his or her speech does not mean that that person uses professional speech. After all, Donald Duck's voice and speech are unique, but most people do not want to sound like him. How differently unique you would be if you were recognized by the excellence of your vocal quality and speech!

Habits can be all-consuming, as you know. The strength of a habit depends on what it is and how long it has existed. Uncle Joey's craving for macadamia nuts began when he returned from his trip to the islands three years ago. His New England speech habits developed many decades before that. It will probably be easier for Uncle Joey to kick his macadamia nut habit than to alter his speech.

Your motivation ought to be influenced by the standard demanded by your chosen career. The theories, discussions, and exercises in this text are designed for students who are planning on careers in which human communication is of vital importance and who want their speech and voice to reflect them accurately. No one wants to be accidentally misunderstood. Nor does one want to give out incorrect cues both verbally and **nonverbally.** If you are angry, you may want to mask it. This course is an opportunity for you not to be misunderstood while you learn to express your emotions.

Yes, your voice and speech ought to reflect you, but they ought to reflect what you want to be reflected. You must be the one in control. Then, and only then, are you truly being reflected by the way you sound. How many times have you heard a voice on the radio or telephone and been shocked, appalled, or pleased when you met or saw the person? In order not to disappoint their audiences, some radio personalities have preferred written contact to physical contact with them. If a radio performer has a pleasant male voice and is personable, we are apt to associate a Robert Redford body with the voice even though it may belong to Don Knotts.

This is perhaps one of the most important courses that you can select for your personal skills. When you have understood, practiced, and habituated yourself to the material, you will be more confident about your communication skills.

STAGES OF DEVELOPMENT

All students studying voice and speech must pass through various stages. Obviously, before you can do anything about modifying and correcting yourself, your vocal response must be analyzed. This is where your teacher's expertise is helpful. The evaluation may be written or oral. Some teachers prefer to make at least two copies of a written evaluation—one for the teacher and the other for the student. That way the student's progress can be monitored easily. It also helps in assigning to a student individual drills. Finally, the list of *problems* that a student must overcome can be added to the evaluation. It is expected that you and your teacher will continue to analyze your progress as your awareness of your speech and voice increases. The evaluation given at the beginning of the term might well become your yardstick for measuring your improvement.

Self-Appraisal Stages

After you are aware of your various problems, you must begin the first and second stages of improvement. These stages will take considerable time and cause much frustration. You must train your ear. In the first stage it is helpful to listen to the voice and speech of others. It will be easier for you to hear errors and changes in the speech of others than in your own. This listening process is critical. In the second stage, you must listen to and then apply voice and speech modifications to yourself. When you focus your listening on yourself, you must not be threatened by the potential change. The most important point is that you be motivated to make the changes necessary so that your speech and vocal skills can be the best possible. You have to be "ripe," so to speak.

It is also important that you trust the expert ear of your teacher. At first, your teacher is in the best position to hear what you actually say. You are going to discover early on that what you think you say may be quite different from what you actually do say. This is why a cassette recorder comes in handy. At times, the teacher will have to prove that you said a word in a particular way. It will take a good while for your mouth to catch up with your mind. The important word is *trust!*

Appraisal of Others

The third stage involves listening to the speech and vocal habits of people around you—your roommates, friends, family, classmates, and, yes, your teachers! The fact that twenty or thirty students are scrutinizing your speech teacher will keep his or her mind on the work at hand. After all, your teacher will set the standard for the class.

Also, be patient with relatives and close friends. It might very well be that they like their speech as it is and do not want career speech. Many family members and friends have gone to war over little Ralph's desire to help by commenting, criticizing, correcting, and, worst of all, imitating their voice and speech. Remember that you are listening to *their* speech only to train *your* ear—not to teach them! As your listening skills improve and you learn more principles of career speech, do not try to save the world's speaking habits. You will find that the responses of others are similar to yours right now: "What's wrong with my speech? I've had it for twenty years—that's the way I am!"

Listen to television, radio, theater, and movie personalities. Why do some of their voices "work"? What turns you off to others? Record yourself on a cassette, play it back, and being as objective as you can, describe the person you see. Now that takes objectivity! What do you really look like according to your voice? Get a true image of yourself. Try to develop auditory accuracy!

Unfortunately, some students are unable to develop the necessary objectivity. Some students continue to be enamored of their own excellence when in reality their voice and speech are not very good; conversely, other students with positive characteristics feel insecure and self-conscious. Try to be objective, and listen to your teacher's feedback!

Practice Situation

The fourth stage is to play around with the corrections and modifications suggested by your teacher. This can be a great deal of fun if you don't take yourself too seriously. (That is a helpful adage all through this course. "Take the work seriously but not yourself!") Try the new skills in the privacy of your boudoir. Use a mirror. See how your mouth looks when you practice the new production or pronunciation. Risk it! It is different, yes. It does feel strange. But how did you feel in your first tuxedo or high heels? You felt awkward and self-conscious, but you knew from Mom and Dad (as well as Uncle Ned and Aunt Maude) that you looked great.

A word of warning! As you are experimenting with changes in your speech and voice, make certain that you do not develop an affected delivery. For example, to New Englanders, it sounds mighty affected to say "Carrrr" instead of the habitual "Caaaaa." New Englanders are prone to making all sorts of grimaces while making certain that they pronounce the /r/ **phoneme** in certain words. (A single phonetic symbol appears between two slashes, / /; letters appear between brackets, [ ].) The affectation is not in the sound but results from the speaker's inability to separate the sound he says habitually from the new sound. The same danger exists when you modify vocal quality, rhythm, inflection, or pitch. Use the mirror so you can make sure that you are not making exaggerated facial expressions. Time will take care of your self-consciousness.

Risk It!

This is the final stage before a speech modification becomes habitual. You must try out the new you on your friends, family, and acquaintances. Try to incorporate each new modification as you are working on it. Concentrate on one thing at a time! This is also the time for trial and error. Yes, you will make mistakes, and you will also be self-conscious. But remember, laugh at yourself before anyone else can laugh at you; take the work seriously but not yourself. Stick with the training that is being done in class. Begin to put it all together in your room in rehearsal rather than during an actual speech occasion.

NEGATIVE PRACTICE

Negative practice is the process of consciously practicing an error. This technique is somewhat controversial, since some communication experts feel that it emphasizes the error and thus should be avoided. However, negative practice, when done properly and consciously, can be very helpful. It should be stressed that the individual practicing negatively must always be aware of the problem and the process. For example, if one of your faults is vocal tension, fluctuating between relaxed and tense sounds underscores the feeling as well as the sound of tension. When used properly, negative practice is a very effective tool.

APPROPRIATENESS

Speech that is clear and readily understood is not necessarily appropriate. You should not be adjusting your speech in a vacuum. There must be a purpose, and you must be convinced that the purpose is justified. No one wants you to sound like a clone or a speech malcontent! You often hear speakers who are partially trained. Their pronunciation is so careful and precise that they become cartoons. Even speech teachers err. How many times have you heard, "Danny, speak up! Pronounce every sound in the word." Let's face it. Not every sound is of equal importance in a word. As a matter of fact, not every word in a sentence is of equal importance.

The word *appropriate* is applicable to all aspects of voice and speech you want to develop. Your pitch, quality, and **volume** ought to be appropriate. Sometimes the appropriateness of speech is called the "working tone." The working tone is the quality that is appropriate for a particular speech occasion. Good taste dictates what is appropriate. When a person communicates with another, regardless of the occasion (a public speech, telephone call, conversation, or theatrical performance), the occasion will determine the choice of vocal and verbal response. You must always be big enough to be seen and loud enough to be heard.

You may ask, "How do you know if you are loud or big enough?" You must begin to tune in to your audience at this point. Read and interpret their expressions and actions. Reading your audience is discussed in detail in Chapter 13.

The basis for all voice and articulation work should be a strong desire to develop **vocal flexibility.** A beautiful, resonating voice is worth little without flexibility. There are voices that have excellent qualities in isolation, but lack any excitement or interest.

As in the acquisition of most habits, it is the repetition that establishes a habit. Thus, to change your speech and voice you must drill, drill, drill; practice, practice, practice; and quite possibly fail, fail, fail. One day your speech will turn around. You will be making fewer and fewer errors. Just when this happens depends on the drilling.

As with dieting, the work may not always be exciting. Do you know anything duller than trying to lose weight? You do the physical exercises a couple of times a day. You take in fewer calories because you know that by eating less and exercising, the pounds will come off. Your poor voice and speech habits "come off" in the same way. You must do those vocal sit-ups and deep knee bends if you expect any change to take place. And, as in physical exercise, it takes a long time to see the effects. But then, all of a sudden, you begin dropping pounds. Likewise, in time your new speech habits will take!

To make progress, you must practice the skills that are the means to the end. By the time an actress is on stage, it is too late for her to be concerned with vocal technique. She must at this point keep her mind on her character. If you are selling a computer package to a company, you cannot concern yourself with proper articulation. This is not the time. Stay with the thought or you will not make that sale.

If you are an anchor doing the evening news, you cannot take the time to think about how to deliver a story. You must stay with that story. Often, if the story is not yours, you must read it at sight and not be the least concerned about the quality of your voice or the presence of a regionalism.

However, all of the good thoughts and intentions in the world will not protect the actress from a bad performance or the salesman from the lack of a sale if their basic speech skills are poor. They must put the time into perfecting those skills beforehand. It has been said that some preachers do not have to spend much time preparing to read the Scriptures because when they ascend the pulpit, the Spirit enters and leads them to read well. But it has also been said, "God helps those who help themselves"—by drilling and preparing.

You should practice frequently but only for a short while. And you must practice every day. Pick a few times of the day when you are alone and have good concentration. Establish those times as your regular voice and speech times. At first, practice no more than fifteen minutes at a time, but do it conscientiously twice or three times a day—after your first cup of coffee in the morning and just before you go to sleep, for instance. Then, add a third time during midday. Eventually you should increase your time periods to twenty minutes, and then to a half-hour. With proper concentration an amazing amount of work can be done in thirty minutes.

The most effective way to teach articulation and enunciation is through the use of the **International Phonetic Alphabet (IPA),** which is an alphabet of sounds. The American-English sounds comprise part of the sounds represented by the IPA; different sounds that occur in other recognized languages comprise the rest. The concept of thinking in sounds rather than letters may be quite challenging until you get used to it. However, it is well worth the time spent because the IPA provides a clear, consistent way to represent sounds. English can be very confusing, since letters can represent multiple sounds or even be silent. Just ask a person who is learning English! In the word *through,* for instance, there are seven letters but only three actual sounds. In the word *plumber* there is a silent letter [b]; in the word *palm* the preferred pronunciation omits the letter [l].

Unless an individual learning English has a facility for hearing and producing speech sounds, he will probably only approximate those English sounds that do not appear in his own language. That is one way we can tell that a person is not a native speaker of English. His **vowels** will resemble those used in the production of his own language.

A few English **consonants** do not exist in other languages, such as the [th] sound. Speakers of German or French who are learning English will substitute /t-d/ or /s-z/, respectively, depending upon their age. This is also true of speakers of Oriental languages; in many Far Eastern cultures, it is not decorous to show the tongue; therefore, there are no [th] sounds.

More examples of the problems confronting a person learning English can be seen and heard in the following English poem.

When the English tongue we speak,
Why is *break* not rhymed with *freak?*
Will you tell me why it's true
We say *sew* but likewise *few;*
And the maker of a verse
Cannot cap his *horse* with *worse?*
Beard sounds not the same as *heard;*
Cord is different from *word;*
Cow is *cow*, but low is *low;*
Shoe is never rhymed with *foe.*
Think of *hose* and *dose* and *lose;*
And think of *goose* and yet of *choose.*
Think of *comb* and *tomb* and *bomb;*
Doll and *roll* and *home* and *some;*
And since *pay* is rhymed with *say,*

Why not *paid* with *said*, I pray?
We have *blood* and *food* and *good;*
Mould is not pronounced like *could.*
Wherefore *done* but *gone* and *lone?*
Is there any reason known?
And, in short, it seems to me
Sounds and letters disagree.

OUR QUEER LANGUAGE *Anonymous*

You are embarking on a very challenging task—altering your voice and speech—two very personal habits. You are going to find it a difficult, humorous, confusing, but most of all frustrating task. Don't give up! The time will come when these changes will become automatic. This is perhaps the most important course you can take for your personal development. Thousands have made it through successfully without lasting scars. The job is considerably easier when you can learn to smile—even howl—at yourself.

EXERCISES FOR THE RECORD

You should purchase at least two blank cassette tapes and record the following selections on both. You should keep one and give the other to your teacher for his or her files. (When you become a celebrity, the teacher can make copies of it and make you pay!) By doing this, you will have a sample of your voice and speech before training. With the use of the tape, your teacher can monitor your progress during the home practice sessions throughout the semester.

On your tape give your name and include some impromptu remarks about yourself. This will be your first performance. Speak to the members of the class in a direct manner, and do not mumble into the recorder. This will give you a better representation of your voice and speech under pressure and the stress of performance!

1. Roll on thou deep and dark blue Ocean—roll!
   Ten thousand fleets sweep over thee in vain;
   Man marks the earth with ruin—his control
   Stops with the shore;—upon the watery plain
   The wrecks are all thy deed, . . .

   FROM CHILDE HAROLD'S PILGRIMAGE *Lord Byron*

2. The following selection presents all of the American-English speech sounds in all positions. Thus, it is helpful in revealing faulty sounds and pronunciations.

A mouse went into a lion's cave by mistake, and before he knew what he was doing, he ran over the nose of the sleeping lion. The lion reached out his paw and caught the mouse and was about to eat him when the mouse said, "Forgive me, King of Beasts, I did not know where I was. I should never have been so proud as to come into this cave if I had known it was yours."

The lion smiled at the poor frightened little mouse and let him go. Not long after this, the lion fell into a rope net left for him by some hunters, and his roars filled the forest. The mouse recognized the voice and ran to see if he could help him. He set to work nibbling the ropes, and soon the lion was free.

THE MOUSE AND THE LION *Aesop*

3. It was the best of times, it was the worst of times, it was the age of wisdom, it was the age of foolishness, it was the epoch of belief, it was the epoch of incredulity, it was the season of Light, it was the season of Darkness, it was the spring of hope, it was the winter of despair, we had everything before us, we had nothing before us, we were all going direct to Heaven, we were all going direct the other way.

From A TALE OF TWO CITIES *Charles Dickens*

2

BREATHING

GLOSSARY

Alveoli Tiny air sacs in the lungs that lead the air to the bloodstream; upon inhalation, oxygen enters the bloodstream; during exhalation, carbon dioxide is released from the bloodstream through the alveoli.

Breathiness A vocal quality characterized by the release of too much breath because the vocal folds are not brought closely enough together during phonation.

Bronchioles Tiny branches at the end of the bronchi that lead the air into the alveoli.

Bronchus (*bronchi,* plural; *bronchial,* adjectival) One of two divisions of the trachea that leads air into the bronchioles.

Buccal Pertaining to the mouth or oral cavity.

Clavicular Breathing Respiration in which the upper chest and shoulders are elevated; named for the clavicles or collarbone.

Diaphragm A dome-shaped muscle that forms the floor of the thorax and the ceiling of the stomach; the most important muscle used in abdominal breathing.

Diaphragmatic Breathing (Abdominal Breathing) Respiration in which the muscles of the abdomen, including the diaphragm, are used; the preferred form of breathing for speech.

Expiration The process of exhalation.

Inspiration The process of inhalation.

Intercostal Muscles   Muscles located between the ribs that elevate the rib cage when contracted; important muscles in diaphragmatic breathing.

Larynx   Commonly called the voice box; composed of five cartilaginous structures and also muscles, including the vocal folds.

Lobe   A curved or rounded projection usually affixed to an organ.

Lung   One of a pair of thoracic organs; the basic organ of respiration.

Nasal Cavity   The cavity above the soft and hard palate that leads to the nose; the entrance but not the size of this cavity can be adjusted.

Oral   Pertaining to the mouth.

Oral Cavity   The buccal or mouth cavity; the size of this cavity can be adjusted.

Pharynx   (*pharyngeal*, adjectival) The throat cavity; the size of this cavity can be adjusted.

Phonation   The vibration of the vocal folds.

Rectus Abdominus   The sheath of muscle going from the sternum down to the pelvis.

Resonance   The amplification of sound. In the production of speech sounds, this amplification occurs in the cavities of the mouth, nose, and throat. The size, shape, and physical makeup of the cavities determine the kind of amplification. In other words, the fundamental tone produced at the vocal folds is "resounded" within these cavities.

Respiration   The process of breathing.

Rib Cage   The bony boundary of the chest or thorax.

Sternum   The breastbone.

Subglottal   Beneath or below the glottis; subglottal breath causes the vocal folds to vibrate.

Thoracic Breathing   Breathing while elevating the sternum and often pulling in the lower ribs.

Thorax   (Thoracic Cavity) The chest or chest cavity.

Trachea   The windpipe.

Turbinates   Three spiral-shaped bones located behind the nose that warm, moisten, and filter the air during vegetative breathing.

Vegetative Breathing   Breathing to sustain life.

Vertebral Column   The spinal column.

Viscera   The soft digestive organs in the stomach.

Vocal Folds   Folds of muscle located within the larynx that, when vibrated by subglottal breath, cause most of the sounds of speech.

Vocal Resonators   The three cavities in which vocal sound should be amplified: mouth, nose, and throat.

If you have ever had singing lessons, you have heard your teacher say, "You must learn to breathe from here," as she pointed toward your abdominal region. No one argues with a singing teacher.

The same principle applies to the speaker. Many students view this statement with more than a little suspicion. Why must we breathe that way all the time? Won't we get tired? Isn't it unnatural? These are common questions that will be answered in this chapter. Keep in mind, however, that the proper development and use of breath are basic to good voice and speech. Breath is the foundation of the voice and the speech pyramid.

For humans, there are two functions of breathing. Many voice and articulation teachers do not like to admit the fact that the major function of breath involves **vegetative** purposes, that is, to keep the organism alive in order to fulfill the second function of speech. Whether one breathes for survival or for speech, the action of the muscles ought to be the same, because breathing is a natural process. Unfortunately, the process does not seem natural to many students studying speech and voice!

In vegetative breathing the inhalation is active and the exhalation is passive. In speech both inhalation and exhalation are strong and controlled and hence active processes.

In vegetative breathing, exhalation and inhalation usually take about the same time for all breaths. However, in breathing for speech, inhalation is usually of relatively short duration, while the duration of exhalation depends on the thought being expressed. In addition, breathing for speech is usually much deeper than breathing to sustain life.

TYPES OF BREATHING

There are three major types of breathing: (1) diaphragmatic (abdominal), (2) clavicular, and (3) thoracic.

1. **Diaphragmatic breathing** (**abdominal breathing**) is recommended for the professional speaker by most trained voice and speech specialists. In this type of breathing, a downward movement of the diaphragm is accompanied by an expansion of the lower ribs. This technique provides easier, more flexible control over exhalation.

2. In **clavicular breathing,** the speaker raises the shoulders and collarbone while inhaling. This can be a very exhausting habit. Since it adds tension to the laryngeal area, the resulting voice is often harsh and high pitched.

3. In **thoracic breathing,** the sternum (breastbone) is elevated during inhalation and often pulls in the lower rib cage.

Swimming coaches often encourage clavicular or thoracic breathing in conjunction with diaphragmatic breathing in order to increase buoyancy. Obviously, this combination would present problems for a speaker. And think of the time wasted for a listener while both breathing processes were used!

Since it is the escaping breath (the exhalation) that produces the sound for speech (as it goes between the **vocal folds**), it is only reasonable to suggest that the best use of breath (and the most natural) ought to be encouraged. This is the diaphragmatic or abdominal breath.

ANATOMY OF RESPIRATION

The **rib cage** is the bony structure of the **thorax,** or chest. It is composed of the spinal column (backbone or **vertebral column**), the **sternum** (breastbone), and twelve pairs of ribs, all of which are attached to the spinal column. The top six pairs of ribs are joined to the sternum in front by cartilage (soft bone). The next four pairs of ribs are attached to the one above by cartilage. The two lower pairs, called the floating ribs, do not connect to anything in the front but are attached to the vertebral column in the back. They can move freely. The sternum can be lifted with the rest of the thorax. The lower ribs can be moved outward and upward, thus allowing the thoracic cavity to enlarge.

In between the ribs are sets of muscles called the superior and inferior **intercostal muscles.** When they contract, they pull the entire rib cage upward and outward, an action that enables the lung capacity to expand.

The **diaphragm** is a dome-shaped muscle that forms the entire floor of the chest and ceiling of the stomach. Like any muscle, the diaphragm can contract or relax. And like any healthy muscle, if it is exercised it will strengthen.

The diaphragm is a large muscle that is attached to the vertebral column in the back, to the sternum in the front, and to the lower ribs along the sides. Obviously, you cannot place your hand directly on your diaphragm without its becoming a very messy process. When you place your hand on your abdomen, you are, in actuality, feeling a sheath of muscle located beneath the layers of skin that goes from the sternum to the pelvic area. This sheath is called the **rectus abdominus.**

The purpose of inhalation is to create as much space as possible in the thoracic cavity so that the lungs can sufficiently fill with air. Therefore, proper inhalation creates the appropriate space. The action of the rib cage is often compared with the action of a bellows. As the handles of the bellows are forced apart, the space is increased and a partial vacuum is created. Since the atmospheric pressure outside is greater than the pressure inside, air rushes into the bellows to equalize the pressure. Similarly, as the rib cage elevates during inhalation, more room is created, a partial vacuum forms, and air rushes in to fill the space. During this process the lungs are passive, like two partially deflated balloons. The central tendon on the diaphragm contracts, causing the diaphragm to descend and press down on the **viscera** below it. If you push down on an inflated balloon, it will expand toward the sides and front. This is similar to the effect on the viscera when it is pushed by the contracting diaphragm. During exhalation the abdominal muscles are contracted and the viscera return to their original position.

During inhalation, as the diaphragm is flattening and creating more space in the lower area of the thorax, the intercostal muscles cause the rib cage to move up and out. This, in turn, creates more space in the thoracic cavity. As the size of the chest cavity increases (both horizontally and vertically), the atmospheric pressure becomes greater outside the body than inside, and therefore, air rushes in to equalize the pressure. The natural advantage to this chest expansion is that the lungs can expand to their capacity. In exhalation the diaphragm and muscles between the ribs relax, allowing the diaphragm and rib cage to return to their original positions (see Figure 2.1).

MAKING USE OF A NATURAL PROCESS

The movements described above are a result of a natural process. For example, look at a baby lying on its back in a bassinet. When the baby takes a breath, the abdominal region rises to an amazing degree. With the exhalation, the abdominal region returns to its passive state. Try to duplicate the baby's inflated stomach. You will probably pull in your stomach and elevate your shoulders. Keep working at it until you can duplicate the natural abdominal process.

FIGURE 2.1   SIDE VIEWS OF RIB CAGE AND DIAPHRAGM

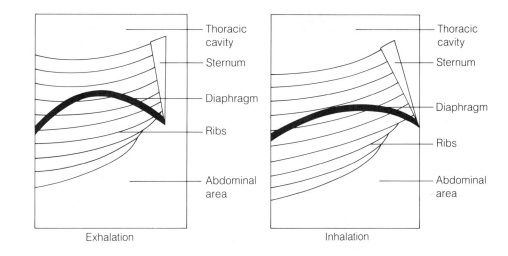

Exhalation   Inhalation

As you continue deep breathing, you may become a little dizzy. This occurs because your bloodstream is not accustomed to so much oxygen at once. This is a frequent complaint of students, but don't be alarmed. You are hyperventilating momentarily. If this occurs, sit down (before you fall down!). Don't let this discourage you from doing your breathing exercises, however. You will build up a tolerance for the increased amount of oxygen in your lungs in no time at all. If you keep in mind that you breathe diaphragmatically in vegetative breathing, the task will not seem so alien.

Posture is important in both breathing and vocal production. Good posture is nothing more than the parts of the body being in their natural alignment. Standing tall makes it easier for the spine to support the body. It is the natural order. If you are stooped while breathing you are inhibiting the diaphragmatic activity. Freedom from tension and full control of the respiratory process are basic to effective breathing.

THE PATHWAY OF BREATH

In vegetative breathing air is taken in through the nose. In speech it is more practical and aesthetic to breathe through the mouth. Try taking a breath through the nose for speech and look in a mirror. You will quickly see why the breath ought to be taken through the mouth—otherwise, your listener thinks he is in need of a shower! Read the following sentence aloud and inhale orally at every slash. Try to visualize the pathway of air from inhalation to exhalation.

/ Mr. President, / I wish to speak today / not as a New Hampshire man, / nor as a Northern man, / but as an American, / and a member of the Senate of the United States.

In vegetative breathing the air passes through the nostrils and enters the three **turbinates**. These are spiral-shaped bones lined with membrane out of which tiny hairs grow. The purpose of the turbinates is to warm the incoming air (done by the spiral-shaped bones), moisten the air (done by the membrane), and filter the air (done by the hairs), thus making inhalation through the nose a healthier process. Whether the breath is taken through the nose into the **nasal cavity** (vegetative breathing), or through the mouth into the **oral** or **buccal cavity** (breathing for speech), the next location for the breath is in the **pharynx** (throat). At this point, the air passes through the **larynx** (or the voice box) and down the **trachea** (more commonly called the windpipe; see Figure 2.2).

The trachea is a tube four or five inches long that is held open by horseshoe-shaped cartilaginous rings approximately three-quarters to one inch in diameter. The open part of the horseshoe is in the back. Across the open end of the carti-laginous rings is a band of muscle, behind which is located the esophagus, or food tube. The open end allows the food tube to have some elasticity, which is necessary in swallowing. The trachea is also capable of getting longer or shorter. Just below these rings the trachea divides, or bifurcates, into the left and right **bronchi.**

The right bronchus is shorter and slightly broader than the left because the right lung has one more lobe than the left and needs more room to expand. Because of this anatomical fact, foreign matter is more apt to be found in the right bronchus. Like the trachea, each bronchus is composed of horseshoe-shaped cartilaginous rings.

The ends of the bronchi branch out into many **bronchioles** (Figure 2.2). Located at the ends of the bronchioles are tiny air sacs called **alveoli** through which oxygen enters the bloodstream. These all work together to form the spongelike **lungs** (Figure 2.3).

There are, of course, two lungs in the thoracic cavity. The right lung has three **lobes** (curved projections); the left lung has only two to allow sufficient room for the heart. The lungs are passive, that is, incapable of moving on their own. When additional space is created within the thoracic cavity, the alveoli are filled with air. At this point oxygen is passed into the bloodstream and carbon dioxide is exchanged into the alveoli for exhalation.

The walls of the thorax and the lungs usually touch. The top of each lung is situated just above the collarbone, and the bottom of each touches the diaphragm. The lungs are coated with a serous, or watery, substance called *pleura*.

FIGURE 2.2   PATHWAY OF BREATH

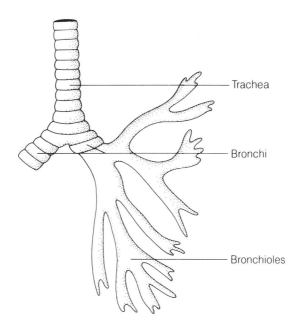

Trachea

Bronchi

Bronchioles

When this coating is attacked by a virus, a very painful condition called pleurisy develops.

Vegetative breathing is involuntary and dictated by the individual's brain stem. Inhalation is active, while exhalation is passive. The amount of air in a person's vegetative inhalations remains about the same. In speech inhalations and controlled exhalations are active, voluntary, and dependent upon the desired message of the speaker. We involuntarily take the amount of air necessary to complete a thought. The depth of inhalation for shouting "Olé!" at a bullfight is significantly different from the amount of air necessary to impress friends with a lengthy tongue twister. This process is closely allied to the psychology of speech, which is a major subject in itself. Inhalation is basically involuntary. However, the professional communicator sometimes takes a deeper breath voluntarily to achieve a desired effect. It is important that the depth of a breath be sufficient to support the intent, thought, or emotion to be conveyed.

VISUALIZING BREATHING

It might be helpful to represent graphically the process of respiration. In Figure 2.4 the vertical scale indicates the depth of the inhalation, and the horizontal scale indicates time. Thus the graph reveals how an inhalation is used or controlled. The top chart illustrates the diaphragmatic breathing of an individual during vegetative breathing, and the bottom chart the thoracic breathing of an

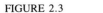

FIGURE 2.3   LUNGS

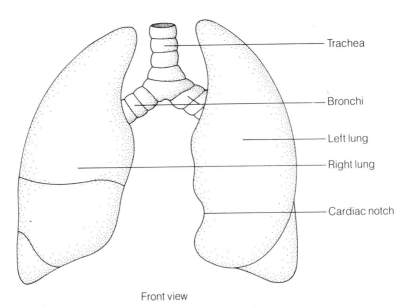

Front view

individual during vegetative breathing.[1] Note that the person breathing diaphragmatically gets more air into the lungs.

During vocal production, the chart for a vocally trained person should look like that in Figure 2.5. Notice that the depth of the inhalation is about the same as that of the exhalation. In addition, because the exhalation is so well controlled, no breath escapes before speech begins. In the thoracic breathing of the untrained speaker's chart, the amount of expended air before **phonation** varies, which greatly affects the quality of the voice.

DIAPHRAGMATIC BREATHING FOR SPEECH

There are many misconceptions about diaphragmatic breathing. Sometimes one hears a director tell a cast member to "breath from the stomach." This is not very helpful unless the director explains the process and underscores the training that is necessary for change. We mentioned earlier that vegetative breathing is natu-

---

[1] Kenneth C. Crannell, "Breathing Patterns of the Individual with a Voice Problem as Compared to the Trained and Untrained Speaker" (Master's thesis, Emerson College, Boston, 1957), 23.

FIGURE 2.4   VEGETATIVE BREATHING

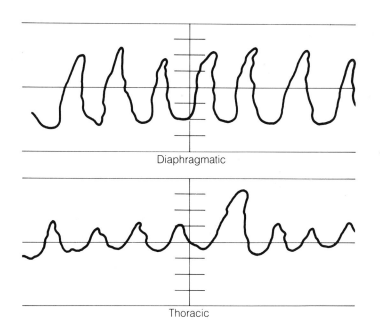

Diaphragmatic

Thoracic

rally diaphragmatic. For some inexplicable reason many untrained speakers (and, unfortunately, even some trained!) shift from diaphragmatic to thoracic breathing when speaking.

To practice diaphragmatic breathing, place your hand on your abdomen and inhale. If your hand moves out on the inhalation and back in on the exhalation, your breathing is diaphragmatic. Now stand up, place your hand on the same spot, and take a deep inhalation. Do your shoulders elevate? Does your hand go in when you inhale and return to the neutral position on the exhalation? If so, you are breathing thoracically. This kind of breathing can have a very negative effect on the speaking voice. The tone of the voice is not sustained, and there are problems with projection. But most important, there is a great deal of tension in the neck and shoulders that tends to spill over into the larynx, creating excessive vocal tension.

Keep in mind that diaphragmatic breathing is natural breathing. However, this does not mean that a speaker automatically uses it. As with speech, one must habituate oneself to diaphragmatic breathing. Since diaphragmatic breathing has a positive effect on amplification, relaxation, and pitch, it is vital to develop good **respiration**.

In time the thoracic breather not only develops poor vocal habits but also tires easily. The abdominal breath is the most natural because the muscles involved in breathing can perform their function without restriction or added ten-

FIGURE 2.5   BREATHING DURING PHONATION

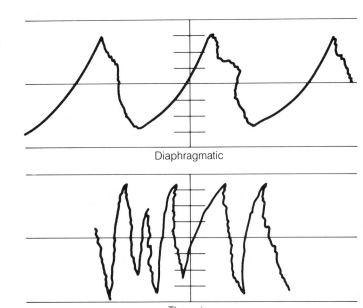

Diaphragmatic

Thoracic

sion. To demonstrate this natural effect of diaphragmatic breathing, do a series of aerobic exercises, push-ups, and sit-ups, or run in place until you are breathing heavily. At that point focus on how you are breathing. It is diaphragmatic. This is the natural way!

You should do the diaphragmatic exercises listed below every day if you want to improve your voice production. Set aside the same time each day. When you first wake up and just before you retire are often practical times. Since some of the exercises do not involve vocal production, they can also be done while you walk to class or work.

The key to making abdominal breathing habitual is to understand why and how the process works. Then you must be highly motivated to do the repetitions necessary for the breathing to become second nature. The length of time required for habituation varies from person to person. In addition, it is important that you do not feel self-conscious. If necessary, do these exercises in the privacy of your boudoir! But the sooner you can do all of the exercises in front of others, such as classmates, friends, or family, the better. Remember that all of your classmates in speech are experiencing similar feelings of inadequacy, hesitancy, and often stupidity.

These are common reactions. You feel as if everyone you meet is viewing you critically and wondering what your problem is. Be careful, however, where you do the exercises, and for your own sanity, develop your sense of humor. Laugh at yourself before anyone else can. It truly makes the process go more speedily, smoothly, and painlessly, and with far less trauma.

EXERCISES FOR DIAPHRAGMATIC BREATHING AND CONTROL

1. Stand up. Place the palm of your hand on your abdomen, stick out your tongue, and pant like a dog. (Remember your classmates feel just as ridiculous as you do!) Feel the diaphragmatic action. When you inhale, the abdominal wall moves out; when you exhale, it returns to the relaxed position. This exercise gives you a good sense of the action of the diaphragm.

2. At home, lie down on your back on a plush Oriental carpet (regular carpets work almost as well!) and place a book on your abdomen. When you inhale slowly through the mouth, make certain that the book is elevated slowly and evenly. When you exhale slowly through the mouth, the book should return evenly to its former position. Do not allow the book to move jerkily. It should return to the neutral position at the same pace as it rose during inhalation.

3. Sit in a straight-back chair without arms. Hold the back legs so that your shoulders cannot be elevated. Breathing through the mouth, take a breath slowly to a silent count of five, hold your breath to a silent count of five, and exhale to a silent count of five. Choose your own rhythm of counting but keep

it consistent. Tension should be on the abdominal region, not on the throat or neck.

4. With your teacher establishing the beat, stand up and repeat the five count as in exercise 3. Your teacher might then count to six, seven, eight, and so on. Make certain that you keep the tension in the abdominal region. Also, be sure that you are inhaling, holding your breath, or exhaling all of the time that the teacher is counting. It is the tension followed by the relaxation that strengthens the diaphragm. Abdominal tension should also be maintained during the "hold" portion of the exercise. Your hand should move outward and inward slowly and evenly during respiration. The teacher might want to alter the rhythm of the counting by increasing the time between each digit. The teacher might set the pace for the class before vocalization begins.

5. This exercise is quite simple. Sit up on the floor with your legs bent. Lie back down slowly, keeping tension in the abdominal region. This reverse sit-up exercise will help strengthen the rectus abdominus.

Note: Make certain that you do not overdo any of these exercises. Obviously, you are exercising muscles and you do not want to injure or strain them.

It is of little use to develop diaphragmatic breathing unless one result is diaphragmatic control. It is the control of the outgoing breath that gives the voice volume, strength, and **resonance**. Proper diaphragmatic habits are essential to a full, resonant voice. To demonstrate the effect that controlling the breath has on the quality of a voice, record the following exercises on a cassette and listen carefully and critically to the results.

6. Take a deep diaphragmatic breath and read the following without controlling the exhalation. Let the air escape as if you were a balloon that was just punctured. Remember, just one breath:

O what can ail thee, Knight-at-arms,
Alone and palely loitering?
The sedge has withered from the Lake
And no birds sing.

From LA BELLE DAME SANS MERCI   *John Keats*

7. Now read the selection in exercise 6 while controlling the output of the diaphragmatic breath. Bring tension to the abdominal area, and just think of filling the room in which you are speaking. If you are controlling the breath properly, there should be a significant difference in the quality of your voice compared with the breathiness of the recording of the uncontrolled exhalation. Remember that both of the inhalations were diaphragmatically controlled, but only the second exercise employed a controlled exhalation. Thus, the inhalation of a diaphragmatic breath is not as important as its controlled exhalation during phonation.

EXERCISES FOR BREATH CONTROL

When practicing these exercises, make certain that your vocalization begins immediately. Keep your loudness and pitch consistent in exercises 1 through 7. These exercises can be done alone or in a group.

Important: During exhalation and speech, your abdominal region must relax gradually. You control its movement back into place. It must return to its relaxed position. Do not try to keep your abdomen out during the entire process. This creates additional tension. The abdomen must return because it is the escaping breath that causes the sound.

1. Stand and place the palm of your hand on your abdomen. With the teacher leading the exercise, take a deep diaphragmatic inhalation, and with a well-projected voice say, "One by one they went away." Exhale the remainder of the air through the mouth. Take another deep diaphragmatic inhalation and say, "One by one and two by two they went away." Repeat the exercise, increasing to "ten by ten they went away." If you begin to feel a little dizzy, sit down. You will gradually build your lung capacity.

2. Stand and place the palm of your hand on your abdomen. With your teacher leading the exercise, take a deep diaphragmatic inhalation. Pick a comfortable pitch and while exhaling produce the vowel "ah" quietly. Increase the volume so that at the end of the exhalation the volume is at its loudest.

3. Complete exercise 2 again, but begin the "ah" at your greatest volume and decrease the projection until you are still sustaining the vowel but at your lowest volume. Make certain that you are bringing muscular tension to the abdominal region.

4. Complete exercise 2 again, but begin the "ah" quietly, build to your greatest volume, and return to the volume at which you began. Keep the tension in the abdominal region.

5. Complete exercise 2 again, but begin the vowel "ah" on the exhalation at your greatest volume, go to your minimal volume, and return to the loudest you can produce.

6. Take a deep diaphragmatic inhalation. At a rhythm determined by the teacher and with a good support of breath and volume, begin counting. When you begin to feel a strain, drop out. Keep a record of your progress.

7. Substitute the alphabet for the numbers in exercise 6.

8. Take a deep diaphragmatic inhalation through the mouth and read the following passages with as few breaths as possible. For your purposes, it is unimportant at present to consider the meaning. Read the selection with good articulation and intensity, if you like. The teacher should set the

rhythm. Keep a daily journal on your progress. How far into the selection can you get before you need to take a new breath? Be sure to keep the abdominal region tense as you speak. Do not force any part of the process. Go as quickly as you like, but make certain that you produce all of the sounds:

a. When you're lying awake with a dismal headache, and repose is ta-
boo'd by anxiety,
I conceive you may use any language you choose to indulge in, without
impropriety;
For your brain is on fire—the bedclothes conspire of usual slumber to
plunder you:
First your counterpane goes, and uncovers your toes, and your sheet
slips demurely from under you;
Then the blanketing tickles—you feel like mixed pickles—so terribly
sharp is the pricking,
And you're hot, and you're cross, and you tumble and toss till there's
nothing 'twixt you and the ticking.
Then the bedclothes all creep to the ground in a heap, and you pick'em
all up in a tangle;
Next your pillow resigns and politely declines to remain at its usual
angle!
Well, you get some repose in the form of a doze, with hot eyeballs and
head ever aching,
But your slumbering teems with such horrible dreams that you'd very
much better be waking.
You're a regular wreck, with a crick in your neck, and no wonder you
snore, for your head's on the floor, and you've needles and pins from
your soles to your shins, and your flesh is a-creep, for your left leg's
asleep, and you've cramp in your toes, and a fly on your nose, and
some fluff in your lung, and a feverish tongue, and a thirst that's intense, and a general sense that you haven't been sleeping in clover;
But the darkness has passed, and it's daylight at last, and the night has
been long—ditto ditto my song—and thank goodness they're both of
them over!

THE NIGHTMARE SONG   *W. S. Gilbert*

b. Rats!
They fought the dogs and killed the cats
And bit the babies in the cradles,
And ate the cheeses out of the vats,
And licked the soup from the cooks' own ladles,
Split open the kegs of salted sprats,
Made nests inside men's Sunday hats,
And even spoiled the women's chats

By drowning their speaking
With shrieking and squeaking
In fifty different sharps and flats.

From THE PIED PIPER OF HAMELIN   *Robert Browning*

9. Take only the diaphragmatic breaths that are indicated by slashes in each reading. Keep a journal on your progress. How long did it take you to finally accomplish this? It can be done! In addition, these exercises are also excellent for articulation.

a./ Do you remember an Inn,
 Miranda?
 Do you remember an Inn?
 And the tedding and the spreading
 Of the straw for a bedding,
 And the fleas that tease in the High Pyrenees,
 And the wine that tasted of the tar?
 And the cheers and the jeers of the young muleteers
 (under the vine of the dark verandah)
 Do you remember an Inn, Miranda,
 Do you remember an Inn?
 And the cheers and the jeers of the young muleteers
 Who hadn't got a penny,
 And who aren't paying any,

/ And the hammer at the doors and the din?
 And the hip! hop! hap!
 Of the clap
 Of the hands to the twirl and the swirl
 Of the girl gone chancing,
 Glancing,
 Dancing, backing, and advancing,
 Snapping of the clapper to the spin
 Out and in—
 And the ting, tong, tang of the guitar!
 Do you remember an Inn,
 Miranda?
 Do you remember an Inn?

/ Never more;
 Miranda,
 Never more.
 Only the high peaks hoar:
 And Aragon a torrent at the door.
 No sound
 In the walls of the halls where falls
 The tread

Of the feet of the dead to the ground,
No sound:
But the boom
Of the far waterfall like doom,

From TARANTELLA   *Hilaire Belloc*

b./ "How does the water
    Come down at Lodore?"
    My little boy asked me
    Thus, once on a time;
    And moreover he tasked me
    To tell him in rhyme.
    Anon, at the word,
    There first came one daughter,
    And then came another,
    To second and third
    The request of their brother,
    And to hear how the water
    Comes down at Lodore,
    With its rush and its roar,
    As many a time
    They had seen it before.
    So I told them in rhyme,
    For of rhymes I had store;
    And 'twas in my vocation
    For their recreation
    That so I should sing;
    Because I was Laureate
    To them and the King.

/ From its sources which well
  In the tarn on the fell;
  From its fountains
  In the mountains,
  Its rills and its gills;
  Through moss and through brake,
  It runs and it creeps
  For a while, till it sleeps
  In its own little lake.
  And thence at departing,
  Awakening and starting,
  It runs through the reeds,
  And away it proceeds,
  Through meadow and glade,
  In sun and in shade,
  And through the wood-shelter,

Among crags in its flurry,
Helter-skelter,
Hurry-skurry.
Here it comes sparkling;
And there it lies darkling;
Now smoking and frothing
Its tumult and wrath in,
Till, in this rapid race
On which it is bent,
It reaches the place
Of its steep descent.

/ The cataract strong
Then plunges along,
Striking and raging
As if a war raging
Its caverns and rocks among;
Rising and leaping,
Sinking and creeping,
Swelling and sweeping,
Showering and springing,
Flying and flinging,
Writhing and ringing,
Eddying and whisking,
Spouting and frisking,
Turning and twisting,
Around and around
With endless rebound:
Smiting and fighting,
A sight to delight in;
Confounding, astounding
Dizzying and deafening the ear with its sound.

/ Dividing and gliding and sliding,
And falling and brawling and sprawling,
And driving and riving and striving,
And sprinkling and twinkling and wrinkling,
And sounding and bounding and rounding,
And bubbling and troubling and doubling,
And grumbling and rumbling and tumbling,
And clattering and battering and shattering;

/ Retreating and beating and meeting and sheeting,
Delaying and straying and playing and spraying,
Advancing and prancing and glancing and dancing,
Recoiling, turmoiling and toiling and boiling,
And gleaming, and streaming and steaming and beaming,

And rushing and flushing and brushing and gushing,
And flapping and rapping and clapping and slapping,
And curling and whirling and purling and twirling,
And thumping and plumping and bumping and jumping,
And dashing and flashing and splashing and clashing;

/ And so never ending, but always descending,
Sounds and motions for ever and ever blending
All at once and all o'er, with a mighty uproar,—
And this way the water comes down at Lodore.

From THE CATARACT OF LODORE   *Robert Southey*

c./ I am the very model of a modern Major-General,
I've information vegetable, animal, and mineral.
I know the kings of England, and I quote the fights historical,
From Marathon to Waterloo, in order categorical;
I'm very well acquainted too with matters mathematical.
I understand equations, both the simple and quadratical,
About binomial theorem I'm teeming with a lot o' news—
With many cheerful facts about the square of the hypotenuse.

/ I'm very good at integral and differential calculus,
I know the scientific names of beings animalculus;
In short, in matters vegetable, animal, and mineral,
I am the very model of a modern Major-General.

From THE PIRATES OF PENZANCE   *W. S. Gilbert*

d./ There is beauty in the bellow of the blast,
There is grandeur in the growling of the gale,
There is eloquent out-pouring
When the lion is a-roaring,
And the tiger is a-lashing of his tail!
Yes, I like to see a tiger
From the Congo or the Niger,
And especially when lashing of his tail!

/ Volcanoes have a splendour that is grim,
And earthquakes only terrify the dolts,
But to him who's scientific
There's nothing that's terrific
In the falling of a flight of thunderbolts!
Yes, in spite of all my meekness,
If I have a little weakness,
It's a passion for a flight of thunderbolts.

From THE MIKADO   *W. S. Gilbert*

e./ Oh! a private buffoon is a light-hearted loon,
If you listen to popular rumour;

From morning to night he's so joyous and bright,
And he bubbles with wit and good humour!
He's so quaint and so terse, both in prose and in verse;
Yet though people forgive his transgression,
There are one or two rules that all Family Fools
Must observe if they love their profession.
There are one or two rules,
Half-a-dozen maybe,
That all family fools,
Of whatever degree,
Must observe if they love their profession.

/ Though your head it may rack with a bilious attack,
And your senses with toothache you're losing,
Don't be mopy and flat—they don't fine you for that,
If you're properly quaint and amusing!
Though your wife ran away with a soldier that day,
And took with her your trifle of money;
Bless your heart, they don't mind—they're exceedingly kind—
They don't blame you—as long as you're funny!
It's a comfort to feel
If your partner should flit,
Though you suffer a deal,
They don't mind it a bit—
They don't blame you—so long as you're funny!

From THE YEOMEN OF THE GUARD   *W. S. Gilbert*

10. Take a diaphragmatic breath through the mouth and read the following selections making certain that you do not allow any breath to escape before you begin speaking. Keep the tone of the voice strong and resonant. These exercises use controlled exhalation more normally. As before, the inserted slash indicates a new diaphragmatic breath.

a. He didn't know which door (or well) or opening in the house to jump at, / to get through / because one was an opening that wasn't a door / and the other was a wall that wasn't an opening, / it was a sanitary cupboard of the same color.

From STUART LITTLE   *E. B. White*

b. It was the best of times, it was the worst of times, / it was the age of wisdom, it was the age of foolishness, / it was the epoch of belief, it was the epoch of incredulity, / it was the season of Light, it was the season of Darkness, / it was the spring of hope, it was the winter of despair, / we had everything before us, we had nothing before us, / we were all going direct to Heaven, we were all going direct the other way.

From A TALE OF TWO CITIES   *Charles Dickens*

c. They tell us, sir, that we are weak—unable to cope with so formidable an adversary. / But when shall we be stronger? Will it be the next week, or the next year? / Will it be when we are totally disarmed, and when a British guard shall be stationed in every house? / Shall we gather strength by irresolution and inaction? / [*Big breath and support it!*] Shall we acquire the means of effectual resistance by lying supinely on our backs, and hugging the delusive phantom of hope, until our enemies shall have bound us hand and foot? / Sir, we are not weak, if we make a proper use of those means which the God of nature hath placed in our power vigilant, the active, the brave. / Besides, sir, we have no election. If we were base enough to desire it, it is now too late to retire from the contest. / There is no retreat, but in submission and slavery! Our chains are forged, their clanking may be heard on the plains of Boston! / The war is inevitable—and let it come! / I repeat, sir, let it come!!! /

It is in vain to extenuate the matter. / Gentlemen may cry, Peace, Peace—but there is no peace. / The war is actually begun! / The next gale that sweeps from the north will bring to our ears the clash of resounding arms! Our brethren are already in the field! / [*Big breath and support it.*] Why stand we here idle? What is it that gentlemen wish? What would they have? Is life so dear, or peace so sweet, as to be purchased at the price of chains and slavery? / Forbid it, Almighty God! / I know not what course others may take; but as for me, give me liberty or give me death!

Patrick Henry

d. Call me Ishmael. / Some years ago—never mind how long precisely—having little or no money in my purse, / and nothing particular to interest me on shore, / I thought I would sail about a little and see the watery part of the world. / It is a way I have of driving off the spleen, and regulating the circulation. / Whenever I find myself growing grim about the mouth; whenever it is a damp, drizzly November in my soul; / [*Big breath and support it!*] whenever I find myself involuntarily pausing before coffin warehouses, and bringing up the rear of every funeral I meet; . . . / then, account it high time to get to sea as soon as I can.

From MOBY DICK *Herman Melville*

e. It is impossible to say how first the idea entered my brain; but once conceived it haunted me day and night. / Object there was none. Passion there was none. I loved the old man. / He had never wronged me. He had never given me insult. For his gold I had no desire. / I think it was his eye! yes, it was this! One of his eyes resembled that of a vulture—a pale blue eye with a film over it. / Whenever it fell upon me, my blood ran cold; and so by degrees—very gradually— / I made up my mind to take the life of the old man, and thus rid myself of the eye for ever. /

Now this is the point. You fancy me mad. Madmen know nothing. / But you should have seen me. You should have seen how wisely I proceeded—with what caution—with what foresight—with what dissimulation I went to work! / I was never kinder to the old man than during the whole week before I killed him. / And every night, about midnight, I turned the latch of his door and opened it—oh so gently! / And then, when I had made an opening sufficient for my head, / I put in a dark lantern, all closed, closed, so that no light shone out, and then I thrust in my head. / Oh, you would have laughed to see how cunningly I thrust it in! / I moved it slowly—very, very slowly, so that I might not disturb the old man's sleep. / It took me an hour to place my whole head within the opening so far that I could see him as he lay upon his bed. / Ha!—would a madman have been as wise as this?

From THE TELL-TALE HEART   *Edgar Allan Poe*

11. Conserve and control the output of breath as you recite this familiar carol; take one deep diaphragmatic breath for each day. Keep the resonance strong to the end of the line. As usual, the slash indicates that you should take an abdominal breath.

/ On the first day of Christmas my true love sent to me a partridge in a pear tree.

/ On the second day of Christmas my true love sent to me two turtle doves, and a partridge in a pear tree.

/ On the third day of Christmas my true love sent to me three French hens, two turtle doves, and a partridge in a pear tree.

/ On the fourth day of Christmas my true love sent to me four calling birds, three French hens, two turtle doves, and a partridge in a pear tree.

/ On the fifth day of Christmas my true love sent to me five golden rings, four calling birds, three French hens, two turtle doves, and a partridge in a pear tree.

/ On the sixth day of Christmas my true love sent to me six geese alaying, five golden rings, four calling birds, three French hens, two turtle doves, and a partridge in a pear tree.

/ On the seventh day of Christmas my true love sent to me seven swans aswimming, six geese alaying, five golden rings, four calling birds, three French hens, two turtle doves, and a partridge in a pear tree.

/ On the eighth day of Christmas my true love sent to me eight maids amilking, seven swans aswimming, six geese alaying, five golden rings, four calling birds, three French hens, two turtle doves, and a partridge in a pear tree.

/ On the ninth day of Christmas my true love sent to me nine ladies dancing, eight maids amilking, seven swans aswimming, six geese alaying, five golden rings, four calling birds, three French hens, two turtle doves, and a partridge in a pear tree.

/ On the tenth day of Christmas my true love sent to me ten lords aleaping, nine ladies dancing, eight maids amilking, seven swans aswimming, six geese alaying, five golden rings, four calling birds, three French hens, two turtle doves, and a partridge in a pear tree.

/ On the eleventh day of Christmas my true love sent to me eleven pipers piping, ten lords aleaping, nine ladies dancing, eight maids amilking, seven swans aswimming, six geese alaying, five golden rings, four calling birds, three French hens, two turtle doves, and a partridge in a pear tree.

/ On the twelfth day of Christmas my true love sent to me twelve drummers drumming, eleven pipers piping, ten lords aleaping, nine ladies dancing, eight maids amilking, seven swans aswimming, six geese alaying, five golden rings, four calling birds, three French hens, two turtle doves, and a partridge in a pear tree.

BREATHINESS

Obviously, much of the vocal characteristic of **breathiness** is eliminated by controlling diaphragmatic breaths and increasing the tension at the vocal folds. There are, however, exercises that should be done in conjunction with controlled exhalation.

To build up tension on initial vowels and diphthongs for the breathy speaker, review the section on glottal shock in Chapter 5. Practice the exercises there. In addition, here is another exercise for strengthening the muscles in your abdomen. Stand a couple of feet from a flat surface (a wall or a door) and lean forward with your hands on the surface. You may have to adjust the distance in order to feel muscular tension in the abdominal region. Then complete a series of vertical push-ups.

A great deal of time has been spent in this chapter explaining how to eliminate the breathy voice by controlling diaphragmatic action with increased phonation. However, there are instances where it might be advantageous to be able to produce a breathy voice. Some of you may be taking voice and articulation as a beginning course to various majors in communication—speech communications, radio, television, or theater. Remember that one of the purposes of this text is to help you develop flexibility of voice and speech. Yes, eliminate the breathiness that is in your personal voice and speech, but realize that the flexible voice is the best voice. The individual who can do many things with his or her voice has more opportunities. As you are well aware, making a commercial or doing a voice-over can be very lucrative.

At any rate, you should be able to make the necessary physiological adjustments to the vocal apparatus so that you can adopt the voice appropriate to the kind of character you wish to present. As an example, if you are an actor in the role of Antigone, you will not want her to sound like the stereotypical weather girl stating that "Rain is expected in the Athens/Piraeus area." No! Antigone is an assertive, definite, now kind of woman, who knows where she is going and what she wants. A breathy quality is often an outward manifestation of a very different sort of character. Antigone's vocal traits ought to reflect these qualities. On the other hand, if you are playing Elvira in Noel Coward's *Blithe Spirit,* you will possibly want to reflect her elegant earthiness partially through the use of a breathy quality. The point is that you want to make your vocal quality appropriate to the character.

The breathy voice is not limited to the female. Most untrained (and, alas, too many trained) male speakers do not control their exhalation, which results in breathiness. The male voice may not sound as breathy as the female because of the differences in pitch and resonance, but the breathiness can still be there. Sometimes you are unaware of breathiness until it has been reduced.

The following exercises have been designed to help you achieve breathiness. Understand why you are doing them. Feel what you are doing. This is a form of negative practice that may well be profitable for you sometime in your career.

EXERCISES FOR BREATHINESS

Take a diaphragmatic breath through the mouth before you read the following sentences and quotations. Let the abdominal region collapse so that the breath rushes out. Then read the exercises with your career speech so that you will not forget what you want to be consciously developing. Record both voices on a cassette so that you also develop your listening acuity. And, as always, concentrate on what is happening to you physically during the process of phonation.

1. It is time to do those dreary exercises.

2. Life is, oh . . . , so very long.

3. After I finished jogging I collapsed into this chair.

4. In Miami the weather is very sunny with 76 degrees.

5. There is sweet music here that softer falls
   Than petals from blown roses on the grass,
   Or night dews on still waters between walls
   Of shadowy granite, in a gleaming pass;
   Music that gentlier on the spirit lies,
   Than tired eyelids upon tired eyes;
   Music that brings sweet sleep down from the blissful skies.

   From THE LOTUS EATERS   *Alfred Lord Tennyson*

6. To be, or not to be—that is the question.
   Whether 'tis nobler in the mind to suffer
   The slings and arrows of outrageous fortune,
   Or to take arms against a sea of troubles
   And by opposing end them. To die, to sleep—
   No more, and by a sleep to say we end
   The heartache and the thousand natural shocks
   That flesh is heir to. 'Tis a consummation
   Devoutly to be wished. To die, to sleep,
   To sleep—perchance to dream. Aye, there's the rub,
   For in that sleep of death what dreams may come
   When we have shuffled off this mortal coil
   Must give us pause. There's the respect
   That makes calamity of so long life.

   From HAMLET   *William Shakespeare*

7. The world is too much with us; late and soon,
   Getting and spending, we lay waste our powers;
   Little we see in Nature that is ours;
   We have given our hearts away, a sordid boon!
   The sea that bares her bosom to the moon;
   The winds that will be howling at all hours,
   And are up-gathered now like sleeping flowers;
   For this, for everything, we are out of tune;
   It moves us not.—God! I'd rather be
   A Pagan suckled in a creed outworn;
   So might I, standing on this pleasant lea,
   Have glimpses that would make me less forlorn.
   Have sight of Proteus rising from the sea;
   Or hear old Triton blow his wreathed horn.

   SONNET   *William Wordsworth*

8. **FS:** Piping down the valleys wild
         Piping songs of pleasant glee
         On a cloud I saw a child
         And he laughing said to me.

   SS: Pipe a song about a Lamb;

   FS: So I piped with merry chear,

   SS: Piper pipe that song again—

   FS: So I piped, he wept to hear.

   SS: Drop thy pipe thy happy pipe
         Sing thy songs of happy chear,

   FS: So I sung the same again
         While he wept with joy to hear

FS (first speaker) more mature voice than SS (second speaker), who is the child.

Obviously, the FS voice would be your career voice and the SS voice would be the breathy voice of a child. Work for the simplicity inherent in the text of the poem.

SS: Piper sit thee down and write
In a book that all may read—

FS: So he vanish'd from my sight.
And I pluck'd a hollow reed.

And I made a rural pen,
And I stain'd the water clear,
And I wrote my happy songs
Every child may joy to hear.

From SONGS OF INNOCENCE
William Blake

9. Little Lamb, who made thee?
Dost thou know who made thee?
Gave thee life, and bid thee feed,
By the stream and o'er the mead;
Gave thee clothing of delight,
Softest clothing, woolly bright;
Gave thee such a tender voice,
Making all the vales rejoice?
Little Lamb, who made thee?
Dost thou know who made thee?

Little Lamb, I'll tell thee,
Little Lamb, I'll tell thee:
He is called by thy name,
For He calls Himself a Lamb.
He is meek, and he is mild;
He became a little child.
I a child, and thou a lamb,
We are called by His name.
Little Lamb, God bless thee!
Little Lamb, God bless thee!

LITTLE LAMB *William Blake*

In this poem a breathy voice could be very effective in creating the child's innocence.

3

THE VOICE

GLOSSARY

Adam's Apple   The bump on the front of the thyroid cartilage.

Arytenoid   One of the two pyramid-shaped cartilages of the larynx.

Cricoid   The signet-ring-shaped cartilage that is the base of, and supports, the larynx.

Epiglottis   The spoon- or leaf-shaped cartilage of the larynx.

Fundamental Tone   The sound produced by the vibration of the vocal folds as a whole unit.

Fused   Blended together.

Glottis   The space between the true vocal folds.

Hyoid Bone   Small bone from which the larynx is suspended.

Laryngectomy   The surgical removal of the larynx.

Larynx   The voice box.

Loudness   The expansiveness of the vibration of sound.

Nasal Resonance   An amplification of the sound in the nose.

Oral Resonance   An amplification of the sound in the mouth.

Partials   (Segmentals, Harmonics) The components of a vibrating agent that are related mathematically. These components are said to be the partials of the fundamental tone produced by that vibrating agent. The partials give the voice its particular quality.

Pharyngeal Resonance   An amplification of the sound in the throat.

Pharynx   The throat.

Pitch   A factor of sound related to the number of vibrations per unit of time.

Processes   Projections.

Quality   A factor of sound determined by the complexity of vibrations per unit of time.

Rate   A factor of sound determined by its duration.

Skeleton   The bony and cartilaginous framework of the body.

Sympathetic Vibration   The vibration of one vibrating agent caused by another vibrating agent without direct contact between them. This is caused when two vibrating agents have the same pitch. This phenomenon is easily observed when one strikes a tuning fork and places it near another that is capable of vibrating at the same pitch; the second fork then vibrates at the same pitch even though there is no direct contact between the two.

Thyroarytenoid Muscles   The vocal folds.

Thyroid   The largest cartilage of the larynx; it is shield shaped.

Thyroid Notch   The Adam's apple.

Tongue   The largest muscle in the mouth.

Vibrating Agent   A physical object that can be vibrated to produce sound; examples are the vocal folds, a reed, and the lips.

Vocal Process   The projection on an arytenoid to which the posterior portion of the vocal fold (thyroarytenoid) is attached.

Before any sound can be produced, there must be an agent capable of being vibrated, that is, a **vibrating agent.** In addition, there must be a force of some sort that is applied to this vibrating agent. If the resulting sound is to be heard easily, there must also be some kind of cavity that can amplify the tone. In a clarinet, the sound is produced by the escaping breath on the vibrating agent, the reed. In the trumpet the escaping breath works on the trumpeter's lips to cause the vibration and thus the sound. In both instruments, the physical shape magnifies and colors the sounds. Rushing breath from between the lips alone would not give Ravel's *Bolero* the same emotional power as it would if an amplifying trumpet were present.

In a piano, the vibrating agents are, of course, the strings with their various tensions and lengths. The force is the amount of power applied to the keys. The pedals also influence the sound. The resonating, or amplifying, cavity of the piano is the area surrounding the strings, and its size varies with the kind of piano: upright, baby grand, or grand.

The sound of musical instruments depends on the quality of the manufactured parts and the subsequent care given them. The same is true of the human voice. You are born with certain anatomical components. These in conjunction with the care you give them will determine the sound of your voice.

In the human voice, the vibrating agents are the folds of muscles called the **thyroarytenoids**. Not too many years ago these vibrating agents were known as the "vocal cords." The word *cords* implied that they were like strings or elastic bands, but the vocal folds are actually folds of muscle. There are two vocal folds, and the inner edges of each can be vibrated by the escaping exhalation. The vocal folds are housed in the **larynx**, commonly called the voice box.

STRUCTURE OF THE LARYNX

Although many voice teachers do not like to admit it, the larynx was not originally designed for beautiful sound. It merely acted as a valve at the opening of the trachea. To demonstrate, if you try to lift yourself off a chair with your hands pushing on the seat, you will feel not only a strong closure at the larynx but also an increase in pressure there. During an effort such as lifting, the vocal folds contract tightly, and air builds up beneath the closure to give the individual more strength. It is interesting to note that a person with a **laryngectomy** (the larynx removed) is physically weaker because such a person no longer has a valve to capture air.

The larynx is composed of five major cartilages as well as muscles other than the vocal folds (Figure 3.1). The five cartilages of the larynx are: the cricoid, the two arytenoids, the thyroid, and the epiglottis. The **hyoid** is a small horseshoe-shaped bone (approximately 1 to 1½ inches long) located horizon-

FIGURE 3.1   CARTILAGES OF THE LARYNX

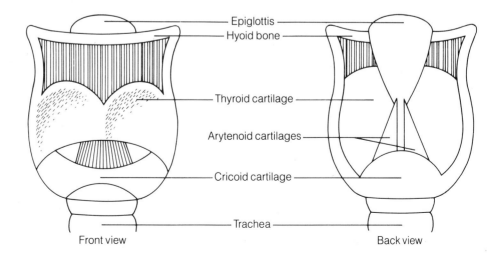

Epiglottis
Hyoid bone
Thyroid cartilage
Arytenoid cartilages
Cricoid cartilage
Trachea

Front view   Back view

tally in the **pharynx** near the base of the tongue (Figure 3.2). The opened end of the horseshoe faces the back. The hyoid bone is considered the only true floating bone in the body, since it is not connected directly to the rest of the **skeleton**. It is held in place by muscles.

In addition, there are many muscles attached to each side of the hyoid that keep it in place. Because of its floating quality, the hyoid is very movable. Its importance to voice production is evident when you realize that the larynx is suspended from this bone. When specific groups of muscles connected to the hyoid contract and relax, the hyoid can move upward or downward. This movement also makes certain sounds easier to produce.

The **cricoid** cartilage is the top ring of the trachea and forms a complete circle. You might remember from an earlier discussion that the other rings of the trachea are three-quarters-closed rings with the opening toward the back. The cricoid is often described as having the shape of a signet ring, with the narrow portion in the front and the wider portion in the back (Figure 3.3). This cartilage is the base of the larynx and gives the larynx some stability.

The two **arytenoids** are paired, pyramid-shaped cartilages whose bases rest on the back portion (posterior) of the cricoid cartilage. They look like a pyramid because they have three sides and a top (apex) (compare Figures 3.4 and 3.5).

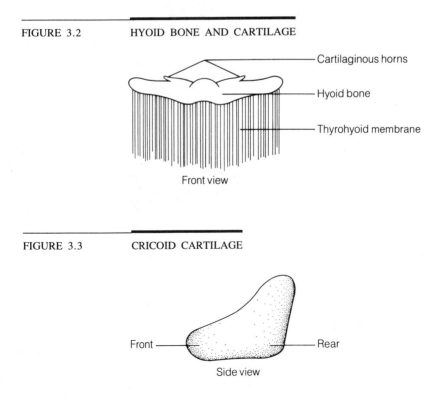

FIGURE 3.2   HYOID BONE AND CARTILAGE

Cartilaginous horns

Hyoid bone

Thyrohyoid membrane

Front view

FIGURE 3.3   CRICOID CARTILAGE

Front —

Rear

Side view

The side corners of each arytenoid (A and B in Figure 3.5) are called the muscular **processes** (projections). To these are attached several important muscles that keep the larynx functioning. Because of the action of these muscles (as well as others), the arytenoids can rotate, move from side to side, and slide forward and backward. The front corner of each arytenoid is called the **vocal process**.

The **thyroid** is a shield-shaped cartilage (composed of two **fused** cartilages) that forms the front and sides of the larynx (Figure 3.6). It is also the largest cartilage of the larynx. The frontal process on the thyroid is commonly called the **Adam's apple**. This **thyroid notch** is important because the vocal folds are located behind it, the front portion (anterior) of the vocal folds being attached to it. The Adam's apple helps to protect the vocal folds.

The vocal folds are fused in the front (just below the thyroid notch) and separate into two strands, or folds, with each posterior end attached to the vocal processes of the arytenoids (Figure 3.7). When the arytenoids slide forward or backward, the length and mass of the vocal folds change. The size of the **glottis** (the space between the true vocal folds) is controlled by the rotation of the arytenoids.

The **epiglottis** is a spoon- or leaf-shaped cartilage that grows upward from

FIGURE 3.4   PYRAMIDS

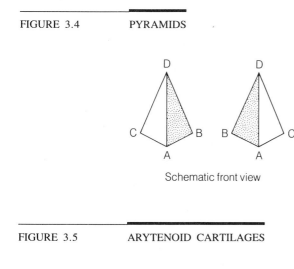

Schematic front view

FIGURE 3.5   ARYTENOID CARTILAGES

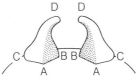

Front view

just above and inside the thyroid notch and rests at the base of the **tongue** (Figure 3.8). When the back of the tongue contracts during swallowing, it presses down on the leaf portion of the epiglottis, making it lean over the glottis (*epiglottis* means "above the glottis") in order to protect it from foreign matter. The epiglottis is not of great importance in the production of sound.

FIGURE 3.6   **THYROID CARTILAGE**

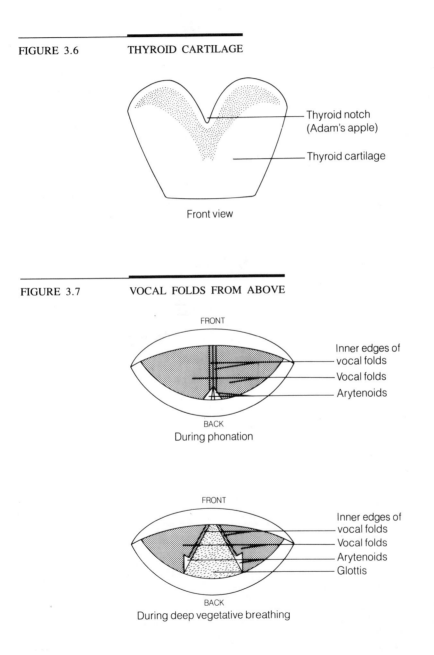

Thyroid notch
(Adam's apple)

Thyroid cartilage

Front view

FIGURE 3.7   **VOCAL FOLDS FROM ABOVE**

FRONT

Inner edges of
vocal folds

Vocal folds

Arytenoids

BACK
During phonation

FRONT

Inner edges of
vocal folds

Vocal folds

Arytenoids

Glottis

BACK
During deep vegetative breathing

SOUND PRODUCTION

The exhaled breath causes vibration when the vocal folds are brought slightly together with just the right amount of tension. The sound that is then produced at the larynx is called the **fundamental tone** and constitutes the general pitch of the voice. At this point in phonation there is little volume or resonance. The sound must be amplified in the cavities of the mouth, throat, or nose with what is called *resonance,* or the *re-sounding* of the fundamental tone, for the voice to have what we call **quality**. A number of factors contribute to how a cavity resonates a basic sound: the size of the cavity, the size of the opening into the cavity, and the condition of the lining of the cavity.

Resonance

There are three kinds of resonance: oral, nasal, and pharyngeal. **Oral resonance** is perhaps the most flexible because the size, shape, and opening of the oral cavity are more easily changed. For example, say the vowel "ah" and move slowly to the "ee" in "see." Feel what the tongue is doing during the transition. The tongue position, the size of the opening (the mouth), and the size of the cavity all change. The fundamental tone remains the same, but through a slight adjustment in the articulatory mechanism a different vowel sound is created.

The least mobile of the cavity resonators is the nose. Only the opening of

FIGURE 3.8   LARYNX

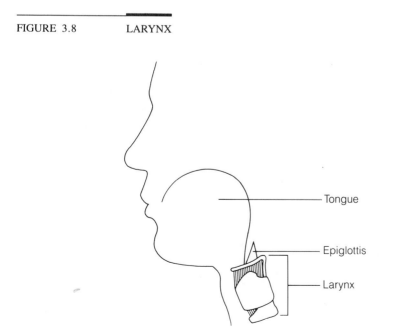

this cavity can be controlled. The only three sounds in the English language that are re-sounded in the nose are /m/, /n/, and the sound of the letters "ng" in "long." Sometimes the nasal opening allows too much **nasal resonance**, or too little. The quality of the voice changes accordingly.

Pharyngeal resonance is perhaps the most important to voice quality. Simple modification of the size and opening into the throat and of tongue placement can change the vocal quality. To get an idea of pharyngeal resonance, constrict the muscles of the throat by making the throat area smaller. Listen to the quality of the voice, which becomes very tense. Now make the throat cavity as large as you can by yawning and producing an overly open throat. The influence on the sound of the voice is unmistakable. Sustain the vowel sound "ee." Slowly modify the sound by producing and sustaining the vowel "oo." You can feel the difference in the amount of tension in the throat and mouth cavities because of the changes in the size and shape of the pharyngeal cavity.

Forced and Sympathetic Vibration

Forced vibration results when one vibrating object is placed directly upon another, causing the second object to vibrate. A forced vibration occurs, for example, when a vibrating tuning fork is placed directly on another tuning fork, causing the second to vibrate. Helen Keller learned the concept of vibration by feeling it in the wood of a piano or the floor upon which she stood. She also felt with her hand the vibration created within the larynx. Since forced vibration cannot be easily controlled, it is not important in developing voice for the average person.

Sympathetic vibration occurs when one frequency is in harmony with another. For example, when one tuning fork at a particular pitch is struck, it can cause another to vibrate at the same frequency without any direct contact. The cause of the vibration of the second tuning fork is indirect. Sympathetic vibration takes place in the three major cavities related to the production of speech sounds: the nose, throat, and mouth. By changing the size of the opening and the shape of the cavity, different choices of resonance can be made.

Factors of Sound

After the fundamental tone is produced at the vocal folds, there are four characteristics that need to be considered. They are frequently called the factors of sound: pitch, rate, loudness, and quality.

Pitch is determined by the number of vibrations per unit of time. In voice, this is determined by the thickness of the vocal folds (the pitch is lowered as the thickness increases), the length of the vocal folds (the pitch is lowered as the length decreases), the density of the vocal folds (the pitch is lowered as density increases), and the amount of tension in the vocal folds (the pitch is raised as the tension increases). The more vibrations there are per unit of time (also called *frequency*), the higher the pitch; the fewer vibrations, the lower the pitch (Figure 3.9). For example, the strings of a piano that produce the higher notes are shorter and thinner than the wires that produce the lower notes.

The second factor is that of **rate**, or duration of sound. A sound must be capable of being prolonged for a certain length of time for it to be heard and the sound understood. If the duration of the sound is increased, the tempo slows. For example, if the vowel sound in the word "man" is prolonged, the tempo of the word is slowed down. When the duration is decreased, the tempo speeds up. One of the common characteristics of poor voice and speech habits, unintelligibility, results from not giving speech sounds (particularly vowels and diphthongs) enough time in production. Controlling the time factor is also used in making inflections, which will be discussed in Chapter 9.

The third characteristic of voice and speech is **loudness**. This involves the expansiveness of the vibration. The greater the vibration, the louder the tone. The amount of power applied to the vibrating agent determines how far the vibrating body moves in its vibration and consequently how loud the sound produced will be. In the production of voice and speech, loudness is determined by the amount of breath during exhalation, the relative condition of the vocal folds, and the amplification by the resonance cavities. Figure 3.10 depicts loudness.

Perhaps the most difficult factor to describe is vocal quality, which is determined by the amplitude and complexity of the vibration. The vocal folds, for

FIGURE 3.9   PITCH

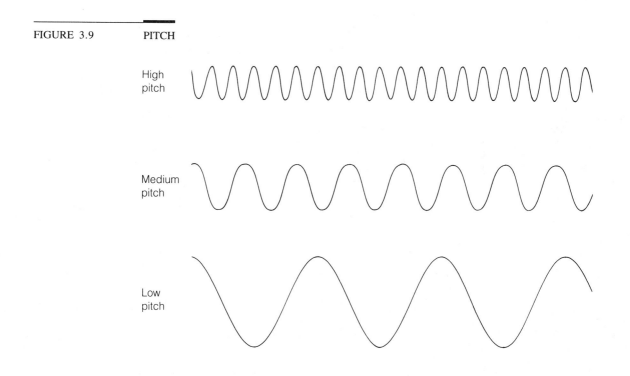

High pitch

Medium pitch

Low pitch

example, vibrate as a whole, giving the aforementioned fundamental tone. The vocal folds also vibrate in *parts* called **partials**, *segmentals,* or *harmonics*. These parts are tuned to, or are in harmony with, different chambers in the resonance cavities. These chambers will select those partials with which they are sympathetic. It is the partials or segmentals that give each voice its unique vibration, thus making voices recognizable. As a matter of fact, the vowels are produced when the cavity sizes change, and they select certain partials to amplify rather than others. Two students may produce the same fundamental tone, but the differences between their voices will be determined by their partials and the resonators.

The anatomical structure of the larynx has been presented here in a most simplistic manner. You must be aware of the basic laryngeal structure if the exercises are to be at all meaningful. If you have the need or the interest, consult Virgil Anderson's *Training the Speaking Voice* and Hilda Fisher's *Improving Voice and Articulation,* both of which describe the anatomy and physiology of speech and voice in greater detail.

FIGURE 3.10   LOUDNESS

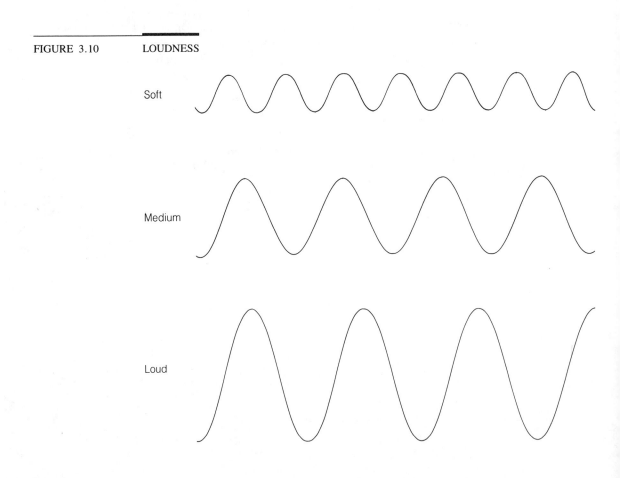

Soft

Medium

Loud

4

VOCAL
RELAXATION

GLOSSARY

Acoustic   Related to the ear.

Habitual Pitch   (Modal Pitch) The pitch that you usually use.

Kinesics   The study or science of movement.

Kinesthetic   The sensory perception of muscular movement.

Medulla Oblongata   The lowest part of the brain, located at the top of vertebral column.

Muscle Memory   The ability to reproduce a remembered muscular activity.

Open Throat   Optimal pharyngeal resonance; a relaxed throat.

Optimum Pitch   The best pitch for your voice, determined by your physical structure.

Overly Open Throat   A voice quality that sounds too relaxed; a yawning quality.

Projection   The act of controlling the loudness.

Tight Throat   Excessive tension in the throat; the opposite of an open throat.

GAINING THE "SOUNDER" VOICE

Human vocal communication can be categorized into three types: (1) conversational, (2) singing, and (3) career or professional. Each communicator can use, in varying degrees, all of these voices. On a continuum, they would be represented in the following way:

conversational ——— career ——— singing

Since conversational speech develops as an individual learns to communicate with another, the conversational voice usually develops accordingly and without the need for concentrated study. Conversational speech is a natural means of communication that is learned through observation and entails a great deal of trial and error.

For instance, say a child wants a drink of milk. He asks his mother for "moo-moo." She laughs, thinks that the expression is cute, and gives him a glass of milk. As long as he gets his milk when he says "moo-moo," why does he need to say the word *milk?* Then years pass. This particular diction (or choice of words) causes more than one raised eyebrow when the now teen-ager asks the football coach for a glass of moo-moo after the big game. Of course, such an expression might be accepted from a person who has speech or linguistic pathology.

However, the singing voice or tone does require study. Since speech differs from song in the same way that walking differs from dance, some people feel that no amount of practice will produce a pleasant singing voice. This may be hard fact about a few people whom you know! Nevertheless, almost any singing voice can be improved through ear training and properly producing the vowel or diphthong, for it is the vowel that gives language its projection and beauty of tone.

Projection is characteristic of the career voice as well as the singing voice. At the basis of projection is the proper use of breath. It is very important to learn to control the exhalation. Besides a very definite difference in volume, controlled exhalation frequently changes the quality of the voice. A steadiness of tone also develops. The voice without diaphragmatic control often wavers and sometimes cracks. This applies to both the singing and speaking voices. The quality of the tone depends upon the use and structure of the resonance cavities (see Chapter 3).

The student is encouraged to pull away from the singing voice in order to get a career voice. The type of public communication, the audience, and the material discussed all determine the speaker's proper voice. A public speech entitled "An End to MTV" would utilize a career voice toward the conversational end of the continuum rather than the singing end. On the other hand, a performance of Dylan Thomas's "Fern Hill" with all of its heightened use of sound might be better served if the performer used career speech that leaned toward the singing end of the continuum.

At any rate, career voice and speech ought to possess a pleasant quality, appropriate projection, and vocal dynamics that suggest a thinking individual. It is important to note that resonance determines quality; breath control determines projection, and mind determines vocal dynamics. If you wish to improve your projection, work on your breath control. If you are unhappy with the quality of your voice because it is nasal, denasal, or thin, develop good resonance. The vocal dynamics that convey your meaning to your listeners depend upon intelligence as well as vocal quality and projection.

OPEN THROAT

A speaker is encouraged to use what is generally called an **open throat**. When the throat is open (relaxed), the sound of the voice is not only more pleasant but can be sustained with the least effort. This does not mean that an open throat ought to be used all of the time. The intention of the thought will dictate the degree of openness. A performer needs to control the degree of relaxation according to the content. If you want to show a relaxed, caring, thoughtful person who is very much at ease in a given situation, the open throat is the sound to use. The open throat has also been called the *working tone*. The working tone is appropriate for the event, the size of the room, the material, and audience. Using a microphone makes choosing the appropriate working tone even more complex.

If as an actor or another type of performer you wish to reveal overt tension, you need to select the degree of tightness. The material dictates the appropriate vocal response.

However, for your habitual sound, the open throat (pharyngeal resonance) is strongly recommended. This is the best voice because when you want to appear relaxed in a tense situation (being interviewed for a job, for example), you want your voice and speech to behave accordingly. It is most unlikely that you will be able to achieve an open throat under pressure if it is not developed and made a habit. You will be too busy with other details, like words! In the same way, ministers or priests cannot use the open throat only in their gospel readings and sermons. The relaxed voice must be made habitual. This is hard work.

The relaxed quality in open throat can be achieved only when the pharynx is relaxed. Muscular tension must be taken away from the laryngeal area and placed in the abdominal region. Part of the vocal tension in most untrained speakers is decreased when they devote proper attention to diaphragmatic breathing.

Your first achievement must be to compare the extremes! Tighten up the voice. Feel how this constriction affects your throat physically. Now relax the throat. Yawn out the sound and feel what your pharyngeal muscles do. This is called **overly open throat**. Granted, this is not the most energetic-sounding quality. It is the sound you make when you talk while yawning. In a relaxed position, take a quick breath through the mouth and quietly vocalize the exhalation. The sound produced is overly open. Yes, there is some tension in the yawning process, but it is not excessive. Now say the following sentence with the same quality of overly open throat: I am speaking with an overly open throat. No, this is not the new professional vocal quality that this text has been espousing. This kind of voice is an extreme but it is not the product of total relaxation! Total relaxation would not be very useful. Become aware of how an overly open throat is produced. Feel what the mouth, throat, and tongue are doing.

Now reverse the extreme again and speak the same material with a very contracted, tense throat. Do you feel the difference? Place your open hand around the front of your neck. While you repeat the exercise, focus on the difference in feeling between the two extremes of tension. Say the exercises with your habitual quality. Toward which end of the continuum do your voice and pharyngeal muscles lean—tight or overly relaxed? Remember that overly open throat is merely an exercise. After you feel more comfortable with the sound of overly open throat and can achieve it at will, you can learn how to pull away from that extreme to gain open throat. For the moment, stick with overly open throat so that you get used to the feeling of reduced muscular tension and the sound of exaggerated vocal relaxation.

What are some of the more positive aspects of a pleasant speaking voice? First, the voice has to be loud enough to be heard easily; thus appropriate projection is necessary. A variation in the rate of speech is also important. Usually an effective speaker slows down when delivering important points and passes over less important material rather quickly. Frequently a lower pitch is also characteristic of good speaking habits because it is more easily heard. Certainly, precise articulation and enunciation are important to good voice and speech. You have already learned the importance of good diaphragmatic breathing habits. The last and perhaps most important factor is the amount of relaxation in the speaker's voice.

Most untrained speakers speak with too much vocal tension. Very little good is achieved in acquiring the positive vocal habits suggested above unless excessive vocal tension is decreased. Therefore, it makes little sense to focus on articulatory problems or good inflection without minimizing the amount of tension first. A speaker may acquire excellent pitch, rate, and projection and still be abrasive if the voice is tense. In general, it is much easier to pull away from the overly open quality (overly relaxed) and gain good open throat than to add good voice and speech characteristics to the voice that is basically tense.

OVERLY OPEN THROAT EXERCISES

There are three ways to achieve overly open throat: (1) taking a quick breath through the mouth, (2) yawning, and (3) vomiting. Of the three possibilities, a quick breath through the mouth seems the most desirable!

Exercises 1 through 4 could be used as warm-up exercises for each class.

1. Begin each relaxation session by stimulating the area at the base of the **medulla oblongata** (the area where the base of the skull meets the vertebral column). With the middle three fingers of each hand, gently massage the area

on each side of the spinal column. You will probably feel little balls of muscle. Gently massage the area until the "crunchies" are minimized.

2. Rotate the left shoulder six times; rotate the right shoulder six times; rotate both shoulders six times. During this procedure it is normal to experience the dreaded "crunchies"!

3. Allow your head to fall forward slowly and gently as if you had no neck. Then slowly rotate your head to the right, all the way back; let your head touch your shoulders; continue all the way left and down in front again. Continue this rotation five times around. Then reverse the direction five times around. Be careful that you do this gently with no jarring or jerky movements. You do not want to end up in a neck brace! *Warning: People with neck problems should not do this exercise!*

4. Shake out both hands! Pretend that you are trying to shake off a sticky piece of candy wrapper from the ends of your fingers. Then shake out your arms in the same manner. (Obviously, it was a bi-i-i-g candy bar!)

5. Now you are ready to yawn. This is a nonverbal preparation for exercise 6. After several yawns, introduce vibration of the vocal folds (this is a vocalized yawn). Then say, "I am yawning." Feel what is happening in the musculature of the pharynx.

6. Place your hands on your abdomen. After taking a quick diaphragmatic breath through the mouth, imitate a popular television cartoon character by saying: "Yogi Baby," "Yabba-dabba doo," and "Hey, Boo Boo." Make sure that you imitate the style of vocal presentation. You are not supposed to sound too intelligent—that is part of the fun in this exercise. Gain the "speak on the yawn" quality. At first, complete this exercise in a group. You will feel less ridiculous!

7. After taking a quick diaphragmatic breath through the mouth, imitate the stereotypical punch-drunk fighter saying, "Gee, ma, it was a great fight!" (Hear that bell ring in the background.)

8. Pretend that you are a graduate of the Ted Baxter School of Broadcasting. Imitate him as he says, "This is Ted Baxter with the latest news." (The more obnoxious you are, the better! And don't forget to use your face and the cocked head.)

9. Give your best ghost imitation as you recite the following passage from *Hamlet*. Use your face and let go with the overly open throat quality:

I am thy father's spirit;
Doom'd for a certain term to walk the night,
And for the day confined to fast in fires,
Till the foul crimes done in my days of nature
Are burnt and purg'd away. But that I am forbid

To tell the secrets of my prison-house,
I could a tale unfold whose lightest word
Would harrow up thy soul, freeze thy young blood,
Make thy two eyes, like stars, start from their spheres,
Thy knotted and combined locks to part
And each particular hair to stand on end,
Like quills upon the fretful porpentine:
But this eternal blazon must not be
To ears of flesh and blood.—List, list, O, list!—
If thou didst ever thy dear father love, . . .
Revenge his foul and most unnatural murder.

Attention! When doing exercise 9, the quality of voice should not be strained or tense. If it is, you are not vocalizing properly. Check with the teacher immediately. Overly open throat should be an easy sound to produce. If you have any doubt about the quality, don't do the exercise until you know you are producing it without strain. Otherwise, you might damage your voice as well as make bad vocal characteristics habitual. Use your cassette recorder to hear the various qualities.

Speaking with an overly open throat becomes easier after using it in group exercises in class. Your teacher will help you attain it and make certain that you can reproduce it before you practice in private. The more frequently you exercise overly open throat, the more quickly you will become accustomed to it.

After you can successfully produce overly open throat, it is time to learn how to pull away from that quality to achieve the desired open throat, or *pharyngeal resonance*. Nasal resonance is also a characteristic of open throat. These are acquired, in part, by applying the rules of good diaphragmatic breathing while increasing the projection. Of course, this stresses the control of the exhalation. Record yourself as you compare and contrast vocal qualities. This will be a very frustrating period for you. At times, you will not know which is which or what is what! This is quite natural. In time, as your **kinesthetic** sense and hearing acuity improve, you will be able to differentiate the vocal qualities.

You can develop the various types of relaxation by doing the following exercise several times a day: Take a diaphragmatic breath. With increased awareness of vowel and consonant production, say "I am speaking with an overly open throat" as you attempt to do so. Then pull away from that quality and say, "I am speaking with an open throat"; then pull away more and say, "I am speaking with a tight throat." Feel the change in vocal and laryngeal tension as you pull more and more away from overly open throat.

In all probability, the pharyngeal resonance in open throat is not characteristic of your habitual voice. Open throat must be made a habit if you want a profession in communication. This new vocal response is not the *you* with whom you are familiar. It is most usual to feel self-conscious, unnatural, and silly, but it will be well worth it to you professionally to take the time necessary to habituate yourself to the new sound that reveals the best elements of your voice. Those elements comprise your *natural* voice.

However, you cannot save open throat for those important moments when you want to sound your best. The faster you incorporate open throat into your own speech patterns, the better. It must be emphasized over and over again that you must tune into the kinesthetic as well as the **acoustic** elements. With open throat, it is particularly important that you feel what the musculature is doing. It stands to reason that muscles that are constantly tense (as in **tight throat**) must affect the quality of the voice.

vocal Tension (Reduce - eliminate)

NASAL RESONANCE EXERCISES

Now that you have open throat, at least theoretically, apply the principles that you have learned to the following exercises for developing good nasal resonance.

1. Produce a good humming sound. Do not clench the teeth. Bring the lips slightly and gently together to prepare for the hum. As you hum, get the sound in the oral as well as the nasal cavity. Feel the vibrating breath trying to get out between the two lips. Make sure that you feel strong vibration in the nasal cavity.

2. Hum the sounds /m/ and /n/ and the sound of the letters "ng," changing from one to the next and then back again. This humming tone amplifies the nasal resonance. This exercise demonstrates that your mouth will open and close without altering the basic fundamental tone.

3. Sing the name of the city in Alaska, Nome, on one note. Prolong each of the sounds individually before going on to the next: /n:o:m:/. (The colon after a sound indicates that the sound is to be prolonged.) A less scientific way of representing it is: NNNNNNOOOOOOMMMMMM. Make sure that you glide from one sound to the next without interfering with the vocal quality.

4. Repeat the exercise above but reverse "Nome" to get "moan."

5. Say the following sound combinations with adequate projection, good open throat, one diaphragmatic breath, and solid nasal resonance on /m/. Try to keep the same feeling throughout the exercise, especially with the vocal attack on the isolated vowel in the final position:

[m "ah"], [z "ah"], [sk "ah"], ["ah"]

The introduction of the consonants in this exercise brings attention to additional articulators besides the nasal and oral cavities: the lips "m," the teeth "z," and the teeth and velum "sk." Also make certain that there is a vocal ease between the last two "ah" vowels. This is also an excellent exercise for developing glottal or vocal shock (see page 81).

6. Read each of the following selections using pharyngeal resonance. Do not worry about articulation or inflection. Simply concentrate on attaining open throat. Vary the tonal qualities intentionally. For example, read an entire selection, alternating the use of overly open throat, open throat, and tight throat line by line. Then, reverse the procedure. Another pattern is to omit tight throat and work exclusively with overly open throat and open throat. In these important exercises, you should be learning to control voluntarily the quality of voice being produced. Finally, read the selections with open throat exclusively and feel the comfort and ease in addition to hearing the difference in quality.

a. Tomorrow, and tomorrow, and tomorrow
   Creeps in this petty pace from day to day
   To the last syllable of recorded time;
   And all our yesterdays have lighted fools
   The way to dusty death. Out, out, brief candle!
   Life's but a walking shadow, a poor player
   That struts and frets his hour upon the stage
   And then is heard no more; it is a tale
   Told by an idiot, full of sound and fury,
   Signifying nothing.

   From MACBETH *Shakespeare*

b. Abou Ben Adhem (may his tribe increase!)
   Awoke one night from a deep dream of peace,
   And saw, within the moonlight in his room,
   Making it rich, and like a lily in bloom,
   An angel writing in a book of gold:—
   Exceeding peace had made Ben Adhem bold,
   And to the presence in the room he said,
   "What writest thou?"—The vision raised its head,
   And with a look made of all sweet accord,
   Answered, "The names of those who love the Lord."
   "And is mine one?" said Abou. "Nay, not so,"
   Replied the angel. Abou spoke more low,
   But cheerily still; and said, "I pray thee then,
   Write me as one that loves his fellow-men."

   The angel wrote, and vanished. The next night
   It came again, with a great awakening light,
   And showed the names whom love of God had blessed,
   And lo! Ben Adhem's name led all the rest!

   ABOU BEN ADHEM *Leigh Hunt*

c. Hear this, all ye people; give ear, all ye inhabitants of the world: Both low and high, rich and poor, together. My mouth shall speak of wisdom; and the meditation of my heart shall be of understanding. I will incline mine ear to a parable: I will open my dark saying upon the harp. Wherefore should I fear in the days of evil, when the iniquity of my heels shall compass me about. They that trust in their wealth, and boast themselves in the multitude of their riches; None of them can by any means redeem his brother, nor give to God a ransom for him.

From PSALM 49

d. One word is too often profaned
   For me to profane it,
   One feeling too falsely disdained
   For thee to disdain it.
   One hope is too like despair
   For prudence to smother,
   And Pity from thee more dear
   Than that from another.

   I can give not what men call love,
   But wilt thou accept not
   The worship the heart lifts above
   And the Heavens reject not:
   The desire of the moth for the star,
   Of the night for the morrow,
   The devotion to something afar
   From the sphere of our sorrow?

   TO _____   *Percy Bysshe Shelley*

e. High on a mountain's highest ridge,
   Where oft the stormy winter gale
   Cuts like a scythe, while through the clouds
   It sweeps from vale to vale;
   Not five yards from the mountain-path,
   This thorn you on your left espy;
   And to the left, three yards beyond,
   You see a little muddy pond
   Of water, never dry;
   I've measured it from side to side:
   'Tis three feet long, and two feet wide.

   From LYRICAL BALLADS   *William Wordsworth*

f. The lunatic, the lover, and the poet
    Are of imagination all compact.
    One sees more devils than vast hell can hold,
    That is the madman. The lover, all as frantic,
    Sees Helen's beauty in a brow of Egypt:
    The poet's eye, in a fine frenzy rolling,
    Doth glance from heaven to earth, from earth to heaven;
    And as imagination bodies forth
    The forms of things unknown, the poet's pen
    Turns them to shapes, and gives airy nothing
    A local habitation and a name.

    From A MIDSUMMER NIGHT'S DREAM   *William Shakespeare*

7. Just how a television reporter interacts within the newsroom depends on many
    variables, such as staff size and even the personality of the reporter.
        For example, in smaller television markets, such as Maine or Montana,
    the news staff would most likely be small and, therefore, the various roles of
    the television reporter would increase. At any given moment, the reporter
    may be asked to shoot, edit, produce, act as assignment editor, or even all of
    these duties at once!

PROJECTION

Appropriate projection, or loudness, is an important vocal component. Projection is discussed here so that during your practice sessions it will be incorporated into open throat. Again, the term *appropriate* is stressed. The volume or intensity of the speaking voice ought to be appropriate to the message, the audience, and the locale. A different kind of projection would be used for an oration than for the reading of an Emily Dickinson poem. The audience must also be considered in choosing projection, for it must always be able to hear (and see) the speaker easily. Nothing is more frustrating to an audience than not being able to hear the speaker. Imagine watching television with the volume off. Conversely, you must not have too much projection and overpower your listeners. Experience and awareness will help you determine the appropriate projection for a communication event. Obviously, an important consideration is your space, which may vary from a small conference room to a church pulpit that has no microphone. Whenever possible, try speaking in your locale in advance.

Be careful when you practice projection exercises! You don't want to injure your voice by increasing muscular tension in the pharyngeal area as you attempt to project. This tension may result in huskiness (sometimes permanent), hoarseness, or vocal strain. Remember how your throat felt (and sounded) after the yelling you did during your school's last big game! In addition to physically abusing the vocal mechanism, pharyngeal tension can also interfere with the aesthetics involved in communication. The emotions evoked by a soothing lyric poem cannot be conveyed with a brash and abrasive voice.

Many vocal factors work together to give appropriate projection. The first thing the speaker must develop is adequate breath control, which is the foundation for all good voice and speech. You have heard this before, right? Proper breath control relates to many characteristics of the voice. To dramatize the influence of breath support on projection and vocal quality, select a wooden door in your classroom, house, or dorm that is in a relatively secluded area. Open it halfway. Plant your feet solidly on either side of the door and with your hands on the doorknobs, place your abdominal area in firm contact with the edge of the door. Take a deep but quick diaphragmatic breath, and while you are consciously controlling the exhalation, pretend that you are in a rather large theater. Having taped the following exercise to the door with masking tape (so you don't damage the paint or stain on the door), read it at full volume:

Roll on, thou deep and dark blue Ocean—roll!
Ten thousand fleets sweep over thee in vain;
Man marks the earth with ruin—his control
Stops with the shore;—upon the watery plain
The wrecks are all thy deeds.

From CHILDE HAROLD'S PILGRIMAGE   *Lord Byron*

Fill that space! You will hear a tremendous difference in the loudness as well as quality of the voice if you are utilizing open throat. If the tension goes from the abdomen to the throat, you are performing the exercise incorrectly.

Another important factor in good projection is how open the mouth is during phonation. All of your exercises should be completed with a conscious effort to articulate well. Don't overarticulate at this point, but do make certain that you are giving enough time to produce the sounds.

While doing the projection exercises below, keep your pitch level in a medium range, neither too low nor too high. Also, make certain that you do not vary the pitch greatly during the exercises. Read them with a good open throat. You will project more easily and comfortably when there is minimal tension in the pharyngeal area.

PROJECTION EXERCISES

After you have become familiar with the following exercises, recite them using the door technique described above. Then reproduce the same vocal strength and ease of tone without the door technique. While practicing, pretend that you are in a large hall and must reach the audience in the last row.

1. O Thou Vast Ocean! ever sounding Sea!
   Thou vast symbol of a drear immensity!
   Thou thing that windest round the solid world,
   Like a huge animal, which downward hurled
   From the black clouds, lies weltering alone,
   Lashing and writhing till its strength be gone.
   Thy voice is like the thunder, and thy sleep
   Is as a giant's slumber, loud and deep.

   ADDRESS TO THE OCEAN   *Bryan W. Proctor*

2. "A merry Christmas, uncle! God save you!" cried a cheerful voice. It was the voice of Scrooge's nephew, who came upon him so quickly that this was the first intimation he had of his approach.

   "Bah!" said Scrooge. "Humbug!"

   He had so heated himself with rapid walking in the fog and frost, this nephew of Scrooge's, that he was all in a glow; his face was ruddy and handsome; his eyes sparkled.

   "Christmas a humbug, uncle!" said Scrooge's nephew. "You don't mean that, I am sure?"

   "I do," said Scrooge. "Merry Christmas! What right have you to be merry? You're poor enough."

   "Come, then," returned the nephew gaily. "What right have you to be dismal? What reason have you to be morose? You're rich enough."

   Scrooge, having no better answer ready on the spur of the moment, said, "Bah!" again; and followed it up with "Humbug."

   From A CHRISTMAS CAROL   *Charles Dickens*

3. Romans, countrymen, and lovers! hear me for my cause; and be silent, that you may hear: believe me for mine honour; and have respect to mine honour, that you may believe: censure me in your wisdom; and awake your senses, that you may the better judge. If there be any in this assembly, any dear friend of Caesar's, to him I say that Brutus' love for Caesar was no less than his.

   From JULIUS CAESAR   *William Shakespeare*

4. Friends, Romans, countrymen, lend me your ears;
   I come to bury Caesar, not to praise him.
   The evil that men do lives after them;
   The good is oft interred with their bones;
   So let it be with Caesar. The noble Brutus
   Hath told you Caesar was ambitious:
   If it were so, it was a grievous fault;
   And grievously hath Caesar answered it.
   Here, under leave of Brutus and the rest,—

For Brutus is an honourable man;
So are they all, all honourable men,—
Come I to speak in Caesar's funeral.
He was my friend, faithful and just to me:
But Brutus says he was ambitious;
And Brutus is an honourable man.
He hath brought many captives home to Rome,
Whose ransoms did the general coffers fill:
Did this in Caesar seem ambitious?

From JULIUS CAESAR   *William Shakespeare*

5. Alice was doubtful whether she ought not to lie down on her face like the three gardeners, but she could not remember ever having heard of such a rule at processions; "And besides, what would be the use of a procession," thought she, "if people had all to lie down on their faces, so that they couldn't see it?" So she stood where she was and waited.

When the procession came opposite to Alice, they all stopped and looked at her, and the Queen said, severely, "Who is that?" She said it to the Knave of Hearts, who only bowed and smiled in reply.

"Idiot!" said the Queen, tossing her head impatiently; and, turning to Alice, she went on: "What's your name, child?"

"My name is Alice, so please your Majesty," said Alice very politely; but she added, to herself, "Why, you're only a pack of cards, after all. I needn't be afraid of them!"

"And who are *these?*" said the Queen, pointing to the three gardeners who were lying round the rose-tree; for, you see, as they were lying on their faces, and the pattern on their backs was the same as the rest of the pack, she could not tell whether they were gardeners, or soldiers, or courtiers, or three of their own children.

"How should *I* know?" said Alice, surprised at her own courage. "It's no business of *mine*."

The Queen turned crimson with fury, and, after glaring at her for a moment like a wild beast, began screaming, "Off with her head! Off with—"

"Nonsense!" said Alice, very loudly and decidedly, and the Queen was silent.

The King laid his hand upon her arm, and timidly said, "Consider, my dear: she is only a child!"

The Queen turned angrily away from him, and said to the Knave, "Turn them over!"

The Knave did so, very carefully, with one foot.

"Get up!" said the Queen in a shrill, loud voice, and the three gardeners instantly jumped up, and began bowing to the King, the Queen, the royal children, and everybody else.

"Leave off that!" screamed the Queen. "You make me giddy." And then, turning to the rose-tree, she went on, "What *have* you been doing here?"

"May it please your Majesty," said Two, in a very humble tone, going down on one knee as he spoke, "we were trying—"

"I see," said the Queen, who had meanwhile been examining the roses. "Off with their heads!" and the procession moved on, three of the soldiers remaining behind to execute the unfortunate gardeners, who ran to Alice for protection.

"You shan't be beheaded!" said Alice, and she put them into a large flower-pot that stood near. The three soldiers wandered about for a minute or two, looking for them, and then quietly marched off after the others.

"Are their heads off?" shouted the Queen.

"Their heads are gone, if it please your Majesty!" the soldiers shouted in reply.

"That's right!" shouted the Queen. "Can you play croquet?"

The soldiers were silent, and looked at Alice, as the question was evidently meant for her.

"Yes," shouted Alice.

"Come on, then!" roared the Queen, and Alice joined the procession wondering very much what would happen next.

From ALICE'S ADVENTURES IN WONDERLAND *Lewis Carroll*

6. Heretofore we women in time of war
   have endured very patiently through it,
   putting up with whatever you men might do,
   for never a peep would you let us
   deliver on your unstatesmanly acts
   no matter how much they upset us,
   but we knew very well, while we sat at home,
   when you'd handled a big issue poorly,
   and we'd ask you then, with a pretty smile
   though our heart would be grieving us sorely,
   "And what were the terms for a truce, my dear,
   you drew up in assembly this morning?"
   "And what's it to you?" says our husband, "Shut up!"
   —so, as ever, at this gentle warning
   I of course would discreetly shut up.

From LYSISTRATA *Aristophanes*

7. Who can be wise, amazed, temperate, and furious,
   Loyal and neutral, in a moment? No man.
   The expedition of my violent love
   Outrun the pauser, reason. Here lay Duncan,
   His silver skin laced with his golden blood,
   And his gash'd stabs look'd like a breach in nature
   For ruin's wasteful entrance; there, the murderers,
   Steep'd in the colors of their trade, their daggers
   Unmannerly breech'd with gore. Who could refrain

That had a heart to love and in that heart
Courage to make's love known?

From MACBETH   *William Shakespeare*

PITCH

Habitual Pitch

Everyone incorporates several pitches when speaking. When under stress, a person usually elevates the pitch. The pitch levels you use most frequently constitute your **habitual pitch**, which is sometimes called *modal pitch*. One usually begins phonation at one's habitual pitch. This pitch is the result of imitation as well as other factors. Basically, an untrained speaker's pitch is habitual rather than natural.

Optimum Pitch

Everyone has a pitch that is naturally best for that person. *Natural* and *best* here mean that the pitch is the most anatomically comfortable for that individual. This pitch is identified as the **optimum pitch**, *optimum* meaning "an inclination to put the most favorable construction upon actions." Webster's definition is most germane to the study of voice when the most favorable "construction" has the least amount of constriction! The optimum pitch is not only the pitch where the speaker is most physically comfortable but also the pitch where muscles in the vocal mechanism function at their best. The most vibrant and resonant tones are produced at the optimum pitch. If there is a marked difference between your modal and optimum pitches, you will be more psychologically comfortable at your modal pitch because it is the pitch that you use most frequently. However, you have learned (we hope) not to mistake the habitual for appropriate or natural.

In addition to gaining comfort, a speaker can gain optimum projection using the optimum pitch. You may remember in an earlier discussion that each resonance cavity selects certain partials with which it is in harmony. When a speaker produces a very tense sound at the habitual rather than optimum pitch, the cavities will amplify those segmentals or partials with which there is sympathy, thus increasing the probability of producing an unpleasant sound. On the other hand, when the optimum pitch is used, the best partials are selected for amplification. Needless to say, it is important that each speaker discover his or her optimum pitch.

Gaining Habitual Pitch

Remember that your habitual pitch is the pitch level that you use most of the time when you are not giving energized meaning to your speech. In other words, your habitual pitch is generally used in speech that has little inflection.

Record the following poem, Shakespeare's Sonnet 18, and highlight those words that are underlined.

1. Shall I compare thee to a summer's day?

2. Thou art more lovely and more temperate:

3. Rough winds do shake the darling buds of May,

4. And summer's lease hath all too short a date:

5. Sometime too hot the eye of heaven shines,

6. And often is his gold complexion dimmed;

7. And every fair from fair sometime declines,

8. By chance or nature's changing course untrimmed;

9. But thy eternal summer shall not fade,

10. Nor lose possession of that fair thou owest;

11. Nor shall Death brag thou wander'st in his shade,

12. When in eternal lines to time thou grow'st;

13. So long as men can breathe, or eyes can see,

14. So long lives this, and this gives life to thee.

As you listen to your recording, become sensitive to the pitch that you use when you are not emphasizing meaning. This particular sonnet was selected because a "color" word often appears at the beginning and end of a line, leaving the middle for you to establish your habitual pitch. Focus your listening acuity on line 1 and lines 5 through 9. See if you can determine your habitual pitch on a piano, guitar, or pitch pipe. Write down the note if you can. Keep in mind that this may or may not be your optimum pitch.

Gaining Optimum Pitch

There are several ways to obtain your optimum pitch. One of the easiest ways is to sing down the scale with the aid of a piano. Don't concentrate on singing. With good open throat, produce the vowel "ah." If you use a tight throat, you will not get your true optimum pitch. At any rate, move down the scale to the lowest comfortable note you can produce with ease and duration. Then go up three or four notes. That should be your optimum pitch. Experiment a little on surrounding notes before you finally decide. You should be able to tell immediately when you have hit your optimum pitch, for there will be a stronger, more resonant, and more physically comfortable sound. Since the optimum pitch is easily heard by a listener, it is often helpful to work with a partner. A pitch pipe or other musical instrument may also help you determine your optimum pitch. The sketch of the piano keyboard in Figure 4.1 should help you duplicate the correct notes. Make a notation of your optimum pitch. In addition, record the note from your piano or pitch pipe onto your cassette tape. Say "This is my optimum pitch" and play that note. You should not be interested in inflection at the moment. Get to the point where you can reproduce your optimum pitch without the aid of the cassette tape.

Of course, it is to your benefit if your modal or habitual pitch is the same or close to your optimum pitch. Many males intentionally lower their pitch during and immediately after that "period of mystery" because they do not want to sound like (ugh!) girls! How many times have you males consciously turned on the macho sound to prove your sexuality? Unfortunately, with these sociological and often self-imposed pressures, males often force the pitch well below the optimum level. Although they may be establishing their masculinity, their voices often sound gravelly and unpleasant.

Sometimes a female voice is too high for similar reasons. Girls are taught to be ladylike, and part of the stereotype includes a soft high-pitched voice.

If there is a discrepancy of a full note or more between your modal and optimum pitches, it is important to make your optimum pitch a habit as quickly as possible. This is accomplished only through practice and conscious effort. Like all modifications, it will not seem natural at first. You will feel very ill at ease and self-conscious until the altered pitch becomes habitual.

OPTIMUM PITCH EXERCISES

Quietly read the following exercises aloud, utilizing your optimum pitch. Include variations of pitch as dictated by the meaning. Concentrate on the sound and feeling while using the optimum pitch. If your **muscle memory** is good, you should be able to reproduce the sound and feeling of the optimum pitch voluntarily.

FIGURE 4.1   SECTION OF PIANO KEYBOARD INDICATING SPEAKING/SINGING RANGE

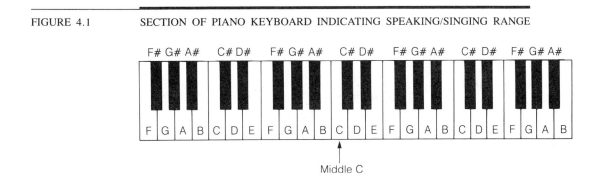

1. The Lord is my light and my salvation; whom shall I fear? the Lord is the strength of my Life; of whom shall I be afraid?

   From PSALM 27

2. He doesn't seem to know what he wants, does he?

3. And now, friends, fellow citizens of Gettysburg and Pennsylvania, and you from remoter States, let me again, as we part, invoke your benediction on these honored graves. You feel, though the occasion is mournful, that it is good to be here.

   From the GETTYSBURG ADDRESS   *Abraham Lincoln*

4. For in that sleep of death what dreams may come
   When we have shuffled off this mortal coil,
   Must give us pause: there's the respect
   That makes calamity of so long life.

   From HAMLET   *William Shakespeare*

5. GOOD MORNING . . . I'M _____ AND THIS IS THE A.M. SPORTS UP-DATE. SAM JONES SCORED A GAME HIGH 29 POINTS—WITH 26 IN THE SECOND HALF ALONE—AS THE *FRIES* PUMMELED THE *FRANKS* 101 TO 86.

   BUT IT WAS THE *FRIES'* DEFENSE THAT ENABLED THEM TO EX-TEND THEIR WINNING STREAK TO NINE GAMES.

   THE GREEN HELD THE *FRANKS* HIGH-FLYING FORWARD BERNARD KITE TO A SEASON LOW 9 POINTS.

   COMBINED WITH THEIR WIN AND THE *FRANKS* LOSS TO MIAMI, THE *FRIES* LEAD OVER SECOND-PLACE BLUES IS NOW FIVE GAMES.

6. Hear the mellow bells—
   Golden bells!
   What a world of happiness their harmony foretells!
   Through the balmy air of night
   How they ring out their delight!

   From THE BELLS   *Edgar Allan Poe*

7. My hair is grey, but not with years,
   Nor grew it white
   In a single night,
   As men's have grown from sudden fears:
   My limbs are bowed, though not with toil,
   But rusted with a vile repose,
   For they have been a dungeon's spoil,
   And mine has been the fate of those
   To whom the goodly earth and air

Are banned, and barred—forbidden fare;
But this was for my father's faith
I suffered chains and courted death;
That father perished at the stake
For tenets he would not forsake;
And for the same his lineal race
In darkness found a dwelling place;
We were seven—who now are one,
Six in youth, and one in age,
Furnished as they had begun,
Proud of Persecution's rage;
One in fire, and two in field,
Their belief with blood have sealed,
Dying as their father died,
For the God their foes denied;—
Three were in a dungeon cast,
Of whom this wreck is left the last.

From THE PRISONER OF CHILLON   *Lord Byron*

By now you have been able to produce a good open throat with your optimum pitch. It is now your responsibility to make it a speech habit. How long it will take depends on you. Yes, you will feel self-conscious at first, but frequent use of the optimum pitch will make it increasingly easy to produce and use. The easy feel in your pharynx ought to encourage you. Your quality of voice is not only more pleasant, but it feels better!

5

COMMON
VOICE
PROBLEMS

GLOSSARY

Alveolar Ridge   The bony ridge behind the upper teeth.

Articulatory Adjustment   The manipulation of the anatomical structure to produce sounds, such as placing the tongue tip on the alveolar ridge and vocalizing, which produces the consonant /l/.

Assimilation   The influence of one speech sound on another.

Assimilation Nasality   Vowels approximating nasal sounds, which take on nasal characteristics.

Bilabial   Pertaining to the two lips.

Cleft Palate Speech   Hypernasality exhibited in the speech of individuals who have palatal problems; excessive nasality.

Denasality   A vocal quality in which not enough voice is resonated in the nose.

Excessive Assimilation Nasality   Too much nasal resonance in vowel production.

Glottal Shock   A vocal quality in which the vocal folds are forced apart by breath that has been held back, resulting in an explosion of sound, usually on an initial vowel or diphthong.

Hard Palate   The first third of the roof of the mouth, composed of bone and membrane.

Hoarseness   A quality of voice caused by strain.

Mandible   The lower jaw.

Maxilla   The upper jaw.

Nasality   A vocal quality in which too much sound vibration escapes through the nose during phonation.

Nasal Spurs   Growths in and around the nasal cavity that interfere with the flow of breath.

Nodule   A kind of polyp.

Septum   The dividing wall of the nose.

Singer's Nodes   Small growths on the vocal folds due to vocal strain; fairly common among singers.

Strident   A quality of voice characterized by harshness and usually high pitch.

Uvula   The hanging tip of the velum.

Velum   The back two-thirds of the palate, composed of muscle and membrane; commonly called the *soft palate*.

Vocal Fry   (Glottal Fry) A quality of voice characterized by a scratchy sound, usually caused by poor breathing habits and characterized by rapid opening and closure of the glottis during phonation.

This chapter deals with common vocal problems among untrained (and sometimes trained) speakers. The first group of errors are due to poor control of the velum. The second group is due to excessive tension in the laryngeal area. Exercises are provided to help minimize and correct the problems described. In addition, there are exercises to help you develop the desirable vocal characteristics needed to replace the vocal problems.

VELIC PROBLEMS

Problems can result when the velum does not make appropriate contact with the pharyngeal wall.

Assimilation

Assimilation in speech is the influence of one sound upon another. Think of articulating the word *bow*. Feel the lips coming together for the closure on the sound /b/. What is the position of the tongue? Because it is not involved in the production of /b/, it is in all probability resting at the bottom of the mouth. Now form the word *brown* but do not pronounce it. The tongue position has changed; instead of being in a relaxed position at the bottom of the mouth, the tongue has anticipated the production of the /r/ coming after the /b/. Now you should be aware that the tip of the tongue is slightly curled toward the roof of the mouth. The tongue is forming the /r/ in *brown* before the /b/ is exploded. Now form the word *blow* without vocalizing it. The tongue tip changes from being slightly curled to touching the ridge behind the upper teeth, anticipating the production of the sound /l/. These are just two examples of how assimilation works.

These actions happen because the second sound in each word can be produced without the two lips. The plosive /b/ is a **bilabial** (made with the two lips) sound. In the first example (*bow*), there are two possible pronunciations: a bow on a dress or a bow of a boat. In either case, the tongue is free to begin the **articulatory adjustment** for the second sound, and there is a difference depending upon which pronunciation you make. There is a slight modification between the /o/ (as in *go*) and the diphthong /aʊ/. Can you feel the difference? The same principle applies to the other two examples, *brown* and *blow*. The adjustment for the /r/ and /l/ are easier to feel because the tongue must be elevated for each sound.

Another example of assimilation occurs in the sentence "I don't have to go." The last sound in the word *have* is not pronounced /v/ but /f/. If the sentence were "I have won," the last sound in *have* would be /v/. In the first example, the /v/ becomes /f/ because in dynamic or conversational speech, the /v/ is often pronounced /f/, depending upon the sound that follows and the amount of stress on the word containing the /v/. If the sound following the /v/ is not vocalized (such as /t/, as in *to*), it is usually pronounced with the unvocalized /f/. The mechanism of the voice adapts to the easier production, whether it is correct or incorrect. Conversely, in the sentence "I have won" the sound /v/ is used because the next sound is the vocalized (/w/). This assimilation process occurs automatically because it is easier for the speaker to produce two voiceless sounds together or two voiced sounds together than to stop and start the vocal machinery each time. It should be made clear, however, that there are numerous exceptions to this generalization.

Nasality

Nasality (sometimes called *hypernasality*) is a vocal quality that occurs when too much sound vibration takes place in the nose. An extreme form is **cleft palate speech,** where the palatal structure allows air to escape through the nose. Since the palate is used to block off the nasal cavity, individuals with a damaged palate often exhibit excessive nasality. People with a normal palate can also have nasal speech, but their degree of nasality is usually less than in cleft palate speech.

Check your own degree of nasality. Place a feather or several small pieces of paper or tissue on cardboard, and place the cardboard above the upper lip and below the nose. Say the following sounds aloud several times: /t/, /d/, /s/, and /z/. The feather or pieces of paper should not move, because the breath ought to escape through the mouth. Now repeat the sounds /m/ and /n/. The objects ought to move, because the vibrating sound escapes through the nose. The good voice contains an appropriate amount of resonance in the nasal cavity. Figure 5.1 shows a side view of the oral, nasal, and pharyngeal cavities.

Place the tip of your tongue just behind the upper teeth on the hard ridge, called the **alveolar ridge.** This ridge, which is composed of bone, is the swelling around the teeth. As the tongue tip leaves the ridge and moves back, it touches the **hard palate,** which is the bony portion of the roof of the mouth. Place the tip of the tongue farther back on the hard palate until you touch the **velum,** or *soft palate*. Because the velum is composed of membrane and muscle, it can move. The hard palate and alveolar ridge are immovable and are extensions of the upper jaw (**maxilla**). At the end of the velum there is a hanging bulb called the **uvula.**

In producing all the speech sounds except the nasals, the velum contracts and moves up and back, while the muscles of the pharynx (throat) contract and

FIGURE 5.1 ORAL AND NASAL CAVITIES DURING VEGETATIVE BREATHING

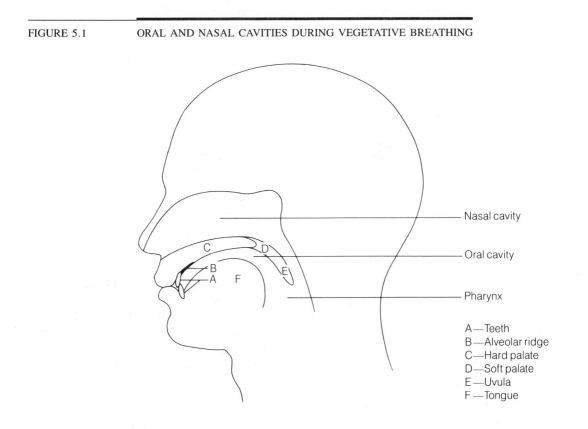

Nasal cavity

Oral cavity

Pharynx

A—Teeth
B—Alveolar ridge
C—Hard palate
D—Soft palate
E—Uvula
F—Tongue

move the pharyngeal wall down and forward, closing off the nasal cavity. On the nasal sounds, the soft palate is actively lowered, allowing the vibrating breath to escape through the nasal cavity and out the nose (Figure 5.2).

Denasality

Denasality occurs when there is insufficient nasal resonance. When you are denasal, you are often told that you have a cold. (The prefix *de-* means "away from"; thus the literal meaning of *denasality* is "away from nasality.") There are many possible causes of denasality. When you have a cold, the mucous linings of the mouth and nose swell, preventing nasal resonance on the nasal sounds. Because of this swelling, the vibrations on these sounds are rerouted and escape through the mouth. That is why you can easily recognize the "cold in the head" quality that is characteristic of denasality.

There are a number of possible organic causes of denasality. Sometimes players of contact sports, such as boxing or wrestling, develop denasality if their

FIGURE 5.2   SOFT PALATE AND PHARYNGEAL MUSCLES

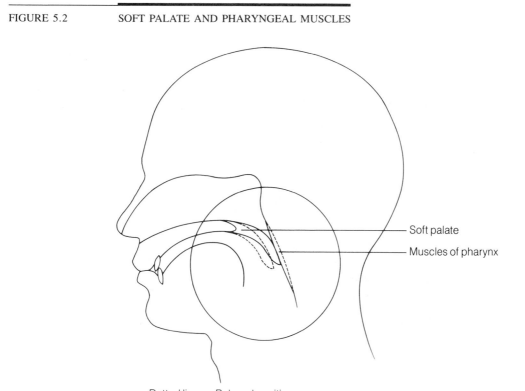

— Soft palate

— Muscles of pharynx

Dotted lines—Relaxed position
Solid lines—Position during production of nonnasal sounds

septum (dividing wall of the nose) becomes deviated. The nasal speech sounds cannot escape through the nose, and the resulting quality is denasal. Other, less violent people can become denasal because of other factors like colds, such as sinus infections and allergies, that cause the nasal membranes to swell. Other possible causes are congestion, **nasal spurs** (growths), and enlarged tonsils or turbinates. Many of these problems must be surgically corrected. However, some people are denasal because of vocal laziness. It is to these individuals that this section of exercises is dedicated.

The following poem emphasizes a lack of nasal resonance. Read it aloud as it is written and you will discover denasality!

No, No

Doe, doe!
I shall dever see her bore!
Dever bore our feet shall rove
The beadows as of your!
Dever bore with byrtle boughs
Her tresses shall I twide—
Dever bore her bellow voice
Bake bellody with bide!
Dever shall we lidger bore,
Abid the flow'rs at dood,
Dever shall we gaze at dight
Upon the tedtder blood!
Ho, doe, doe!
Those berry tibes have flowd,
Ad I shall dever see her bore,
By beautiful! by owd!
Ho, doe, doe!
I shall dever see her bore,
She will forget be id a bonth,
(Bost probably before)—
She will forget the byrtle boughs,
The flow'rs we plucked at dood,
Our beetigs by the tedtder stars.
Our gazigs at the bood.
Ad I shall dever see agaid
The Lily and the Rose;
The dabask cheek! the sdowy brow!
The perfect bouth ad dose!
Ho, doe, doe!
Those berry tibes have flowd—
Ad I shall dever see her bore,
By beautiful! by owd!!

LAY OF THE DESERTED INFLUENZAED   *Henry Cholmondeley-Pennell*

EXERCISES FOR ELIMINATING DENASALITY

Lambert itis

1. Become aware of the action of the velum and uvula by alternating quickly between the letters "ng" as in "song" (/ŋ/) and the vowel "ah" (/ɑ/) ten times. Feel, hear, and visualize the muscular action.

2. The humming and nasal resonance drills in Chapter 4 are excellent for denasality because they exercise the velum and allow the opening into the nasal cavity to open and close (see pages 57–60).

3. Place small pieces of tissue or cut up paper on a piece of cardboard (as in testing for nasality) and place it just under the nostrils. Hum a quiet, sustained tone. Try to keep the pieces of paper on the cardboard rather than forcing them off in a spurt.

4. Read the following passage and prolong the underlined nasal sounds. Make certain that the transition to and from the nasal consonant is produced with as much nasal resonance as possible:

And now, friends, fellow citizens of Gettysburg and Pennsylvania, and you from remoter States, let me again, as we part, invoke your benediction on these honored graves. You feel, though the occasion is mournful, that it is good to be here. . . . You now feel it a new bond of union, that they shall lie side by side, till a clarion, louder than that which marshalled them to the combat, shall awake their slumbers. God bless the Union;—it is dearer to us for the blood of brave men which has been shed in its defence. The spots on which they stood and fell; these pleasant heights; the fertile plain beneath them; the thriving village whose streets so lately rang with the strange din of war; the fields beyond the ridge, where the noble Reynolds held the advancing foe at bay; and, while he gave up his own life, assured by his forethought and self-sacrifice the triumph of the two succeeding days; the little streams which wind through the hills, on whose banks in after times the wondering plough-man will turn up, with the rude weapons of savage warfare, the fearful missiles of modern artillery; Seminary Ridge, the Peach Orchard, Cemetery, Culp, and Wolf Hill, Round Top, Little Round Top, humble names, henceforward dear and famous,—no lapse of time, no distance of space, shall cause you to be forgotten. But they, I am sure, will join us in saying, as we bid farewell to the dust of these martyr-heroes, that wheresoever throughout the civilized world the accounts of this great warfare are read, and down to the latest period of recorded time, in the glorious annals of our common country there will be no brighter page than that which relates the battles of Gettysburg.

Abraham Lincoln

Assimilation Nasality

Assimilation and nasality have been discussed in detail. Used together, they create a rather common vocal quality that, when excessive, is quite unpleasant. **Excessive assimilation nasality** is not limited to any particular regional dialect, although it is quite typical of Eastern U.S. speech. Say the words *apple* and *man*. Do the vowels in both words sound the same to you? If you were to look them up in a pronouncing dictionary, you would discover that both words contain the vowel /æ/, as in *cat*. However, to most people the vowels in the two words sound different. The reason is that the vowel in *man* is surrounded by two nasal sounds.

We identified the velum as the controller of the air and sound waves into the nasal cavity, and we noted that the velum contracts on all English sounds other than the three nasals. Since there are no nasal sounds in *apple*, the velum remains contracted. However, in *man* the velum must first be actively lowered, allowing the sound vibrations to escape through the nose on /m/. For the next sound, /æ/, the velum must contract upwards, closing off the entrance into the nasal cavity; on the third sound, /n/, the velum must be lowered again. Since this movement is very rapid, a bit of nasal vibration normally escapes into the vowel. If the speaker is careless with this closure, the vowel absorbs too much nasal resonance and becomes too nasalized. That is why the vowels in *apple* and *man* sound slightly different. It is the assimilation, or the influence of the nasal on the vowel, that produces the nasality, which must also be present in the good speaking voice. A good voice exhibits the proper degree of nasality. **Assimilation nasality** often occurs when a vowel sound comes before or after nasal sounds.

Excessive Assimilation Nasality

Assimilation nasality is common. When it is excessive, the sound is most unpleasant. At this point, it is considered a quality problem. Since we are essentially lazy beings, the velum is often too relaxed during normal assimilation nasality. Therefore, too much vibrating air escapes through the nose, causing the vowel to contain excessive nasality. Although this condition may occur with any vowel or diphthong, the phoneme /æ/ as in *cat* is a particular favorite. Thus the exercises below focus on that vowel in combination with the nasal sounds. Excessive assimilation nasality is corrected by dropping the lower jaw (**mandible**) considerably and flattening the tongue for the low-front production of the vowel /æ/. You must make certain, however, that you are producing the same vowel. The common error is to substitute the /ɑ/ (as in *father*) for the /æ/ (as in *cat*). To be clear, do not hesitate to overdo the production of the correct sound. As a matter of fact, such exaggeration is to be encouraged. When the exaggerated movement is easy, it is a simple task to pull away and produce the sound appropriately. Don't forget to work with negative practice.

EXERCISES FOR ELIMINATING EXCESSIVE ASSIMILATION NASALITY

1. In pronouncing the following words, drop the lower jaw and flatten the tongue with a tongue depressor or spoon, if necessary, on the vowel /æ/. Make certain that the underlined vowel is produced in the front of the mouth. Employ negative practice by reading the three columns across for each word. "Career" indicates career speech. You will notice that all of the words contain /æ/. This is so you can feel and hear the error. It must be repeated, however, that excessive assimilation nasality may occur in conjunction with other vowels.

	Career	*Error*	*Career*
man	[mæn]	[mæ̃n][1]	[mæn]
and	[ænd]	[æ̃nd]	[ænd]
handle	[hændl̩]	[hæ̃ndl̩]	[hændl̩]
Flannery	[flænɚɪ]	[flæ̃nɚɪ]	[flænɚɪ]
mammal	[mæml̩]	[mæ̃ml̩]	[mæml̩]
family	[fæməlɪ]	[fæ̃məlɪ]	[fæməlɪ]
scandal	[skændl̩]	[skæ̃ndl̩]	[skændl̩]
animal	[ænəml̩]	[æ̃nəml̩]	[ænəml̩]
understand	[əndɚstænd]	[əndɚstæ̃nd]	[əndɚstænd]
jam	[dʒæm]	[dʒæ̃m]	[dʒæm]
ant	[ænt]	[æ̃nt]	[ænt]
lamb	[læm]	[læ̃m]	[læm]
Danny	[dænɪ]	[dæ̃nɪ]	[dænɪ]
Vangy	[vændʒɪ]	[væ̃ndʒɪ]	[vændʒɪ]
nag	[næg]	[næ̃g]	[næg]
ran	[ræn]	[ræ̃n]	[ræn]
panda	[pændə]	[pæ̃ndə]	[pændə]

    Since negative practice is quite valuable, go back and produce each word with exaggerated assimilation nasality, and then immediately say the word again with appropriate assimilation nasality. This should give you a contrast between a careless and a professional production of the vowel sound.

---

[1] /˜/ indicates nasality.

2. In the following sentences, make certain that you drop the lower jaw and flatten the tongue on the underlined vowels.

   a. Nancy, hand the man the dandy candy.

   b. His name is Stanley and he comes from Manchester, New Hampshire.

   c. Don't raise the banner with your left hand, Randall.

   d. Samantha is living on Hancock Street.

   e. Rant and rave all you want.

   f. Vangy never crammed for her examination.

   g. Sandra smelled the rancid cheese.

   h. Do you have a Handy Andy in your pocket?

   i. Mandy, handle the candle carefully.

   j. Frannie, do you like candied yams with your ham?

   Now read the sentences using negative practice. Say the sentences properly, then with excessive assimilation nasality, and then properly again. Feel and hear the contrasting production of sounds.

3. In the following poems, pay close attention to the words that are underlined. Remember to drop your jaw and keep the tongue position flat. After you have read the poems with appropriate assimilation nasality, read them again using negative practice (that is, say them properly, then with excessive assimilation nasality, and then properly again).

   a. I met a traveller from an antique land
         Who said: "Two vast and trunkless legs of stone
         Stand on the desert. Near them, on the sand
         Half sunk, a shattered visage lies, whose frown
         And wrinkled lip and sneer of cold command
         Tell that its sculptor well those passions read
         Which yet survive, stamped on these lifeless things.
         The hand that mocked them and the heart that fed.
         And on the pedestal these words appear:
         'My name is Ozymandias, king of kings:
         Look on my works, ye Mighty, and despair!'
         Nothing beside remains. Round the decay
         Of that colossal wreck, boundless and bare,
         The lone and level sands stretch far away."

   OZYMANDIAS   *Percy Bysshe Shelley*

   b. My heart leaps up when I behold
         A rainbow in the sky:

So was it when my life <u>began</u>;
So is it now I <u>am</u> a <u>man</u>;
So be it when <u>I</u> shall grow old,
Or let me die!
The Child is father of the <u>Man</u>;
And I could wish my days <u>to</u> be
Bound each to each by natural piety.

        MY HEART LEAPS UP   *William Wordsworth*

c. Thy summer's play,
  My thoughtless <u>hand</u>
  Has brushed away.
  <u>Am</u> I not
  <u>A</u> fly like thee?
  Or art not thou
  A <u>man</u> like me?
  For <u>I</u> dance
  <u>And</u> <u>drink</u> <u>and</u> sing.

        LITTLE FLY   *William Blake*

EXCESSIVE VOCAL TENSION

Glottal Shock

Glottal shock is a voice problem often caused by poor breathing habits. It occurs when the subglottal breath (breath below the opening between the vocal folds) does not escape evenly because of tension at the vocal folds. The tension is most easily heard during the production of initial vowels and diphthongs. Breathiness could be considered the opposite of glottal shock. In breathiness, because there is a lack of tension at the vocal folds, the air escapes with no perceptible tension. To get the feel of glottal shock, bring the vocal folds together as in the beginning of a cough. Habitual glottal shock may cause severe vocal problems. When there is glottal shock, there is usually tight throat. The sound produced is harsh and strident. However, used carefully and purposefully, glottal shock can add color to your speech.

Elimination of Glottal Shock

To eliminate glottal shock, you have to get rid of the tension in the vocal area that is causing the problem. This can be easily accomplished by incorporating the /h/ consonant, which is produced by breath escaping through the glottis. Since it is a completely aspirated sound, there is little tension in its production.

    Read the following list of words using negative practice. Increase the tension on the vowel of the word that appears in the first column. Cause a slight explosion or click of breath on the initial vowel. Feel what is happening. This is glottal shock! Does it feel at all natural or habitual? Do you identify glottal shock as part of your speech? Is there any in your voice and speech? You probably have glottal shock to some degree. Place an aspirated /h/ before the initial vowel sound. *Apple* becomes *happle*. Feel the release of the breath and the reduction in tension at the vocal area. Then say the word in the third column, attempting to duplicate the feeling of the second column but without the /h/.

apple	/h/apple	apple
even	/h/even	even
Ida	/h/Ida	Ida
owl	/h/owl	owl
aim	/h/aim	aim
earth	/h/earth	earth
under	/h/under	under
open	/h/open	open

EXERCISES FOR ELIMINATING GLOTTAL SHOCK

Read the following sentences and lines of poetry in the same way using negative practice. The first time you read them, concentrate on the feeling of tension in the larynx. You might even consciously build up the pressure in the larynx before uttering the first word to underscore the production of glottal shock. During the second reading, place the /h/ on the initial vowels, then remove it on the third reading but maintain a similar feeling.

1. Even Edna couldn't tell him everything.
   /h/Even /h/Edna couldn't tell him /h/everything.
   Even Edna couldn't tell him everything.

2. The aim of the course was to interest everyone.
   The /h/aim /h/of the course was to /h/interest /h/everyone.
   The aim of the course was to interest everyone.

3. How awful it is to eat everything!
   How /h/awful /h/it /h/is to /h/eat /h/everything!
   How awful it is to eat everything!

4. Oil is oozing under our oven.
   /h/Oil /h/is /h/oozing /h/under /h/our /h/oven.
   Oil is oozing under our oven.

5. Amy admires Arthur more than anyone else.
   /h/Amy /h/admires /h/Arthur more than /h/anyone /h/else.
   Amy admires Arthur more than anyone else.

6. He always acts that way.
   He /h/always /h/acts that way.
   He always acts that way.

7. I never admit when I am wrong.
   /h/I never /h/admit when /h/I /h/am wrong.
   I never admit when I am wrong.

8. Everyone arrived at the party early and upset Agnes.
   /h/Everyone /h/arrived /h/at the party /h/early /h/and /h/upset /h/Agnes.
   Everyone arrived at the party early and upset Agnes.

9. Keep your eye on "Edgy Al" all the time.
   Keep your /h/eye /h/on /h/Edgy /h/Al /h/all the time.
   Keep your eye on "Edgy Al" all the time.

10. I was born an American; I live an American; I shall die an American; and I
    intend to perform the duties incumbent upon me in that character to the end
    of my career.

    Daniel Webster

    /h/I was born /h/an /h/American; /h/I live /h/an /h/American; /h/I shall die
    /h/an /h/American; /h/and /h/I /h/intend to perform the duties /h/incumbent
    /h/upon me /h/in that character to the /h/end /h/of my career.

    I was born an American; I live an American; I shall die an American; and I
    intend to perform the duties incumbent upon me in that character to the end
    of my career.

11. In the afternoon they came unto a land
    In which it seemed always afternoon.

    From THE LOTUS-EATERS   *Alfred Lord Tennyson*

    /h/In the /h/afternoon they came /h/unto /h/a land
    /h/In which /h/it seemed /h/always /h/afternoon.

    In the afternoon they came unto a land
    In which it seemed always afternoon.

12. O Jehovah, our Lord,
    How excellent is thy name in all the earth.

    From PSALM 8

    /h/O Jehovah, /h/our Lord,
    How /h/excellent /h/is thy name /h/in /h/all the /h/earth.

    O Jehovah, our Lord,
    How excellent is thy name in all the earth.

13. Out of the mouth of babes and sucklings hast thou established strength.

    From PSALM 8

    /h/Out /h/of the mouth /h/of babes /h/and sucklings hast thou /h/established strength.

    Out of the mouth of babes and sucklings hast thou established strength.

Producing Glottal Shock

Glottal shock used sparingly and intentionally can support your verbal communication. In your acting career you might need to create a character who has glottal shock. For example, a Scottish dialect requires glottal shock. Know when you are using glottal shock.

GLOTTAL SHOCK EXERCISES

In the following exercises, produce a glottal shock or attack on the underlined vowels and diphthongs. Remember that the larynx is meant primarily as a valve. Allow the pressure to build up a bit and force the vocal folds apart in a short spurt or click of air.

1. I told you to get out of my sight!

2. Under the bamboo bamboo bamboo
   Under the bamboo tree

   From FRAGMENT OF AN AGON   *T. S. Eliot*

3. It was an awful automobile accident.

4. Everyone knows everything about it.

5. Always—I tell you this they learned—
   Always at night when they returned

   From THE HILLWIFE   *Robert Frost*

6. It stuck in a barb wire snare.
   Ich, ich, ich, ich,
   I could hardly speak.

   From DADDY   *Sylvia Plath*

7. By folly, error, stinginess, and vice
   our flesh is worked, our souls inhabited,
   and all our dear remorses are well fed,
   as beggars nourish their own fleas and lice.

   From NOUVELLES FLEURS DU MAL   *Charles Baudelaire*

8. <u>OOOOOOO</u>, but he was <u>a</u> tight fisted hand <u>at</u> the grindstone, Scrooge!

From A CHRISTMAS CAROL *Charles Dickens*

Vocal Fry

Vocal fry is generally caused by improper breathing. The speaker runs out of breath before the speech is finished and creates excessive tension at the vocal folds. Fry is characterized by a lowering of pitch (sometimes up to a full octave) at the end of a thought, and the quality of the voice is often described as scratchy and unsustained. The name came from the sound of hot frying grease. Excessive vocal fry can cause vocal damage. Since vocal fry is a breath problem, continue to develop your breath control.

EXERCISES FOR ELIMINATING VOCAL FRY

Read the following exercises aloud, sustaining your voice to the next inhalation mark (the slash). Follow the inhalation marks, even though they may not agree with your interpretation of the selection. As you work at your own pace, you may find that you need to take more inhalations than are indicated; that is perfectly acceptable. Build up your capacity. Remember, it is very important to keep your tone strong throughout the thought. Control your exhalation.

1. A squeezing, wrenching, grasping, scraping, clutching, covetous old sinner. / Hard and sharp as flint, / from whom no steel had ever struck out generous fire; / secret and self-contained and solitary as an oyster. / The cold within him froze his old features, / nipped his pointed nose, shrivelled his cheek, stiffened his gait, made his eyes red, his thick lips blue; / and spoke out shrewdly in his grating voice.

From A CHRISTMAS CAROL *Charles Dickens*

2. When, / in disgrace with fortune and men's eyes, /
I all alone beweep my outcaste state, /
And trouble deaf heaven with my bootless cries, /
And look upon myself, and curse my fate, /
Wishing me like to one more rich in hope, /
Featured like him, like him with friends possessed, /
Desiring this man's art and that man's scope,
With what I most enjoy contented least; /
Yet in these thoughts myself almost despising,
Haply I think on thee; / and then my state,
Like to the lark at break of day arising
From sullen earth, / sings hymns at heaven's gate; /

For thy sweet love remembered such wealth brings
That then I scorn to change my state with kings.

SONNET 29   *William Shakespeare*

3. The Lord is my shepherd; / I shall not want. / He makes me to lie down in green pastures; / he leads me beside still waters. / He restores my soul; / he leads me in paths of righteousness / for his name's sake. / Even though I walk through the valley of the shadow of death, / I fear no evil; / for thou art with me. / Thy rod and thy staff they comfort me. / Thou preparest a table before me / in the presence of my enemies; / thou anointest my head with oil. / My cup overflows. / Surely goodness and mercy / shall follow me all the days of my life, / and I shall dwell in the house of the Lord forever.

PSALM 23

4. No doubt I now grew very pale. / But I talked more fluently / and with a heightened voice. / Yet the sound increased / —and what could I do? / It was a low, dull, quick sound— / much like the sound a watch makes when enveloped in cotton. / I gasped for breath / and yet the officers heard it not. / I talked more quickly, / more vehemently, / but the noise steadily increased. / I arose and argued about trifles, / in a high key and with violent gesticulations, / but the noise steadily increased. / Why would they not be gone? / I paced the floor to and fro with heavy strides, / as if excited to fury by the observation of the men— / but the noise steadily increased, / O God! / What could I do? / I foamed— / I raved— / I swore! / I swung the chair upon which I had been sitting, / and grated it upon the boards, / but the noise arose overall and continually increased. It grew louder— / louder— / louder—! / And still the men chatted pleasantly, / and smiled. / Was it possible they heard not? / Almighty God! / —no, no. / They heard! / They suspected! / They were making mockery of my horror! / But anything was better than this agony! / Anything was more tolerable than this derision! / I could bear those hypocritical smiles no longer! / I felt that I must scream or die! / And now— / again! / Hark! / Louder! / Louder! / Louder! / Louder! / "Villains!" I shrieked, / "dissemble no more! / I admit the deed! / Tear up the planks! / Here, / here! / It is the beating of his hideous heart!"

FROM THE TELL-TALE HEART   *Edgar Allan Poe*

Producing Vocal Fry

There are many comedians who use vocal fry for their characters. Many of the cartoon voices created by the great Mel Blanc (the voice of Bugs Bunny and many other characters) gain much of their impact through the use of vocal fry. A character like Gloria Upson, the narrator of the unforgettable Ping Pong match in *Auntie Mame,* or even Agnes Gooch from the same play, incorporate much vocal fry in their vocal responses. Vocal fry sounds like the voice of the wonderful Margaret Hamilton, who played the Wicked Witch in *The Wizard of Oz.* Remember "I'm m-e-e-l-l-l-t-t-i-i-i-n-n-n-n-g-g-g-g!"

Imitate the stereotypical witch with the three witches from Shakespeare's *Macbeth:*

1 Witch: When shall we three meet again
In thunder, lightning, or in rain?

2 Witch: When the hurlyburly's done,
When the battle's lost and won.

3 Witch: That will be ere the set of sun.

1 Witch: Where the place?

2 Witch: Upon the heath.

3 Witch: There to meet with Macbeth. . . .

All: Fair is foul and foul is fair:
Hover through the fog and filthy air.

Edwin Arlington Robinson, in "Mr. Flood's Party," presents a very long opening primary cadence (sentence):

Old Eben Flood, / climbing alone one night
Over the hill between the town below
And the forsaken upland hermitage
That held as much as he should ever know
On earth again of home, / paused warily.

The poet helps the performer achieve Mr. Flood's spent and tired physical state by forcing the effective inhalation before "paused warily." A performer might support the tone with some vocal fry at the end ("On earth again of home").

Record the following description of the creation of the first four days of the world from the *Torah* (Genesis 1). As you listen to the playback, note whether you used vocal fry to enhance and amplify the meaning.

When God began to create the heaven and the earth—the earth being unformed and void, with darkness over the surface of the deep and a wind from God sweeping over the water—God said, "Let there be light"; and there was light. God saw that the light was good, and God separated the light from the darkness. God called the light Day, and the darkness He called Night. And there was evening and there was morning, a first day.

God said, "Let there be an expanse in the midst of the water, that it may separate water from water." God made the expanse, and it separated the water which was below the expanse from the water which was above the expanse. And it was so. God called the expanse Sky. And there was evening and there was morning, a second day.

God said, "Let the water below the sky be gathered into one area, that the dry land may appear." And it was so. God called the dry land Earth, and the gathering of the waters He called Seas. And God saw that this was good. And

God said, "Let the earth sprout vegetation: seed-bearing plants, fruit trees of every kind on earth that bear fruit with the seed in it." And it was so. The earth brought forth vegetation: seed-bearing plants of every kind, and trees of every kind bearing fruit with the seed in it. And God saw that this was good. And there was evening and there was morning, a third day.

God said, "Let there be lights in the expanse of the sky to separate day from night; they shall serve as signs for the set times—the days and the years; and they shall serve as lights in the expanse of the sky to shine upon the earth." And it was so. God made the two great lights, the greater light to dominate the day and the lesser light to dominate the night, and the stars. And God set them in the expanse of the sky to shine upon the earth, to dominate the day and the night, and to separate light from darkness. And God saw that this was good. And there was evening and there was morning, a fourth day.

Hoarseness

Hoarseness is a kind of breathiness caused by strain. A common source of hoarseness is laryngitis, which is caused by a severe cold. There is, however, a kind of hoarseness that is caused by vocal abuse. Remember what your cheerleaders sounded like after the big game? Their voices probably had that strained sound of hoarseness. If they spoke little afterwards, their voices healed until the next Saturday, when the misuse and abuse began again. In some cases the abuse that causes hoarseness can injure the voice permanently.

Hoarseness results because the vocal folds cannot close the glottis effectively and the vocal muscles are strained. When vocal rest does not clear up hoarseness, see a laryngologist or voice therapist. With the advent of rock and roll and of singers who brag that they have never had a singing lesson and can be heard easily over the guitars, there has been a marked increase in the incidence of hoarseness. This hoarseness can be momentary or chronic.

Sometimes this kind of vocal abuse creates **nodules** on or near the vocal folds. Nodules are types of polyps and are benign rather than malignant. They are caused by excessive strain or friction. Often called **singer's nodes,** such nodules continue to grow as long as the abuse continues. Nodules can be removed surgically if necessary, but they grow back if the speech habits continue that create tension. Therefore, it is of great importance that a speech pathologist be consulted so that bad vocal habits can be eliminated.

Characteristics of the hoarse voice are an unsteady pitch that favors the lower registers, a weak voice, and frequent cracking of the voice.

Stridency

A **strident** voice is harsh, unpleasant, tinny, and generally high pitched. The person with a strident voice is stereotypically neurotic, whether male or female. Another group of individuals who often have strident voices are the hearing impaired. Many speakers with a hearing loss cannot hear their stridency.

It may be professionally advantageous to produce a strident voice. However, do not use it for a long time or at high volume.

The following exercises will help correct hoarse and strident voices: Exercises for Breath Control (pp. 27–36), Overly Open Throat Exercises (pp. 54–56), Nasal Resonance Exercises (pp. 57–60), and Optimum Pitch Exercises (pp. 67–69).

PART

II

SPEECH

6

ARTICULATION— THE PRODUCTION OF CONSONANTS

GLOSSARY

Affricate   A speech sound composed of a plosive and a fricative.

Allophone   A variation of a phoneme.

Articulation   The production of sounds, particularly consonants.

Aspirate   A sound composed predominantly of breath.

Auditory Discrimination   The ability to hear differences among sounds.

Auditory Sense   The sense of hearing.

Cognate Pairs   Two sounds having the same articulatory adjustment where one is voiceless and the other is voiced.

Dental   Pertaining to the teeth.

Dentalization   The articulation error resulting when the teeth are inappropriately used in the production of a sound.

Fricative   A speech sound in which breath or sound waves pass through a narrow opening so as to create frictional noises.

Kinesthetic Sense   The sense of small muscular movements.

Lambda   An /l/ allophone made with the tongue tip resting behind the lower front teeth.

Lateralization   The improper escape of air from the sides of the mouth and over the sides of the tongue, as in a lateralized sibilant.

Linguaalveolar   Pertaining to the tongue and alveolar ridge.

Linguapalatal   Pertaining to the tongue and the palate.

Linguavelar   Pertaining to the tongue and the velum.

Nasal   Pertaining to the nose or to a speech sound in which the vibrating air resonates in the nose.

Phoneme   A sound family.

Phonetics   The science of speech sounds.

Plosive   A speech sound in which breath under pressure reaches a peak point in the articulatory adjustment and is released in a small puff of air when the articulators are relaxed.

Schwa   The most-used vowel in English; any unstressed vowel can become a schwa.

Semivowel   A speech sound in which there is a gliding movement of the tongue, the lips, or both.

Sibilant   A speech sound in which breath passes through a narrow opening so as to create a hissing noise.

Tactile Sense   The sense of touch.

Visual Sense   The sense of sight.

Voiced Sound   A sound produced by the vibration of the vocal folds; also called a sonant, tonic, phonating, or vibrating sound.

Voiceless Sound   A sound produced with no vibration of the vocal folds; also called a surd, atonic, nonphonating, or nonvibrating sound.

In Chapter 1 we mentioned how misleading letters can be. That is the reason why the IPA (International Phonetic Alphabet), dealing exclusively with sounds, was developed in 1888 at an international convention of language teachers. Although the traditional alphabet can be used to create words and therefore meaning, it can be very confusing. The IPA is a common system of notation that simplifies our study of the sound of language. This study is called **phonetics,** the science of speech sounds.

Before we isolate English speech sounds and determine their symbols in the phonetic alphabet, we must clarify a few terms. Speech sounds are composed of phonemes. A **phoneme** is the smallest unit of recognizable speech sound; it is a sound family. Not everyone produces a phoneme in the same exact way. In addition, as indicated in the discussion on assimilation, the location of sounds in a word and the transition from one sound to another is also relevant. In the words *theme, seat, bean,* and *peach,* the only similarity is that all of the words contain the same vowel phoneme. Each consonant phoneme in the words is different. There are a number of ways to produce a phoneme, depending on the sounds that surround it and the capability of the speaker. The /d/ in *deal* is not produced exactly the same as the /d/ in *drown.* You can easily feel the difference between the sound productions by going back and forth between the two words. These varieties of the phoneme /d/ are called allophones. An **allophone** is a variation of a phoneme; an allophone can be acceptable or unacceptable, depending on the standard for the particular dialect or profession in question.

SENSE STIMULI

There are four senses of particular importance in developing good articulation and enunciation: the auditory, visual, tactile, and kinesthetic senses. Everyone has a favorite sense, through which much information can be obtained. All can be developed, however.

Because of the printing press, many people believe that the strongest sense is the **visual sense.** For many others, the **auditory sense** is the most important because it prevailed before printed material arose. Both the visual and auditory senses are important in the production of speech, but hearing the difference between sounds is particularly valuable. After all, you distinguish the difference between /o/ (as in *go*) and /u/ (as in *true*) through auditory discrimination rather than visual.

Visualization is used not only in the production of the sound but also—and more importantly—in the communicative process as a whole. Much of the information received by a listener is visual, including sound production (such as the difference between /f/ as in *fun* and /θ/ as in *thing*), gestures, and attitude.

The **tactile sense** concerns touch and the sensation of physical contact. The differences between suede, burlap, and cashmere are most dramatically perceived through the tactile sense. When you buy fruit or vegetables, it is recommended (but not by the store owner!) that you touch and gently squeeze as well as smell the item. In sound production, it is often very helpful to feel what your tongue is doing when you articulate an /l/ or /t/. The tactile sense is especially useful in producing consonant sounds.

The **kinesthetic sense** involves the feeling or tension of the muscles and the awareness of the resulting movement. (The word is from the Greek *kine* meaning "muscle" and *thesis* meaning "concept"). For example, you can tell whether your lips are rounded in the production of /u/ (as in *true*).

The four senses work together, of course. Although you sometimes favor one or two of the senses, all four are very helpful in learning and distinguishing sound production. They are also very helpful in the general communication process.

ARTICULATION

Articulation as used in this text refers to the production of consonant sounds. There is certainly a strong relationship between this definition and the more usual definitions, such as the ability to speak clearly and skillfully. However, we have chosen this usage because the term also means "to join." Since consonants need more precise production than vowels, with articulators "joining," or interacting with each other, the term *articulation* has been chosen. The term *enunciation* (Chapter 7) will be used in discussing the production of vowel sounds.

The articulators that are responsible for producing consonants and vowels can be divided into active (those that are capable of moving) and passive (those that are immovable) (see Figure 6.1):

Active	*Passive*
Tongue (largest and most active articulator)	Maxilla (upper jaw)
	Alveolar Ridge

FIGURE 6.1　　PARTS OF THE TONGUE

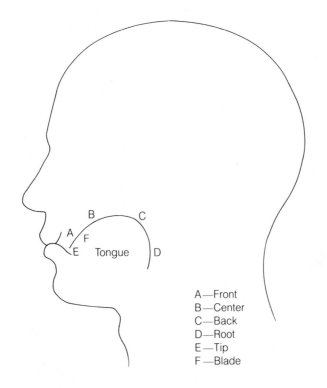

A—Front
B—Center
C—Back
D—Root
E—Tip
F—Blade

Velum   Teeth (passive in most cases!)

Muscles of the Cheeks   Hard Palate

Muscles of the Pharynx

Lips

Mandible (lower jaw)

Usually one of these articulators comes in contact with another in producing a speech sound.

All sounds, whether they are consonants, vowels, or diphthongs, are composed of either (1) breath (with no vibration of the vocal folds) or (2) vibration of the vocal folds. Breath must be present to produce all sounds, whether voiced or voiceless. One of the classifications of English sounds is based on whether the vocal folds vibrate. If just breath is used with no vibration of the vocal folds, the sound is referred to as **voiceless,** surd, atonic (without tone), nonphonating, or nonvibrating. If the sound is produced with breath plus vibration, it is referred to as **voiced,** sonant, tonic, phonating, or vibrating.

Two sounds, one voiced and one unvoiced, having the same articulatory adjustment are called **cognate pairs.** In other words, these sounds are made in the same way, but in one the vocal folds vibrate and in the other there is just breath (/v/ and /f/, for example). Two classifications of consonant sounds contain cognate pairs: plosives and fricatives.

CONSONANT CLASSIFICATIONS

Plosives

An American-English sound is either a continuant (capable of being prolonged) or a plosive. If it is a **plosive,** there is breath under pressure, which is at a peak in the articulatory mold and is released in a small puff of sound when the articulators are relaxed. There are eight plosives, composed of four cognate pairs. All of the remaining sounds in English are continuants.

Articulatory Adjustment	*Voiceless*	*Voiced*
Bilabial (two lips)	/p/ as in *put*	/b/ as in *bad*
Linguaalveolar (tip of tongue on alveolar ridge)	/t/ as in *take*	/d/ as in *day*
Linguavelar (back of tongue and velum)	/k/ as in *cake*	/g/ as in *gun*
Linguaalveolar and **Linguapalatal** (tongue against front and sides of palate)	/tʃ/ as in *chain*	/dʒ/ as in *joint*

Remember that each pair of sounds /p-b/, /t-d/, /k-g/, and /tʃ-ʤ/ have the same articulatory adjustment and differ only in the presence of vibration of the vocal folds.

Although the major heading for the plosives /tʃ/ and /ʤ/ is plosive, they are also known as **affricates**, a combination of a plosive and fricative.

The following word list presents each plosive in the three possible positions in a word:

	Initial	*Medial*	*Final*
/p/	pout, punch, pick	apply, apart, apple	slap, step, clip
/b/	but, bunch, back	about, rubble, mobbing	slab, sub, crab
/t/	toy, talk, tub	matter, hurting, plotter	sweet, night, mint
/d/	dine, deal, den	toddler, middle, rudder	add, tied, fled
/k/	keep, kill, kind	picket, pocket, ankle	hawk, book, track
/g/	get, gone, game	ago, beggar, anger	bag, pig, drag
/tʃ/	chip, check, chop	butcher, catcher, matches	birch, witch, etch
/ʤ/	jump, Jim, juggle	agile, angel, budget	age, garbage, rampage

Fricatives

A **fricative** is a speech sound in which breath passes through such a narrow opening in the articulatory mold so as to create frictional noises. Most fricatives occur as cognate pairs. The last four fricatives are also known as sibilants. A **sibilant** is a type of sound, not a production error. Thus, it is redundant to say that someone has a "sibilant /s/." All /s/ phonemes are sibilants. A speaker with a whistling /s/ is sometimes described incorrectly as having a sibilant /s/.

Articulatory Adjustment		*Voiceless*	*Voiced*
Labiodental (lower lip and upper teeth)	/f/	as in *fun*	/v/ as in *vine*
Linguadental (tongue between upper and lower teeth)	/θ/	as in *thing*	/ð/ as in *them*
Glottal (takes on articulatory characteristics of sound that follows)	/h/	as in *hop*	
Bilabial	/ʍ/	as in *while*	
Linguaalveolar	/s/	as in *save*	/z/ as in *zoo*
Linguapalatal	/ʃ/	as in *shape*	/ʒ/ as in *treasure*

ınds /s/, /z/, /ʃ/, and /ʒ/ are also called sibilants.

Initial	*Medial*	*Final*
fine, fit, phone	after, afraid, offer	hoof, half, beef
vouch, very, vain	average, avenue, cover	stove, cave, above
theme, thought, Thursday	author, birthday, anything	sheath, birth, breath
there, that, thou	bathing, bother, other	clothe, writhe, breathe
hoe, hay, home	ahoy, behind, bee-hive	(does not occur)
where, when, white	meanwhile, any-where, everywhere	(does not occur)
say, sail, sign	asleep, basket, faster	class, face, chess
zebra, zipper, zero	hazel, razor, amazed	as, phase, bruise
ship, shell, shore	lashing, ashes, brushes	blush, crash, dish
(does not occur)	azure, leisure, measure	garage, mirage, es-pionage

Lateral

There is one lateral speech sound, /l/ as in *leg*. It is produced with the tip of the tongue against the alveolar ridge with the sides of the tongue free from contact. It can appear in any position within a word:

	Initial	*Medial*	*Final*
/l/	lie, lick, lamp	along, allow, alibi	fill, while, hole

Semivowels

A **semivowel** is a speech sound in which there is a gliding movement of the tongue, the lips, or both. Because of the gliding movement, the semivowels maintain characteristics of the vowel (see Chapter 7). There are three semivowels: /r/, /w/, and /j/. There are no cognate pairs among the semivowels, since all of them are voiced.

Articulatory Adjustment	*Phoneme*
Gliding movement of lips and tongue	/r/ as in *red*
Gliding movement of lips	/w/ as in *way*
Gliding movement of tongue	/j/ as in *yet*

	Initial	*Medial*	*Final*
/r/	run, rig, robbed	arrange, around, carriage	tar, bore, fear
/w/	wedge, willow, web	aware, forward, coward	(does not occur)[1]
/j/	yonder, yell, young	billiard, beyond, lawyer	(does not occur)

Nasals

A **nasal** sound is a speech sound in which the vibrating breath escapes through the nose because the velum is relaxed. All nasal sounds are sonant, so there are no cognate pairs. The three nasal sounds are /m/, /n/, and /ŋ/. The last nasal is the sound that corresponds to the pronunciation of the two letters "ng." This sound is particularly problematic for the person learning English, and it also poses difficulties for American-born speakers.

Articulatory Adjustment	*Phoneme*
Bilabial with relaxed velum	/m/ as in *mit*
Linguaalveolar with relaxed velum	/n/ as in *no*
Linguavelar with relaxed velum (back of tongue against velum)	/ŋ/ as in *ring*

	Initial	*Medial*	*Final*
/m/	may, marsh, mug	amid, camel, camera	same, crumb, clam
/n/	nice, knife, numb	annoy, annual, candle	tan, sane, been
/ŋ/	(does not occur)	singer, hanger, length	rang, fling, lung

Each sound will be presented and discussed in terms of articulatory production, frequent problems in production of the sound, and exercises for improvement.

---

[1] Some words end in the letter *w* (*slow, how*), but it is not accompanied by a /w/ sound.

PLOSIVES

/p/ and /b/

Production

Both /p/ and /b/ are made with the lips coming together and the teeth slightly apart. Pressure is built up behind the lips; when they are pushed apart so that the air or sound waves escape, sound is produced. The sound produced varies with the amount of air expended and the amount of pressure built up behind the lips. Another variable is the location of the sound within the words. For example, there is more pressure in the initial /p/ (as in *Pat*) than the final (*up*). Also, there is more pressure in the initial /b/ (*ball*) than the medial /b/ in *robbed*.

Problems

The phonemes /p/ and /b/ are usually not problematic unless there is some difficulty with the bite. If there is a fairly severe overbite, for example, the upper teeth may touch the lower lip when /p/ and /b/ are produced. (This **dental** problem would affect the production of other sounds as well.) Make certain that your lips touch when you say these phonemes. Use a mirror in addition to employing the tactile and kinesthetic senses.

EXERCISES FOR /p/ AND /b/

1. Read the following word lists with an exaggerated production of /p/ and /b/. Build up the pressure so that you can feel and see in the mirror the production of the sounds. Make certain that when you pull away from the exaggerated sound to articulate more appropriately you don't pull away too much. Chances are you are an underarticulator!

Initial	*Medial*	*Final*
pot	clapping	top
pay	apart	cup
paid	report	tape
paste	stepping	strap
pray	rupture	hope
bought	above	dab
base	rebound	disturb

back	stable	crab
beggar	rebel	slab
blame	habit	stub

Read aloud the following selections.

2. It is never any good dwelling on goodbyes. It is not the being together that it prolongs, it is the parting.

3. If you pick up a starving dog and make him prosperous, he will not bite you. That is the principal difference between a dog and a man.

4. Bring a bit of buttered, brown, bran bread.

5. Betty Botter bought a bit of butter. "But," she said, "this butter's bitter. If I put it in my batter, it will make my batter bitter." So Betty Botter bought a bit of better butter, and it made her batter better.

6. Bloom, beauteous blossoms, budding bowers beneath!
   Behold, Boreas' bitter blast by brief
   Bright beams becalmed; balmy breezes breathe,
   Banishing blight, bring bliss beyond belief.

7. Peter Piper picked a peck of pickled peppers,
   A peck of pickled peppers Peter Piper picked.
   If Peter Piper picked a peck of pickled peppers,
   Where's the peck of pickled peppers Peter Piper picked?

8. Beauty without virtue, is like a flower without perfume.

9. Joakim was a tool of Egypt and permitted many of the worse forms of religious syncretism to come into his country. He was a despot with little concern for the people. Jeremiah, the prophet, reproached him for his deeds—impoverishing the land through levies, compulsory labor, extortion, illegal death sentences, and deterioration of the religious worship of Yahweh.
   THE BIBLE

10. The bleak breeze blighted the bright broom blossoms.

11. Better beans and bacon in peace than cakes and ale in fear.
    Aesop

/t/ and /d/

Production

Both /t/ and /d/ are made with the tip of the tongue against the alveolar ridge behind the upper teeth. Pressure is built up between the tongue tip and alveolar ridge, and the sound is produced when the tongue tip is dropped. The sound produced varies with the amount of air expended and the amount of pressure behind the ridge. There is more pressure when the sound is produced in the initial (*tale*) than in the final (*eight*) position.

Problems

The most common problem in the production of /t/ and /d/ is contact of the tongue or blade of the tongue with the back of the upper teeth rather than with the gum ridge. Thus, these sounds are linguaalveolar but are often made linguadentally. The problem sound that is produced is said to be **dentalized** and is transcribed as /t̪/ and /d̪/, respectively. Instead of saying *toot* /tut/ or *dude* /dud/ with just the tongue tip, the person who dentalizes says /t̪ut̪/ or /d̪ud̪/ by placing the blade of the tongue on the back of the upper teeth. This is how many a New Yorker sounds. Use a mirror to see what dentalization looks like.

A major problem for the Southern speaker (especially young girls) is the substitution of the glottal stop [ʔ] for the /t/ and /d/ in the medial position in the contraction of "did not" and "could not." However, this error is not limited only to the South! If this is one of your errors, see the section on implosion and explosion in Chapter 8.

EXERCISES FOR /t/ AND /d/

1. Read the following word lists exaggerating your production of /t/ and /d/. Build up the pressure so that you can feel and see in a mirror the production of the sounds. Make certain that when you pull away from the exaggerated sound to articulate more appropriately you do not pull away too much.

Initial	*Medial*	*Final*
tongue	sweater	polite
toll	lettuce	fruit
tree	sitter	clapped
towel	lately	dirt
television	painting	boat
diety	adding	side
dare	buddy	learned
Danny	android	find
donor	feeder	signed
divine	wedding	avid

Read aloud the following selections. Many of them are also good for breath control.

2. This exercise is also good for the articulation of the /l/ phoneme as well as breath control. Make certain that you do not substitute the /d/ phoneme for the /t/ in words such as "Waterloo," "categorical," and "matters mathematical."

I am the very model of a modern Major-General,
I've information vegetable, animal, and mineral.
I know the kings of England, and I quote the fights historical,
From Marathon to Waterloo, in order categorical;
I'm very well acquainted too with matters mathematical.
I understand equations, both the simple and quadratical,
About binomial theorem I'm teeming with a lot o' news—
With many cheerful facts about the square of the hypotenuse.
I'm very good at integral and differential calculus,
I know the scientific names of beings animalculus;
In short, in matters vegetable, animal, and mineral,
I am the very model of a modern Major-General.

From THE PIRATES OF PENZANCE   *W. S. Gilbert*

3. He didn't say he wouldn't, and he didn't say he couldn't, or shouldn't but he didn't.

4. Teasing Tom was a very bad boy;
A great big squirt was his favorite toy;
He put live shrimps in his father's boots,
And sewed up the sleeves of his Sunday suits;
He punched his poor little sisters' heads,
And cayenne-peppered their four-post beds;
He plastered their hair with cobbler's wax
And dropped hot half-pennies down their backs.

TEASING TOM   *W. S. Gilbert*

5. Oh, somewhere in this favored land the sun is shining bright;
The Band is playing somewhere, and somewhere hearts are light.

From CASEY AT THE BAT   *Ernest Lawrence Thayer*

6. Deep into that darkness peering, long I stood there, wondering, fearing,
Doubting, dreaming dreams no mortal ever dared to dream before;
But the silence was unbroken, and the stillness gave no token,
And the only word there spoken was the whispered word "Lenore!"
This I whispered, and an echo murmured back the word "Lenore!"
Merely this and nothing more.

From THE RAVEN   *Edgar Allan Poe*

7. A silly young fellow named Hyde
   In a funeral procession was spied;
   When asked, "Who is dead?"
   He giggled and said,
   "I don't know; I just came for the ride."

8. Thomas Tattertoot took taut twine to tie ten twigs to two tall trees.

9. When a twiner a-twisting will twist him a twist.
   For the twining has twist he three times doth untwist;
   But if one of the twines of the twist do untwist,
   The twine that untwineth, untwineth the twist.

10. If you pick up a starving dog and make him prosperous, he will not bite you.
    This is the principal difference between a dog and a man.

11. I go to books and to nature as a bee goes to the flower, for a nectar that I can
    make into my own honey.

/k/ *and* /g/

Production

Both /k/ and /g/ are made with the back of the tongue firmly against the velum.
Pressure should be built up between the tongue and velum; when the tongue is
relaxed and the air escapes, the sounds are produced.

Problems

The two most frequent difficulties in producing /k/ and /g/ are: (1) failure to make
firm contact between the tongue and the velum and (2) the omission of the /k/
in certain words ("breafast" for *breakfast*) and in conversational speech ("Don't
ass questions!"), giving a street quality to the speech.

EXERCISES FOR /k/ AND /g/

1. *Weakness in Contact.* Read the following word lists with an exaggerated
   production of /k/ and /g/. Build up the pressure so that you can feel and see
   in the mirror the production of the sounds. This is more difficult than in /p/
   and /b/, because the production of those sounds is easier to see. Make certain
   that when you pull away from the exaggerated to articulate more appropriately you don't pull away too much.

Initial	*Medial*	*Final*
count	lucky	back
care	bunker	book

crunch	become	fork
chemical	looking	bake
quite	turkey	stork
goose	begin	bag
guess	forget	rig
guard	regulate	vague
goat	trigger	iceberg
gift	beggar	intrigue

2. *Omission of* /k/. Read and record the following list of words and phrases aloud, making certain that all of the sounds in the words are produced. For the present purposes, you should explode all of the underlined /k/ sounds so that you feel the production of the sound. Use negative practice, and make sure that you omit the /k/ phoneme in the second pronunciation. In career speech, you would use implosion, which is discussed in Chapter 8.

asked him	desktop	risks everything
Masked Marvel	disk drive	white tusks
car flasks	heavy tasks	asks him

Read aloud the following selections.

3. I know the Kings of England, and I quote the fights historical.
   From Marathon to Waterloo, in order categorical.

   From THE PIRATES OF PENZANCE *W. S. Gilbert*

4. Children begin by loving their parents; after a time they judge them; rarely, if ever, do they forgive them.

5. I can't help detesting my relations, I suppose it comes from the fact that we can't stand other people having the same faults as ourselves.

6. The sea is calm to-night,
   The tide is full, the moon lies fair
   Upon the Straits;—on the French coast, the light
   Gleams, and is gone; the cliffs of England stand,
   Glimmering and vast, out in the tranquil bay.
   Come to the window, sweet is the night air!

   From DOVER BEACH *Matthew Arnold*

7. A fancy young dandy from Niger
   Went out for a ride on a tiger.
   They returned from the ride

With the dandy inside
And a smile on the face of the tiger.

8. Good men, the last wave by, crying how bright
Their frail deeds might have danced in a green bay.

From DO NOT GO GENTLE INTO THAT GOOD NIGHT   *Dylan Thomas*

9. Give me a condor's quill! Give me Vesuvius' crater for an inkstand! . . . To
produce a mighty book, you must choose a mighty theme.

From MOBY DICK   *Herman Melville*

10. There was a young lady of Crete
Who was exceedingly neat.
When she got out of bed
She stood on her head
To make sure of not soiling her feet.

11. I saw a peacock with a fiery tail
I saw a blazing comet drop down hail
I saw a cloud wrapped with ivy round
I saw an oak creep on along the ground
I saw a pismire swallow up a whale
I saw the sea brimful of ale
I saw a Venice glass full fathom deep
I saw a well full of men's tears that weep
I saw red eyes all of a flaming fire
I saw a house bigger than the moon and higher
I saw the sun at twelve o'clock at night
I saw the man that saw this wondrous sight.

Anonymous

12. As I was playing on the green
A little book it chanced I seen.
Carlyle's *Essay on Burns* was the edition;
I left it laying in the same position.

Anonymous

/tʃ/ and /dʒ/

Production

The phonemes /tʃ/ and /dʒ/ are made with the tip and the blade of the tongue
firmly against the alveolar ridge. The sides of the tongue touch the inner edges
of the upper back teeth along the palate. Pressure is built up behind the tongue,
and the sound is produced when the air escapes and the tip and blade of the

tongue drop down, causing a small groove. The sides of the tongue remain along the inner edges of the palate and upper teeth to prevent air from escaping over the sides of the tongue.

Problems

The biggest problem in the production of /tʃ/ and /dʒ/ is the escape of air over the sides of the tongue rather than over the tip. This problem is called **lateralization**. Make believe that you are going to phonate the consonant /l/. Place the tip of your tongue on the alveolar ridge and blow air over the sides of the tongue. This is lateralization. The problem arises in the production of /ʃ/ and /ʒ/ rather than /t/ and /d/.

EXERCISES FOR /tʃ/ AND /dʒ/

1. To correct lateralization, a good exercise is to increase the feeling of linguaalveolar closure. As in the other exercises for initial plosives, exaggerate the buildup of pressure as you read aloud the following word lists. Round the lips as you exaggerate the production of the sound. Using a mirror, pay attention to the visual aspects of the production of the sounds.[2]

Initial	*Medial*	*Final*
cheerful	butcher	pitch
chase	benches	batch
chin	beaches	witch
chopping	matches	beach
chain	furniture	match
jail	besieged	average
jump	stranger	Madge
joke	regent	lunge
jelly	major	dirge
gem	plunging	marriage

Read aloud the following selections.

---

[2] These affricates are particularly difficult for foreign speakers learning English. Because many languages do not contain /tʃ/ and /dʒ/, foreign speakers substitute the fricatives /ʃ/ and /ʒ/. These are discussed in detail on page 22. A German or Frenchman is apt to say "sheet" for *cheat* and "ship" for *chip*. Further difficulty stems from the inconsistency in the English spelling of the sound /dʒ/: soldier, rage, general, jump, grandeur, and major.

2. A cheap, changeable, childlike chimpanzee champion playing checkers with Charles.

3. The angels wrote down the strategy for the ancient major.

4. The lunatic, the lover, and the poet
   Are of imagination all compact.
   One sees more devils than vast hell can hold,
   That is the madman. The lover, all as frantic,
   Sees Helen's beauty in a brow of Egypt:
   The poet's eye, in a fine frenzy rolling,
   Doth glance from heaven to earth, from earth to heaven;
   And as imagination bodies forth
   The forms of things unknown, the poet's pen
   Turns them to shapes, and gives to airy nothing
   A local habitation and a name.

   From A MIDSUMMER NIGHT'S DREAM   *William Shakespeare*

5. If a woodchuck could chuck wood, how much wood would a woodchuck chuck if a woodchuck could or would? But if a woodchuck could and would chuck wood, no reason why he should, how much wood would a woodchuck chuck if a woodchuck could and would chuck wood?

6. Madge and Jim jammed George and Geraldine into the Volkswagen.

7. Cheddar and Jack cheese can be cheap.

8. The gym teacher jumped at the chance to coach the gymnastics team.

9. Christianity and Judaism are compatible religions.

10. Speech teachers are often accused of teaching gibberish.

11. Jenny kissed me when we met,
    Jumping from the chair she sat in;
    Time, you thief, who loves to get
    Sweets into your list, put that in:

    Say I'm weary, say I'm sad,
    Say that health and wealth have missed me,
    Say I'm growing old, but add
    Jenny kissed me.

    JENNY KISSED ME   *Leigh Hunt*

/f/ and /v/

Production

Both /f/ and /v/ sounds are made by bringing the inner edges of the lower lip against the upper teeth. The sounds are produced when the breath or voice escapes through a narrow opening between the upper teeth and lower lip.

Problems

The most common error in the production of /f/ and /v/ is too much or too little contact between the upper teeth and the lower lip. If there is too much contact and a pressing down of the teeth on the lip, the sounds resemble plosive sounds. If there is too little contact or the teeth touch too low on the lip, the sounds become "slushy."

EXERCISES FOR /f/ AND /v/

In the following word lists and exercises, exaggerate the articulation before you attempt to pull away. Using a mirror, watch the formation of the sounds; maintain good articulation when you pull away.

1. *Initial* *Medial* *Final*

Initial	Medial	Final
fame	infamous	belief
ferment	influence	cliff
photo	telephone	laugh
food	coffee	cough
funny	chauffeur	enough
vanity	evil	eve
Venus	devil	groove
victory	David	shelve
valley	prevent	stove
vain	avoid	love

2. The flesh of freshly dried flying fish.

3. Fanny Finch fried five floundering fish for Francis Fowler's father Fred.

4. Five flippy Frenchmen foolishly fanning fainting flies.

5. Pillow'd upon my fair love's ripening breast,
   To feel for ever its soft fall and swell,
   Awake for ever in a sweet unrest,
   Still, still to hear her tender-taken breath,
   And so live ever—or else swoon to death.

   From BRIGHT STAR *John Keats*

6. Hearts just as pure and fair
   May beat in Belgrave Square

As in the lowly air
Of Seven Dials.

From IOLANTHE   *W. S. Gilbert*

7. The holy passion of Friendship is of so sweet and steady and loyal and enduring a nature that it will last through a whole lifetime, if not asked to lend
money.

From PUDD'NHEAD WILSON   *Mark Twain*

8. Our minds are finite, and yet even in these circumstances of finitude we are
surrounded by possibilities that we are infinite, and the purpose of human
life is to grasp as much as we can out of that infinitude.

From DIALOGUES   *Alfred North Whitehead*

9. Christian endeavor is notoriously hard on female pulchritude.

From THE AESTHETIC RECOIL   *H. L. Mencken*

10. Faint heart never won fair lady!
Nothing venture, nothing win—
Blood is thick, but water's thin—
In for a penny, in for a pound—
It's Love that makes the world go round!

From IOLANTHE   *W. S. Gilbert*

11. The prophesying business is like writing fugues; it is fatal to every one save
the man of absolute genius.

From PREJUDICES   *H. L. Mencken*

/θ/ *and* /ð/

Production

Both /θ/ and /ð/ are produced with the tip of the tongue lightly placed against the
upper front teeth. The breath or voice that escapes through the space between
the tongue and the teeth causes the frictional noise.

Problems

The major problems in producing these phonemes are (1) the substitution of /t/
or /d/ for /θ/ and /ð/, respectively, and (2) their omission. For example, the
stereotypical street kid says, "Ya bedda go wid me!" substituting the /d/ plosive
for the /ð/ fricative. In words like *widths, sixths, baths,* and *clothes,* you don't
have to be a thug to omit /θ/ and /ð/—care is necessary to articulate all of the
sounds. Career speech requires this kind of precision. Carefully articulating
some of these words will probably make you feel somewhat self-conscious. It's
almost like learning a foreign language.

These fricative sounds can be problematic for individuals learning English as a second language. In many languages, including German, French, Italian, and Spanish, there are no /θ/ and /ð/ sounds. When these people learn English, they usually substitute /t-d/ or /s-z/.

EXERCISES FOR /θ/ AND /ð/

1. Read the following word lists with exaggerated articulation. Take the time to feel and see the production of all of the sounds, particularly /θ/ and /ð/.

Initial	*Medial*	*Final*
theme	bathroom	breath
thought	pathetic	wrath
think	Catholic	mouth
thanks	pathway	cloth
thin	youthful	bath
them	father	tithe
those	leather	breathe
though	either	soothe
there	weather	lithe
that	feather	with

2. Read the following pairs of words with exaggerated articulation. Take the time to feel and see the production of the fricative sounds both without and with the sibilant. Repeat the words with appropriate articulation, making certain that you do not pull away too much from overarticulation.

myth, myths	wreath, wreaths[3] ∿
breathe, breathes	wreathe, wreathes ✓
teethe, teethes	writhe, writhes
clothe, clothes	depth, depths
lathe, lathes	earth, earths
length, lengths	north, norths

Read aloud the following selections.

---

[3] Pronounced /riðz/.

3. The sea ceaseth—it sufficeth sufficiently that the sea ceaseth.

4. Theophilus Thistledown the thistle sifter sifted a sieve of unsifted thistles. If Theophilus Thistledown the thistle sifter sifted a sieve of unsifted thistles, where is the sieve of unsifted thistles Theophilus Thistledown the thistle sifter sifted?

5. A certain soap is said to be ninety-nine and forty-four one hundredths percent pure.

6. The sixth sheik's sixth sheep's sick.

7. A thatcher of Thatchwood went to Thatchet a-thatching;
Did a thatcher of Thatchwood go to Thatchet a-thatching?
If a thatcher of Thatchwood went to Thatchet a-thatching,
Where's that thatching the thatcher of Thatchwood has thatched?

8. Helen, thy beauty is to me
Like those Nicean barks of yore,
That gently, o'er a perfumed sea,
The weary, wayworn wanderer bore
To his own native shore.

TO HELEN   *Edgar Allan Poe*

9. The minister gave out his text and droned along monotonously through an argument that was so prosy that many a head by and by began to nod—and yet it was an argument that dealt in limitless fire and brimstone and thinned the predestined elect down to a company so small as to be hardly worth the saving.

From THE ADVENTURES OF TOM SAWYER   *Mark Twain*

10. When I hear people say they have not found the world and life so agreeable or interesting as to be in love with it, or that they look with equanimity to its end, I am apt to think they have never been properly alive nor seen with clear vision the world they think so meanly of, or anything in it—not a blade of grass.

From FAR AWAY AND LONG AGO   *W. H. Hudson*

11. Whose wreathed friezes intertwine
The viol, the violet, and the vine.

From THE CITY IN THE SEA   *Edgar Allan Poe*

12. Though I am old with wandering
Through hollow lands and hilly lands.

From THE SONG OF WANDERING AENGUS   *William Butler Yeats*

13. Rejoice not when thine enemy falleth, and let not thine heart be glad when he stumbleth.

/h/

Production

Since the glottal sound /h/ has no articulatory adjustment, it takes on the adjustment of the vowel or diphthong that follows. The frictional sound is produced at the glottis with slight tension but no vibration of the vocal folds.

Problems

Difficulties with /h/ are rare for the native American. Most problems are found among people learning English as a second language. Sometimes the letter "h" is silent, as in words like *honor* or *hour*. Some words like *humor* or *human* can be said with or without the phoneme /h/.

EXERCISES FOR /h/

1. Read the following word lists aloud with exaggerated articulation. Take the time to feel and see the assimilation that takes place during the production of /h/. Don't pull away too much when you read the exercises with appropriate articulation. Be guided more by your visual rather than the kinesthetic sense.

Initial	*Medial*	*Final*
home	somehow	(does not occur)
who	inhuman	
honey	behave	
hill	beehive	
half	bohemian	
hear	unheard	
head	prehistorical	
hair	exhale	
hospital	unholy	
hall	cohort	

2. The following is a partial list of words that may be pronounced with or without the /h/ phoneme according to Webster's *International Dictionary*. However, in professional speech, the /h/ should be pronounced.

humanity	humane	humidify
huge	humor	humiliate
humid	humorist	humble
humidor	Hugh	homage
human	humorous	

Read aloud the following selections.

3. Whose woods these are I think I know.
   His house is in the village though.

   From STOPPING BY WOODS ON A SNOWY EVENING   *Robert Frost*

4. Heap high the farmer's wintry hoard!
   Heap high the golden corn!
   No richer gift has Autumn poured
   From out her lavish horn!

   From THE CORN SONG   *John Greenleaf Whittier*

5. But oh! shipmates! on the starboard hand of every woe, there is a sure delight; and higher the top of that delight, than the bottom of the woe is deep.
   Is not the main-truck higher than the kelson is low? Delight is to him—a
   far, far upward, and inward delight—who against the proud gods and commodores of this earth, ever stands forth his own inexorable self.

   From MOBY DICK   *Herman Melville*

6. It must be remembered that the point of honour which decrees that a man
   must not under any circumstances accept money from a woman with whom
   he is on certain terms, is of very modern growth, and is still tempered by
   the proviso that he may take as much as he likes or can get from his wife.

   From the Preface to TOM JONES   *George Saintsbury*

7. The hawthorn hedge puts forth its buds,
   And my heart puts forth its pain.

   From ALL SUDDENLY THE SPRING   *Rupert Brooke*

8. Here comes a candle to light you to bed,
   Here comes a chopper to chop off your head.

9. Saul hath slain his thousands, and David his ten thousands.

   1 SAMUEL

10. He that trusteth in his own heart is a fool.

    PROVERBS

11. All say, "How hard it is that we have to die"—a strange complaint to come
    from the mouths of people who have had to live.

/ʍ/

Production

The phoneme /ʍ/ is sometimes transcribed /hw/. However, the sound should not be separated into /h/ and /w/, because the latter component is voiced while /h/ is unvoiced. Notice that the symbol looks something like the nasal /m/, with which it is often confused. In this text, /ʍ/ is classified as an unvoiced fricative having the **aspirate** characteristics of the /h/ phoneme. Like /h/, the phoneme /ʍ/ is influenced by the vowel or diphthong that it precedes. The sound is produced as the breath escapes between the slightly tensed vocal folds, which causes the frictional sound. In addition, upon production, round the lips and blow out the cheeks slightly. This adjustment of the cheeks feels most alien to the American, but it is one of those professional characteristics that you are strongly encouraged to make into a habit.

Problems

Many Americans do not use this sound in their speech because they do not know that it exists. Instead, they use only the phoneme /w/. Others, because of sloppy articulation, poor auditory discrimination, or both, use the semivowel /w/ instead of /ʍ/. Believe it or not, there is a difference in the pronunciation as well as the meaning between *weather* and *whether*. The phoneme /ʍ/ is truly an endangered sound.

Bing Crosby sang this way

EXERCISES FOR /ʍ/

In the following exercises, it is natural to feel self-conscious while you learn how to produce an English sound you never realized existed! Use a mirror and make certain that when the sound is produced, the cheeks blow out a bit. Light a cigarette lighter or candle and hold it ten to twelve inches from your mouth. Make the flame waver as you pronounce the /ʍ/ words. If you are producing the sound properly, you can see the action of the cheeks clearly. If you are beginning to look like Dizzy Gillespie, the trumpeter, you are overinflating your cheeks. However, that is a fine way to feel the sensation necessary to the production.

1. In the following pairs, "Gillespie-ize" the second word, which contains the /ʍ/ phoneme. As in all introductory exercises, overdo the articulation. This sound, incidentally, occurs only in front of a vowel or diphthong. Make certain that when you pull back from overarticulation, you maintain the same accuracy of articulation.

witch, which	wear, where
wen, when	wit, whit
wine, whine	way, whey
wite, white	wail, whale
wile, while	we'll, wheel
wig, Whig	world, whirled
woe, whoa	wax, whacks
Y, why	word, whirred

[handwritten margin notes: "Blow out cheeks" ; "interrogative pronouns"; "Wen- cold n nose   Margret mitchell"; "Wart   wizard noz"]

In the remaining exercises, compare /ʍ/ with /w/. The double underline is under the phoneme /ʍ/; the single underline, under the /w/. Remember to blow out the cheeks!

2. What whim lead "Whitey" White to whittle, whistle, whisper, and whimper near the wharf where a whale might wheel and whirl?

3. To the Windmills said the Millwheel:
   "When the wind wills do you still the wheel?"
   "Yes, we still wheel when the wind wills!"
   To the Millwheel said the Windmills.

4. Oh, what a tangled web we weave,
   When first we practice to deceive!

   Sir Walter Scott

5. They are accustomed to deliberate on matters of the highest moment when warm with wine; but whatever they in this situation may determine is again proposed to them on the morrow, in their cooler moments, by the person in whose house they had before assembled. If at this time meet their approbation, it is executed; otherwise it is rejected. Whatever also, they discuss when sober, is always a second time examined after they have been drinking.

   BOOK 1 CLIO   *Herodotus*

6. What will you say when the world is dying?
   What, when the last wild midnight falls.

   Alfred Noyes

7. Ah, what is more blessed than to put cares away, when the mind lays by its burden, and tired with labor of far travel we have come to our own home and rest on the couch we longed for? This it is which alone is worth all these toils.

   ODES   *Catullus*

8. <u>Wh</u>y art thou cast down, O my soul?
and <u>wh</u>y art thou dis<u>qu</u>ieted <u>w</u>ithin
me? hope thou in God: for I shall
yet praise him, who is the health of my
countenance, and my God.

PSALMS

9. But be contented: <u>wh</u>en that fell arrest
<u>W</u>ithout all shall carry me a<u>w</u>ay,
My life hath in this line some interest,
<u>Wh</u>ich for memorial still <u>w</u>ith thee shall stay.
<u>Wh</u>en thou reviewest this, thou dost review
The very part <u>w</u>as consecrate to thee:
The earth can have but earth, <u>wh</u>ich is his due;
My spirit is thine, the better part of me:
So then thou hast but lost the dregs of life,
The prey of <u>w</u>orms, my body being dead;
The co<u>w</u>ard con<u>qu</u>est of a wretch's knife,
Too base of thee to be remembered.
The <u>w</u>orth of that <u>wh</u>ich it contains,
And that is this, and this <u>w</u>ith thee remains.

SONNET 74   *William Shakespeare*

10. I'll <u>w</u>alk <u>wh</u>ere my own nature <u>w</u>ould be leading—
It vexes me to choose another guide—
<u>Wh</u>ere the grey flocks in ferny glens are feeding,
<u>Wh</u>ere the <u>w</u>ild <u>w</u>ind blows on the mountain-side.

From OFTEN REBUKED   *Emily Bronte*

11. <u>Wh</u>y tarry the <u>wh</u>eels of his chariot?

2 JUDGES

12. This is the <u>w</u>ay the <u>w</u>orld ends
Not <u>w</u>ith a bang but a <u>wh</u>imper.

From THE HOLLOW MEN   *T. S. Eliot*

13. <u>Wh</u>ither, O splendid ship, thy <u>wh</u>ite sails crowing,
Leaning across the bosom of the urgent <u>W</u>est, . . .
<u>Wh</u>ither a<u>w</u>ay, fair rover, and <u>wh</u>at thy <u>qu</u>est?

A PASSER-BY   *Robert Bridges*

FRICATIVE SIBILANTS

/s/ and /z/

Production

The cognates /s/ and /z/ are made with the blade of the tongue contacting the alveolar ridge. In addition, the sides of the tongue touch the inner edges of the upper teeth. A small groove is created down the middle of the tongue over which the escaping breath or voice is forced, causing the frictional sound. Some speakers produce the sounds with the tongue tip raised, others with the tongue tip remaining behind the lower teeth. The preferred production depends on the surrounding sounds.

Problems

There are perhaps more difficulties in the production of these cognates than in the production of any other sounds. Although the sounds are not classified as dental, the teeth are essential for proper production. Thus, a child learns to "thpeak" long before the permanent front teeth come in. As a result, the child develops a frontal lisp, the substitution of /θ/ and /ð/ for /s/ and /z/.

If for the /s/ or /z/ the child produces the /l/ formation and blows out the air over the sides of the tongue, he or she is exhibiting lateralization.

In producing /s/ or /z/, some people bring the top and bottom teeth together and make the groove down the center of the tongue too narrow, causing the sound to be too sharp. In males, the resulting sound is considered effeminate.

Another common error is the whistling /s/. If this is a problem, shorten the length of the sound during production. The whistle often results from the groove down the blade of the tongue being too narrow.

All too often a speaker touches the lower lip to the upper teeth in producing /s/ or /z/. This is another form of dentalizing. The lip should not be used in the formation of the sibilants.

EXERCISES FOR /s/ AND /z/

Read the following exercises with overarticulation. Use a mirror to see how you produce the sounds. When you pull away from overarticulation, make certain to produce your sounds precisely. To develop flexibility in producing /s/ and /z/, you might also read the exercises with (1) a frontal lisp, (2) a lateral lisp, (3) with the top and bottom teeth together, and (4) using the lower lip. In creating characterizations, these faulty productions of /s/ and /z/ might prove helpful.

1. *Initial*   *Medial*   *Final*

Initial	Medial	Final
seem	answer	notice
Sunday	useful	house
suddenly	excited	grass
soon	excellent	nice
circle	hospital	juice
zipper	seizing	phase
zoo	lazy	chaise
xylophone	razor	craze
zink	sneezing	pays
zany	buzzing	prize

2. Slippery sleds slide smoothly down the sluiceway.

3. Moses supposes his toeses aren't roses
   But Moses supposes amiss.
   For Moses he knoses his toeses aren't roses
   As Moses supposes his toeses is.

4. A snifter of snuff is enough snuff for a sniff for the snuff sniffer.

5. The little Reed, bending to the force of the wind, soon stood upright again
   when the storm had passed over.

   Aesop

6. O, no! it is an ever-fixed mark,
   That looks on tempests and is never shaken;
   It is the star to ever wandering bark.

   SONNET *William Shakespeare*

7. Susan Simpson strolled sedately,
   Stifling sobs, suppressing sighs,
   Seeing Stephen Slocum, stately,
   She stopped, showing some surprise.

   "Say," said Stephen, "Sweetest sigher,
   Say, shall Stephen spouseless stay?"
   Susan, seeming somewhat shyer,
   Showed submissiveness straightaway.

   Summer's season slowly stretches,
   Susan Simpson Slocum she—
   So she signed some simple sketches—
   Soul sought soul successfully.

Six Septembers Susan swelters;
Six sharp seasons snow supplies;
Susan's satin sofa shelters
Six small Slocums side by side.

Anonymous

8. Left to herself, Salomy Jane stared a long while at the coffeepot, and then called the two squaws who assisted her in her household duties, to clear away the things while she went up to her own room to make her bed.

Bret Harte

9. God's gift was not a spirit of timidity, but the Spirit of power, and love, and self-control. . . . You have been trusted to look after something precious; guard it with the help of the Holy Spirit who lives in us.

From 2 TIMOTHY

10. He will lead me into luxuriant pastures,
    as befits his name.
    Even though I should walk
    in the midst of total darkness,
    I shall fear no danger
    since you are with me.

From PSALM 23

11. The world is too much with us; late and soon,
    Getting and spending, we lay waste our powers;
    Little we see in Nature that is ours;
    We have given our hearts away, a sordid boon!
    The sea that bares her bosom to the moon;
    The winds that will be howling at all hours,
    And are up-gathered now like sleeping flowers;
    For this, for everything, we are out of tune;
    It moves us not.—Great God! I'd rather be
    A Pagan suckled in a creed outworn;
    So might I, standing on this pleasant lea,
    Have glimpses that would make me less forlorn;
    Have sight of Proteus rising from the sea;
    Or hear old Triton blow his wreathed horn.

THE WORLD IS TOO MUCH WITH US   *William Wordsworth*

12. Six, slick, slim, slippery, slimy, sleek, slender saplings.

13. The sea ceaseth—it sufficeth sufficiently that the sea ceaseth.

14. A skunk stood on a stump. The stump thunk the skunk stunk, but the skunk thunk the stump stunk.

/ʃ/ *and* /ʒ/

Production

The cognates /ʃ/ and /ʒ/ are made by placing the tongue farther back in the mouth than for the production of /s/ and /z/ and bringing the sides of the tongue in direct contact with the upper back teeth. The blade of the tongue almost touches the area of the palate just behind the alveolar ridge. When the breath or voice is forced through a groove down the center of the tongue and out between a narrow aperture between the upper and lower teeth, a frictional sound results. The lips should be slightly rounded.

Problems

Check the discussions of problems in articulating the fricative sibilants /s/ and /z/ and the plosive affricates /tʃ/ and /dʒ/. Many of the same errors in producing those sounds are applicable here, including lateralization, whistling, and lower lip action.

EXERCISES FOR /ʃ/ AND /ʒ/

1. Read the following word lists with an exaggerated production of /ʃ/ and /ʒ/. Make certain that when you pull away from the exaggerated sound to articulate the sounds appropriately you do not pull away too much.

Initial	*Medial*	*Final*
ship	assure	wash
sheet	fissure	crash
Chicago	patient	mash
shack	cashier	leash
shirt	precious	dish
	treasure	garage
	lesion	corsage
(No English words	casual	mirage
begin with /ʒ/.)	confusion	camouflage
	occasion	barrage

Exaggerate the articulation in the following exercises. However, make certain that you do not pull away too much to achieve a professional standard of articulation.

2. This harsh and untimely interruption of summer is brought to you by Middlesex Bank. If your house could use a little ventilation and winterizing, summer is the time to do it.

3. Shop for furnishings at Chicago's newest shopping mall.

4. Gustave Aschenbach—or von Aschenbach, as he had been known officially since his fiftieth birthday—had set out alone from his house in Prince Regent Street, Munich, for an extended walk.

   From DEATH IN VENICE   *Thomas Mann*

5. Suspicion always haunts the guilty mind;
   The thief doth fear each bush an officer.

   From KING HENRY VI   *William Shakespeare*

6. We shall not flag or fail. We shall fight in France, we shall fight on the seas and oceans, we shall fight with growing confidence and growing strength in the air, we shall defend our island, whatever the cost may be, we shall fight on the beaches, we shall fight on the landing grounds, we shall fight in the fields and in the streets, we shall fight in the hills; we shall never surrender.

   DUNKIRK   *Winston Churchill*

7. Bob and Vangy put Zaza's leash in the garage.

8. The people that walked in darkness have seen a great light: they that dwell in the land of the shadow of death, upon them hath the light shined.

   From ISAIAH

9. He shall feed his flock like a shepherd: he shall gather the lambs with his arm, and carry them in his bosom, and shall gently lead those that are with young.

   From ISAIAH

10. At Blair's leisure he ordered a corsage for Beverly.

LATERAL

/l/

Production

In the production of the voiced lateral /l/, the tip of the tongue touches the alveolar ridge and the sound escapes over the sides of the tongue. The /l/ phoneme is deceptive because its production cannot be easily seen.

There are two allophones of the phoneme /l/, a fact that complicates the situation even further. These are called the light or clear /l/ and dark /l/. The dark /l/ is formed with the tongue farther back and lower than in the production of the light /l/. The light /l/ is used when the sound appears initially and is followed by a front vowel or diphthong. The dark /l/ is used in the medial and final positions or preceding a back vowel, as in the words *lower* and *Louis*.

Problems

Sometimes /w/ is substituted for /l/ ("wion" for *lion*), although this pronunciation is rather rare among college-age students. Of course, another problem is the mixture of clear and dark allophones. This occurs more frequently among speakers learning English than among native speakers.

A fairly common error is to produce /l/ with the tip of the tongue behind the lower front teeth instead of touching the alveolar ridge. This unacceptable allophone of /l/ is called **lambda**.

EXERCISES FOR /l/   Tom Brokaw
Jerry

1. In reading the following word lists aloud, exaggerate the articulation, making certain that you do not pull away too much when you then articulate appropriately.

Initial	*Medial*	*Final*
laugh	alone	broil
long	alas	mill
languid	follow	kneel
late	hailed	motel
lawn	squalor	deal
lower	squealer	keel
lucky	believe	hall
learn	balloon	style
lunch	below	cruel
liver	bellow	pill

Read the above lists again, but this time use the lambda by keeping the tongue tip down behind the lower front teeth during the production of the sound. Feel what the tongue is doing and listen to the sound that the error produces. It has no place in career speech, even though some national communicators have the speech defect. As Captain Hook maintains, "It is the canker that g-naws!"

Read aloud the following selections.

2. Lea and Lew are lovely people.

3. To the gods alone
   Belongs it never to be old or die,
   But all things else melt with all-powerful Time.

   From OEDIPUS AT COLONUS   *Sophocles*

4. Really, universally, relations stop nowhere, and the exquisite problem of the artist is eternally but to draw, by a geometry of his own, the circle within which they shall happily "appear" to do so.

   From RODERICK HUDSON   *Henry James*

5. All ambitions are lawful except those which climb upward on the miseries or credulities of mankind.

   From A PERSONAL RECORD   *Joseph Conrad*

6. You do not need to leave your room. Remain sitting at your table and listen. Do not even listen, simply wait. Do not even wait, be quite still and solitary. The world will freely offer itself to you to be unmasked, it has no choice, it will roll in ecstasy at your feet.

   From THE GREAT WALL OF CHINA   *Franz Kafka*

7. To be loved, be lovable!

   From THE ART OF LOVE   *Ovid*

8. Whither, O splendid ship, thy white sails crowding,
   Leaning across the bosom of the urgent West.

   From A PASSER-BY   *Robert Bridges*

9. I shall remember while the light lives yet
   And in the night-time I shall not forget.
   Though (as thou wilt) thou leave me ere life leave,
   I will not, for thy love I will not, grieve.

   From EROTION   *Algernon Swinburne*

10. Ah, what is more blessed than to put cares away, when the mind lays by its burden, and tired with labor of far travel we have come to our own home and rest on the couch we longed for? This is it which alone is worth all these toils.

    From ODES   *Catullus*

11. Big blue jeans in a brown blown bladder.

12. Slippery sleds slide smoothly down the sluiceway.

13. Eight eager, earnest, eccentric Englishmen eating eleven elusive eagles.

14. Six, slick, slim, slippery, slimy, sleek, slender saplings.

15. Our eyes met; several seconds elapsed, till our glances still mingled, I extended my hand and turned the lamp out. . . . He was still lingering . . . in the greatness of his zeal, giving a rub-up to a plated cruet sgand.

From THE SECRET SHARER   *Joseph Conrad*

16. His room, a regular human bedroom, only rather too small, lay quiet between the four familiar walls.

From THE METAMORPHOSIS   *Franz Kafka*

17. Mrs. Shortley recalled a newsreel she had seen once of a small room piled high with bodies of dead naked people all in a heap.

Flannery O'Connor

18. The dull light fell more faintly upon the page whereon another equation began to unfold itself slowly and to spread abroad its widening tail.

From A PORTRAIT OF THE ARTIST AS A YOUNG MAN   *James Joyce*

19. Fine leather sofas, lounge chairs are on sale at 25 percent off. Lamps, end tables, occasional chairs, and desks—all on sale at prices you have to see to believe.

SEMIVOWELS

/r/

Production

The phoneme /r/ is a voiced semivowel produced with tension in the center of the tongue; the tongue tip is elevated toward the hard palate, and the lips are slightly rounded.

Problems

One of the reasons that /r/ is problematic for many speakers is that to produce the sound properly, there must be a gliding movement of the tongue and lips. The tongue tip is elevated toward the alveolar ridge and glides downward when the sound is completed. The lips are slightly pursed at the beginning of production and are relaxed when the sound is completed. It is impossible to put the articulators in a set position and produce the sound, as in /p/ or /v/. Another cause of difficulty is that the sound cannot be seen in production. The action of the tongue can only be described.

Some speakers curl the tongue tip too much toward the hard palate, giving a very heavy-sounding /r/. This is quite characteristic of some Midwesterners. If you have this heavy-sounding /r/, bring the tongue tip forward but not down.

Other speakers produce the /r/ phoneme with the tongue tip down behind the lower front teeth. The difficulty is in getting the speaker to feel the action of the tongue since the only portion of the sound's production that can be observed is the slight rounding of the lips. Often the sound becomes labialized through the excessive use of the lips in producing the sound. This is particularly evident in some Eastern speech. This articulation certainly has its advantages in creating a character type—a character that does not reflect professional speech.

New Englanders (as well as others) tend to make other errors relating to the /r/ phoneme. These speakers frequently add or omit the /r/. These characteristics will be discussed in a later chapter.

EXERCISES FOR /r/

Read the following exercises without the accustomed exaggerated articulation. Since the production of the sound is obstructed visually and an exaggeration of the sound might promote the heavy Midwestern /r/, you should articulate the phoneme appropriately. However, your habitual production of the sound may be inappropriate. If so, get used to increasing the articulatory movements.

1. The first time you read the word lists below, add the "er" vowel sound before each word in the first column. Feel, visualize, and listen to the production of the sound.

Initial	*Medial*	*Final*
ripe	arrive	care
rent	carrion	hear
really	carriage	wear
rant	horrible	jar
rim	around	liar
right	garbage	par
rave	very	scare
rotten	bearing	there
rough	barren	tour
rhyme	oral	four

2. Because the phoneme /r/ is such a rascal, the following word lists include the consonant blends involving the phoneme. As with the word lists above, the first time you read the exercise exaggerate the /r/ to get the feeling of the blend, although you are actually producing the vowel /ɝ/ (as in *her*). For example, in the word *trip,* produce "ter-r-r-r-rip" while paying attention to

the feel of the sound. If you produce the vowel correctly, you will have little trouble getting the feel of the semivowel.

/pr/	/br/	/tr/	/dr/	/kr/
proud	brown	trip	drip	cream
print	brought	trump	drum	cringe
prom	bright	trick	droop	crime
problem	brim	trim	dram	crone
pram	brash	troop	drawn	crown
promote	bring	truck	dreary	crag
prim	Bret	trollop	draft	crunch
pronto	brag	tray	dream	cream
preppy	bray	trunk	dragon	crime
prattle	brother	tram	dry	craft

/gr/	/fr/	/θr/	/str/
grim	frown	thrive	strong
ground	frame	thrill	struggle
great	frump	throne	streak
grant	Frances	threat	stroll
grudge	frill	thrust	street
green	front	throttle	strip
grand	frame	through	stripe
greet	French	throb	stream
graft	freeze	thrown	strict
grown	fragile	thrash	strap

Read aloud the following selections.

3. Around the rough and rugged rocks the ragged rascal ran.

4. The bleak breeze blighted the bright broom blossoms.

5. Strong Stephen Strangelove struggled with the strings of the stranger's racket.

6. All religion, all life, all art, all expression come down to this: to the effort of the human soul to break through its barrier of loneliness, of intolerable loneliness, and make some contact with another seeking soul.

From CHAPTERS FOR THE ORTHODOX   *Donald Marquis*

7. Carole raced around the room arranging the chairs.

8. Bread of deceit is sweet to a man; but afterwards his mouth shall be filled with gravel.

   From PROVERBS

9. The lion and the unicorn
   Were fighting for the crown;
   The lion beat the unicorn
   All round the town.
   Some gave them white bread,
   And some gave them brown;
   Some gave them plum cake,
   And sent them out to town.

   Anonymous

10. Gentlemen always seem to remember blondes. Also, a girl never really looks as well as she does on board a steamship, or even a yacht.

    From GENTLEMEN PREFER BLONDES   *Anita Loos*

11. Four be the things I'd be better without:
    Love, curiosity, freckles, and doubt.

    Dorothy Parker

12. In the following excerpt, many of the instances of the letter "r" are vowel sounds and not the consonant /r/.

    The writer must teach himself that the basest of all things is to be afraid; and, teaching himself that, forget it forever, leaving no room in his workshop for anything but the old verities and truths of the heart, the old universal truths lacking which any story is ephemeral and doomed—love and honor and pity and pride and compassion and sacrifice.

    William Faulkner

13. Such horses are
    The jewels of the horseman's hands and thighs,
    They go by the word and hardly need the rein.

    From JOHN BROWN'S BODY   *Stephen Vincent Benet*

14. Dancing is wonderful training for girls, it's the first way you learn to guess what a man is going to do before he does it.

    From KITTY FOYLE   *Christopher Morley*

/w/

Production

The bilabial, voiced /w/ is made with a gliding movement of the lips that is similar to the pursed position of the lips in producing the vowel /u/, as in *true*. The tongue is elevated toward the back.

Problems

The phoneme /w/ is not a difficult sound to produce or teach. The major difficulty with the sound occurs when it is substituted for the voiceless /ʍ/. Reread aloud the exercises for discriminating between /w/ and /ʍ/ on pp. 116–118.

In addition, nonnative speakers sometimes substitute /v/ for /w/ ("vade" for *wade*).

EXERCISES FOR /w/

Read the following exercises with exaggerated articulation before pulling away to the appropriate articulation.

1. *Initial*   *Medial*   *Final*

Initial	Medial	Final
witty	upward	(does not occur)
walk	awake	
worm	award	
wife	unwind	
wash	anyone	
wonder	liquid	
weigh	highway	
woman	inquest	
with	require	
wall	unworthy	

2. Those who have wealth must be watchful and wary.

   From I'D BE A BUTTERFLY   *Thomas Bayly*

3. The witch said she was from Walla Walla, Washington.

4. If I am not worth the wooing, I surely am not worth the winning.

   From THE COURTSHIP OF MILES STANDISH   *Henry Wadsworth Longfellow*

5. I know that one is able to win people far more by the spoken than by the
written word, and that every great movement on this globe owes its rise to
the great speakers and not to the great writers.

    From MEIN KAMPF   *Adolf Hitler*

6. There never was a war that was not inward.

    From IN DISTRUST OF MERITS   *Marianne Moore*

7. But there's wisdom in women, of more than they have known,
And thoughts go blowing through them, are wiser than their own.

    From THERE'S WISDOM IN WOMEN   *Rupert Brooke*

8. Was ever woman in this humour wooed?
Was ever woman in this humour won?

    RICHARD III   *William Shakespeare*

9. Brief words, when actions wait, are well.

    From ADDRESS   *Bret Harte*

10. If love were what the rose is,
And I were like the leaf,
Our lives would grow together
In sad or singing weather.

    A MATCH   *Algernon Swinburne*

11. He went through the Wet Wild Woods, waving his wild tail, and walking
by his wild lone. But he never told anybody.

    From THE CAT THAT WALKED BY HIMSELF   *Rudyard Kipling*

12. The passengers would crowd to the windows and go out onto the open gang-
way at the end of the carriages to find out whether the track was under repair.

    Aleksandr Solzhenitsyn

/j/

Production

The voiced semivowel /j/ glides from the /i/ position (as in *see*) toward the following vowel. The front portion of the tongue is elevated and tense. In English
/j/, like /w/, is found only before a vowel sound.

Problems

Most of the problems associated with the production of this sound are found
among nonnative speakers of English.

EXERCISES

Read the following exercises aloud and overarticulate. For your own speech standard, make certain that you don't pull away too much.

1. | *Initial* | *Medial* | *Final* |
   |---|---|---|
   | yard | onion | (does not occur) |
   | yet | companion | |
   | yellow | junior | |
   | yawn | million | |
   | Europe | canyon | |
   | Yankee | union | |
   | youth | bunion | |
   | yesterday | stallion | |
   | year | beyond | |
   | yes | genius | |

2. Yesterday, William Junior was yearning for a bigger backyard.

3. In winter I get up at night
   And dress by yellow candle-light.

   From BED IN SUMMER   *Robert Louis Stevenson*

4. Children of yesterday,
   Heirs of tomorrow.

   From SONG OF HOPE   *Mary Lathbury*

5. Oh, yer's yer good old whiskey,
   Drink it down.

   From TWO MEN OF SANDY BAR   *Bret Harte*

6. Bards of Passion and of Mirth,
   Ye have left your souls on earth!
   Have ye souls in heaven too?

   From ODE/BEAUMONT   *John Keats*

7. Young Love may go,
   For aught I care,
   To Jerico!

NASALS

/m/

Production

This voiced nasal sound is made by closing the lips and relaxing the velum, allowing the sound to resonate through the nose. In the production of /m/, the teeth are slightly apart.

Problems

The main difficulty in the production of the /m/ phoneme is an obstruction interfering with the nasal emission of breath. A physician should be consulted. The exercises for denasality might also prove helpful (pp. 76–77).

EXERCISES

Read the exercises below with exaggerated articulation. Feel what is occurring as the nasal sound is produced. Remember—do not pull away too much for appropriate articulation.

1.

Initial	*Medial*	*Final*
mate	demean	form
middle	demolish	climb
mine	someday	home
Monday	cement	column
make	terminal	game
march	umbrella	groom
month	semester	autumn
mob	comfortable	phlegm
myth	teamwork	foam
murder	humanity	grime

2. Are you copperbottoming 'em, man? No, I'm aluminizing 'em, ma'am.

3. The art of medicine in Egypt is thus exercised: one physician is confined to the study and management of one disease; there are of course a great number who practice this art; some attend to the disorders of the eyes, mind, head, and bowels; whilst many attend to the cure of maladies which are less conspicuous.

   From EUTERPE *Herodotus*

4. From that day onwards one had the impression that all cars were moving in circles.

From THE PLAGUE   *Albert Camus*

5. Call me Ishmael. Some years ago—never mind how long precisely—having little or no money in my purse, and nothing particular to interest me on shore, I thought I would sail about a little and see the watery part of the world.

From MOBY DICK   *Herman Melville*

6. A gentleman friend and I were dining at the Ritz last evening and he said that if I took a pencil and a paper and put down all of my thoughts it would make a book. This almost made me smile as what it would really make would be a whole row of encyclopedias. I mean I seem to be thinking practically all of the time.

From GENTLEMEN PREFER BLONDES   *Anita Loos*

7. On my right hand there were lines of fishing-stakes resembling a mysterious system of half-submerged bamboo fences, incomprehensible in its division of the domain of tropical fishes, and crazy of aspect as if abandoned for ever by some normal tribe of fishermen now gone to the other end of the ocean; for there was no sign of human habitation as far as the eye could reach.

From THE SECRET SHARER   *Joseph Conrad*

8. Matryona made me try the village again, and when I arrived the second time she made countless excuses.

Aleksandr Solzhenitsyn

9. A time for giving birth,
   a time for dying;
   a time for planting,
   a time for uprooting what has been planted.
   a time for killing,
   a time for healing;
   a time for knocking down,
   a time for building.
   a time for tears,
   a time for laughter;
   a time for mourning,
   a time for dancing.
   a time for throwing stones away,
   a time for gathering them up;
   a time for embracing,
   a time to refrain from embracing.

ECCLESIASTES

10. As Gregor Samsa awoke one morning from uneasy dreams he found himself transformed in his bed into a gigantic insect. He was lying on his hand, as if it were armor-plated, back and when he lifted his head a little he could see his dome-like brown belly divided into stiff arched segments on top of which the quilt could hardly keep in position and was about to slide off completely. His numerous legs, which were pitifully thin compared to the rest of his bulk, waved helplessly before his eyes.

   From THE METAMORPHOSIS   *Franz Kafka*

11. The young man's impression of his prospective pupil, who had first come into the room, as if to see for himself, as soon as Pemberton was admitted, was not quite the soft solicitation the visitor had taken for granted. . . . Pemberton was modest—he was even timid; and the chance that his small scholar might prove cleverer than himself had quite figured, to his nervousness, among the dangers of an untried experiment.

   From THE PUPIL   *Henry James*

12. No human thing is of serious importance. . . . The soul of man is immortal and imperishable.

   From THE REPUBLIC   *Plato*

13. Tossing his mane of snows in wildest eddies and tangles,
    Lion-like March cometh in, hoarse, with tempestuous breath.

    From EARLIEST SPRING   *William Dean Howells*

/n/

Production

This voiced nasal sound is made with a closure created by the tongue tip touching the alveolar ridge; the relaxed velum allows the breath to escape through the nose.

Problems

In some words the letter "n" is pronounced with the phoneme /m/. This assimilation takes place because the sound that follows is a bilabial and imprecise articulation is easier for the vocal mechanism. Examples of such words include the following:

unpleasant	unblessed	unpatriotic
unbutton	unborn	unbolt
unpardonable	unburden	unpolished

un<u>b</u>ind	un<u>b</u>aptized	un<u>b</u>ridled
un<u>b</u>ending	un<u>b</u>leached	un<u>b</u>olt

Sometimes the linguavelar nasal /ŋ/ should be substituted for /n/, but sometimes it is substituted erroneously. In all these instances, the /n/ phoneme is followed by either /k/ or /g/, which, except for the nasality, has the same articulatory adjustment as /ŋ/. Check with your dictionary to determine whether /ŋ/ should be used. Again, because of assimilation, it is easier to pronounce these words using /ŋ/, whether it is correct or not. Using negative practice, exaggerate the incorrect pronunciation and then exaggerate the proper pronunciation:

co<u>ng</u>ressional[4]	i<u>nc</u>lude
co<u>ng</u>ruent[5]	i<u>nc</u>apacity
co<u>ng</u>ratulate	i<u>nc</u>antation
i<u>nc</u>omplete	i<u>nc</u>line
e<u>nc</u>lose	i<u>nc</u>lement
i<u>nc</u>lusive	i<u>nc</u>oherent
i<u>nc</u>ognito	i<u>nc</u>ome

Often the /n/ phoneme turns into a dentalized /m/ when followed by a labiodental /f/ or /v/. Feel how easy it is to say *imfant* for *infant*. The symbol [m̪] indicates an /m/ with dentalization. Therefore, the word *infant* would be transcribed as /ɪm̪fənt/. Using negative practice, say the following list of words exaggerating the error and then exaggerating the articulation:

co<u>nf</u>er	i<u>nf</u>ernal	i<u>nv</u>ade
co<u>nf</u>ess	i<u>nf</u>ant	i<u>nv</u>eigle
co<u>nf</u>etti	i<u>nf</u>antile	i<u>nv</u>ert
co<u>nf</u>ident	i<u>nf</u>ect	i<u>nv</u>est
co<u>nf</u>ine	i<u>nf</u>est	i<u>nv</u>isible
co<u>nf</u>irm	i<u>nf</u>inite	i<u>nv</u>ite

Sometimes /n/ is omitted, particularly when /n/ is followed by /m/. This is one of the sound combinations that you ought to develop if you desire a professional standard of speech. Exaggerate the wrong articulation in negative practice of the following list of words. Feel what is wrong as you intentionally exaggerate the error. Then repeat the list producing the correct sound with exaggeration.

---

[4] Notice that *congress* maintains the /ŋ/ phoneme.

[5] The word *congruent* may be pronounced with /n/ or /ŋ/.

When you pull away, make certain that you don't underarticulate the production of the word.

government	adjournment
environment	assignment
lean more	adornment
earn more	consignment
can make	corn meal
an(d) make	

EXERCISES FOR /n/

1. Overarticulate the correct pronunciation of the following word list. Then pull away, but not too much!

Initial	*Medial*	*Final*
knowledge	grinning	spoon
knit	announce	open
nimble	annual	heaven
neck	demand	crown
nice	Donny	began
nothing	fence	token
nail	funny	scene
nasal	standing	main
natural	bench	spoon
nothing	blond	burn

2. Once upon a sunny morning a man who sat in a breakfast nook looked up from his scrambled eggs to see a white unicorn with a gold horn quietly cropping the roses in the garden.

   From THE UNICORN IN THE GARDEN   *James Thurber*

3. No man is an island, entire of itself; every man is a piece of the continent, a part of the main.

   From DEVOTIONS   *John Donne*

4. More than an end to war, we want an end to the beginnings of all wars.

   Franklin Delano Roosevelt

5. And now there came both mist and snow,
   And it grew wondrous cold:
   And ice, mast-high, came floating by,
   As green as emerald.

   From THE ANCIENT MARINER   *Samuel Taylor Coleridge*

6. When all the world is young, lad,
   And all the trees are green;
   And every goose a swan, lad,
   And every lass a queen;
   Then hey for boot and horse, lad,
   And round the world away:
   Young blood must have its course, lad,
   And every dog his day.

   From WATER BABIES   *Charles Kingsley*

7. The beginnings and endings of all human undertakings are untidy, the building of a house, the writing of a novel, the demolition of a bridge, and,
   eminently, the finish of a voyage.

   From OVER THE RIVER   *John Galsworthy*

8. Blessed is the man that endureth temptation; for when he is tried, he shall
   receive the crown of life.

   BOOK OF JAMES

9. An honest man, like the true religion, appeals to the understanding, or mod-
   estly confides in the internal evidence of his conscience. The imposter employs force instead of argument, imposes silence where he cannot convince,
   and propagates his character by the sword.

   Anonymous

10. I want live things in their pride to remain.
    I will not kill one grasshopper vain.

    From THE SANTA FE TRAIL   *Vachel Lindsay*

11. Nothing is more dangerous in wartime than to live in the temperamental
    atmosphere of a Gallup Poll, always feeling one's pulse and taking one's
    temperature.

    Winston Churchill

12. My apple trees will never get across
    And eat the cones under his pines, I tell him.

    From MENDING WALL   *Robert Frost*

/ŋ/

Production

This is a voiced nasal with strong contact between the back of the tongue and the velum. The velum is relaxed, allowing the sound to resonate through the nose.

Problems Adam

The nasal /ŋ/ (as in *ring*) is a single sound, like /m/ or /n/. The most common confusion in its production stems from its expression as two letters, "n" and "g." However, there is no sound of the phoneme /n/ in the phoneme /ŋ/, nor of the phoneme /g/.

Closet gupping

no g or

finger

fener

Jews—
parents dropped
g for their
prior to school
eliminate it
altogether

There are three common errors in the production of /ŋ/. Many untrained speakers (and, alas, even some trained) make the first error: substituting /n/ for /ŋ/. Such speech thugs say "goin'" for *going* and "comin'" for *coming*. Unfortunately, the error is so prevalent that writers indicate the substituted sound with the apostrophe. But you are not leaving off the "g"—you are using a full-fledged sound-for-sound substitution!

The second error is to pronounce the /ŋ/ (as in *ring*) and then add the plosive /g/, as in "He is a singer's singer" (/hi ɪz ə sɪŋɡɚz sɪŋɡɚ/). This is caused partly by a misconception of the sound and partly from the bad habit of producing a sound as the tongue drops down from the velum. The letters "ng" are misleading (especially to someone who is learning English) because they imply two sounds where only one exists. This error is *never* accepted in career speech. In fact, the error sometimes arouses ethnic prejudice, even though no one ethnic or religious group makes this error more than another. Generally, anyone who has learned English as a second language makes the error, which can be passed along to the following generations. As has been mentioned time and time again, habit is immeasurably strong!

The third error involves the substitution of /ɪn/ for /ɪŋ/ in the "ing" combination. This is true particularly when the sound combination occurs in the final position.

EXERCISES FOR /ŋ/

1. *Substitution of* /n/ *for* /ŋ/. Use negative practice when you pronounce each word in the middle column below. Exaggerate the pronunciations, and make certain that you do not pull back too much to gain the appropriate articulation.

	Career	*Error*	*Career*
going	/goɪŋ/	/goɪn/ /goən/	/goɪŋ/
doing	/duɪŋ/	/duɪn/ /duən/	/duɪŋ/
walking	/wɔkɪŋ/	/wɔkɪn/ /wɔkən/	/wɔkɪŋ/
following	/fɑloɪŋ/	/fɑloɪn/ /fɑloən/	/fɑloɪŋ/
jumping	/dʒʌmpɪŋ/	/dʒʌmpɪn/ /dʒʌmpən/	/dʒʌmpɪŋ/

2. *Addition of* /g/. In order to understand the kinesics involved, make a strong closure in producing /ŋ/ and then add the /g/ after you have held the nasal for a few seconds. Repeat this several times. Feel the addition of the /g/ each time. (This pronunciation is transcribed as /ŋ:g/.)

/ŋ: -------------g/

/ŋ: ------------g/

/ŋ: ------------g/

/ŋ: ------------g/

/ŋ: ------------g/

3. The correct pronunciation of /ŋ/ is made more complicated by the fact that there are a few words in which a /g/ *should* follow /ŋ/. After you overarticulate and use negative practice in pronouncing the following comparative adjectives, repeat the exercise with appropriate articulation. Remember not to pull away too much.

	Career	*Error*	*Career*
strong	/strɔŋ/	/strɔŋg/	/strɔŋ/
stronger	/strɔŋgɚ/	/strɔŋɚ/	/strɔŋgɚ/
strongest	/strɔŋgɪst/	/strɔŋɪst/	/strɔŋgɪst/
long	/lɔŋ/	/lɔŋg/	/lɔŋ/
longer	/lɔŋgɚ/	/lɔŋɚ/	/lɔŋgɚ/
longest	/lɔŋgɪst/	/lɔŋɪst/	lɔŋgɪst/
young	/jʌŋ/	/jʌŋg/	/jʌŋ/
younger	/jʌŋgɚ/	/jʌŋɚ/	/jʌŋgɚ/
youngest	/jʌŋgɪst/	/jʌŋɪst/	/jʌŋgɪst/

4. When a suffix is added to a root word, the /g/ is not added. In the word *ringer,* the suffix is added to the root word *ring,* which is a recognizable English word. Therefore, /g/ is not added to the /ŋ/. Use negative practice and overarticulation in the pronunciation of the following words; then repeat with good articulation.

	Career	*Error*	*Career*
longing	/lɔŋɪŋ/	/lɔŋgɪŋ/	/lɔŋɪŋ/
singer	/sɪŋɚ/	/sɪŋgɚ/	/sɪŋɚ/
coat hanger	/kot hæŋɚ/	/kot hæŋgɚ/	/kot hæŋɚ/
swinger	/swɪŋɚ/	/swɪŋgɚ/	/swɪŋɚ/
bringer	/brɪŋɚ/	/brɪŋgɚ/	/brɪŋɚ/
laughing	/læfɪŋ/	/læfɪŋg/	/læfɪŋ/
coaxing	/koksɪŋ/	/koksɪŋg/	/koksɪŋ/

5. If a suffix is added to a syllable that is not recognizable in English, the /g/ is added to the /ŋ/; an example is the word *linger.* Use negative practice and overarticulation in the following word lists. Then repeat the exercise with appropriate articulation.

	Career	*Error*	*Career*
linger	/lɪŋgɚ/	/lɪŋɚ/	/lɪŋgɚ/
finger	/fɪŋgɚ/	/fɪŋɚ/	/fɪŋgɚ/
mangle	/mæŋgl̩/	/mæŋl̩/	/mæŋgl̩/
Congress	/kɑŋgrəs/	/kɑŋrəs/	/kɑŋgrəs/
tangle	/tæŋgl̩/	/tæŋl̩/	/tæŋgl̩/
penguin[6]	/pɛŋgwɪn/	/pɛŋwɪn/	/pɛŋgwɪn/
wrangle	/ræŋgl̩/	/ræŋl̩/	/ræŋgl̩/
bingo	/bɪŋgo/	/bɪŋo/	/bɪŋgo/
shingle	/ʃɪŋgl̩/	/ʃɪŋl̩/	/ʃɪŋgl̩/
Singapore[7]	/sɪŋgəpor/	/sɪŋəpor/	/sɪŋgəpor/

6. Use negative practice and overarticulation as you read aloud the following phrases. Then repeat the exercise with appropriate articulation. Feel what is happening in the production of the various sounds.

---

[6] A secondary pronunciation.

[7] Yes, this is the preferred pronunciation.

	Career	*Error*	*Career*
going out	/goɪŋ aʊt/	/goɪŋgaʊt/	/goɪŋ aʊt/
Long Island	/lɔŋ aɪlənd/	/lɔŋgaɪlənd/	/lɔŋ aɪlənd/
coming in	/kʌmɪŋ ɪn/	/kʌmɪŋgɪn/	/kʌmɪŋ ɪn/
singing a song	/sɪŋɪŋ ə sɔŋ/	/sɪŋgɪŋgəsɔŋg/	/sɪŋɪŋ ə sɔŋ/
running along	/rʌnɪŋ əlɔŋ/	/rʌnɪŋgəlɔŋg/	/rʌnɪŋ əlɔŋ/

7. *Substitution of* /in/ *for* /ɪŋ/. Use overarticulation and negative practice in producing the following sound combinations; the second production is incorrect for the "ing" combination: /ɪŋ/, /in/, /ɪŋ/. Repeat this several times.

8. Use negative practice and overarticulation in reading aloud the following words. The middle pronunciation is the substitution of /in/ for /ɪŋ/. Then repeat the exercise with appropriate articulation.

	Career	*Error*	*Career*
going	/goɪŋ/	/goin/	/goɪŋ/
doing	/duɪŋ/	/duin/	/duɪŋ/
singing	/sɪŋɪŋ/	/sɪŋin/	/sɪŋɪŋ/
following	/faloɪŋ/	/faloin/	/faloɪŋ/
sitting	/sɪtɪŋ/	/sɪtin/	/sɪtɪŋ/
walking	/wɔkɪŋ/	/wɔkin/	/wɔkɪŋ/
flinging	/flɪŋɪŋ/	/flɪŋin/	/flɪŋɪŋ/

	retreating and beating and meeting and sheeting
Career:	/rɪtritɪŋ ænd bitɪŋ ænd mitɪŋ ænd ʃitɪŋ/
Error:	/rɪtritin ænd bitin ænd mitin ænd ʃitin/
Career:	/rɪtritɪŋ ænd bitɪŋ ænd mitɪŋ ænd ʃitɪŋ/

Read aloud the following selections.

9. The cataract strong
   Then plunges along,
   Striking and raging
   As if a war waging
   Its caverns and rocks among;
   Rising and leaping,
   Sinking and creeping,
   Swelling and sweeping,
   Showering and springing,
   Flying and flinging,
   Writhing and ringing,
   Eddying and whisking,

Spouting and frisking,
Turning and twisting,
Around and around
With endless rebound
Smiting and fighting,
A sight to delight in;
Confounding, astounding,
Dizzying and deafening the ear with its sound.

From THE CATARACT OF LODORE   *Robert Southey*

10. I'm sure I'm no ascetic; I'm as pleasant as can be;
You'll always find me ready with a crushing repartee,
I've an irritating chuckle, I've a celebrated sneer,
I've an entertaining snigger, I've a fascinating leer.
To everybody's prejudice I know a thing or two;
I can tell a woman's age in half a minute—and I do.
But although I try to make myself as pleasant as I can,
Yet everybody says I am a disagreeable man!
And I can't think why!

From PRINCESS IDA   *W. S. Gilbert*

SYLLABIC CONSONANTS

Sometimes the consonants /l/, /m/, and /n/ form syllables without the aid of a full vowel. These consonants are called *syllabic* and are identified by a mark underneath the sound: /l̩/, m̩/, and /n̩/. In the word *button* there is a slight vowel component between /t/ and /n/. If the syllable were prolonged, it would contain the **schwa**, or /ə/ (as in *about*). Listen and develop **auditory discrimination** in the following words in which the full vowel and the syllabic consonant are compared.

	Full Vowel	*Syllabic Consonant*
bottle	/bɑtəl/	/bɑtl̩/
bottom	/bɑtəm/	/bɑtm̩/
button	/bʌtən/	/bʌtn̩/
single	/sɪŋgəl/	/sɪŋgl̩/
cycle	/saɪkəl/	/saɪkl̩/
prison	/prɪzən/	/prɪzn̩/
mitten	/mɪtən/	/mɪtn̩/
Latin	/lætən/	/lætn̩/

The use of the syllabic consonant is quite appropriate in career speech and in some circles is preferred, especially in words where the syllabic sound follows /t/, such as *cotton* (/kɑtṇ/) and *little* (/lɪtḷ/).

GENERAL ARTICULATION EXERCISES

In practicing these exercises do not forget the technique of overarticulating and then pulling away for appropriate articulation. Too many speakers revert back to their habitual production, which as a rule, is underarticulated. In the following selections by W. S. Gilbert, keep up the pace and stay with the rhythm. Then increase your pace.

1. In the selection below there are three primary, or heavy, stresses in each line. Maintain the heavy stress and your pace will increase. However, remember this exercise is for articulation, so keep your concentration on your sound production.

   I'm the sláve of the góds, neck and heéls,
   And I'm boúnd to obéy, though I ráte at 'em;
   And I not ónly órder their méals,
   But I coók 'em, sérve 'em, and wáit at 'em.
   Then I máke all their néctar—I dó—
   (Which a térrible líquor to ráck us is)
   And whenéver I míx them a bréw,
   Why áll the thanksgívings are Bácchus's!

   THESPIS   *W. S. Gilbert*

2. In this selection, the rhythm alternates between four stresses in the odd-numbered lines and three in the even-numbered.

   In Westmínster Háll I dánced a dánce,
   Like a sémi-despóndent fúry;
   For I thóught I should néver hít on a chánce
   Of addréssing a Brítish Júry—
   But I sóon got tíred of thírd-class jóurneys,
   And dínners of bréad and wáter;
   So I féll in lóve with a rích attórney's
   Élderly, úgly daúghter.

   (Mark the accents in the next stanza yourself.)

   The rich attorney, he jumped with joy,
   And replied to my fond profession:

"You shall reap the reward of your pluck, my boy
At the Bailey and Middlesex Sessions.
You'll soon get used to her looks," said he,
"And a very nice girl you'll find her!
She may very well pass for forty-three
In the dusk, with a light behind her!"

From TRIAL BY JURY   *W. S. Gilbert*

3. The rhythm in this selection is slightly different from that in the selections above. Each line has four primary stresses. Keep up the pace and rhythm, but do not forget that the purpose of these exercises is to improve your articulation. Mark the stressed syllables in the lines.

When I was a lad I served a term
As office boy at an Attorney's firm.
I cleaned the windows and I swept up the floor,
And I polished up the handle of the big front door.
I polished up that handle so carefullee,
That now I am the Ruler of the Queen's Navee!

As office boy I made such a mark
That they gave me the post of a junior clerk.
I served the writs with a smile so bland,
And I copied all the letters in a big round hand—
I copied all the letters in a hand so free,
That now I am the Ruler of the Queen's Navee!

In serving writs I made such a name
That an articled clerk I soon became;
I wore clean collars and a brand-new suit
For the pass examination at the Institute,
And that pass examination did so well for me,
That now I am the Ruler of the Queen's Navee! . . .

I grew so rich that I was sent
By a pocket borough into Parliament.
I always voted at my party's call,
And I never thought of thinking for myself at all.
I thought so little, they rewarded me
By making me the Ruler of the Queen's Navee!

From H.M.S. PINAFORE   *W. S. Gilbert*

4. In the following selection, the rhythm is determined by the four primary stresses in lines 1 through 3 followed by three major stresses in line 4.

It's a song of merryman, moping mum,
Whose soul was sad, and whose glance was glum,

Who sipped no sup, and who craved no crumb,
As he sighed for the love of a ladye.

From THE YEOMEN OF THE GUARD   *W. S. Gilbert*

5. Notice in the following selection that there is only one major stress in lines
1 through 4.

That celebrated,
Cultivated,
Underrated,
Nobleman,
The Duke of Plaza Toro!

From THE GONDOLIERS   *W. S. Gilbert*

6. Unlike the selections above, the rhythm in the following selection is less
structured.

You must lie upon the daisies and discourse in novel phrases
of your complicated state of mind,
The meaning doesn't matter if it's only idle chatter of a
transcendental kind.
And everyone will say,
As you walk your mystic way,
"If this young man expresses himself in terms too deep for me,
Why, what a very singularly deep young man this deep young man must be!"

From PATIENCE   *W. S. Gilbert*

7. The following poem is a fine example of the figure of speech called conso-
nance, which is the use of the same or similar consonant sounds with differ-
ing vowels. For those of you who think that a poet is governed by inspiration
exclusive of perspiration, this poem ought to be of some interest. (It is a
little labored, though, isn't it!)

Leaves
Murmuring by myriads in the shimmering trees.
Lives
Wakening with wonder in the Pyrenees.
Birds
Cheerily chirping in the early day.
Bees
Shaking the heavy dews from bloom and frond.
Boys
Bursting the surface of the ebony pond.
Flashes
Of swimmers carving thro' the sparkling cold.
Fleshes

Gleaming with wetness to the morning gold.
A mead
Bordered about with warbling water brooks.
A maid
Laughing the love-laugh with me; proud of looks.
The heat
Throbbing between the upland and the peak.
Her heart
Quivering with passion to my pressed cheek.
Braiding
Of floating flames across the mountain brow.
Brooding
Of stillness; and a sighing of the bough.
Stirs
Of leaflets in the gloom; soft petal-showers;
Stars
Expanding with the starr'd nocturnal flowers.

From MY DIARY, JULY 1914   *Wilfred Owen*

In the next four selections, play with the repetitions.

8. Between two hawks, which flies the higher pitch;
   Between two dogs, which hath the deeper mouth;
   Between two blades, which bears the better temper;
   Between two horses, which doth bear him best;
   Between two girls, which hath the merriest eye;
   I have, perhaps, some shallow spirit of judgment;
   But in these nice sharp quillets of the law,
   Good faith, I am no wiser than a daw.

   From HENRY VI, PART 1   *William Shakespeare*

9. From birth to age eighteen, a girl needs good parents. From eighteen to
   thirty-five, she needs good looks. From thirty-five to fifty-five, she needs a
   good personality. From fifty-five on, she needs good cash.

   Sophie Tucker

10. For winter's rains and ruins are over,
    And all the season of snows and sins;
    The days dividing lover and lover,
    The light that loses, the night that wins;
    And time remembered is grief forgotten.
    And frosts are slain and flowers begotten,
    And in green underwood and cover
    Blossom by blossom the spring begins.

    ATLANTA IN CALYDON   *Algernon Swinburne*

11. He shall feed his flock like a shepherd: he shall gather the lambs with his arm, and carry them in his bosom, and shall gently lead those that are with young.

    From ISAIAH

12. If you are to be successful with the following classic mouthful, it would be a good idea to look up the meanings as well as pronunciations of those words that are new to you. Then, pray a lot! This makes a fine oral examination for articulation. It is also a good challenge for your classroom professional—the professor!

    In promulgating your esoteric cogitations, or articulating your superficial sentimentalities, and amicable, philosophical, or psychological observations, beware of platitudinous ponderosity. Let your conversational communications possess a clarified conciseness, a compacted comprehensibleness, coalescent consistency, and a concatenated cogency. Eschew all conglomerations of flatulent garrulity, jejune babblement, and asinine affectations. Let your extemporaneous descantings and unpremeditated expatiations have intelligibility and voracious vivacity, without thrasonical bombast. Sedulously avoid all polysyllabic profundity, pompous prolixity, ventriloquial verbosity, and vain vapidity. In other words, say what you mean and mean what you say, and don't use big words.

    Anonymous

7

ENUNCIATION

GLOSSARY

Connotation   A verbal association evoked by a word (for instance, connotations for *horse* could be "stallion," "mount," and "horsey").

Diphthong   A sound composed of two vowels coming together in the same syllable.

Dynamic Speech   Conversational or performance speech.

Enunciation   The production of sounds, especially the vowels and diphthongs.

Habitual   Accustomed through repetition.

Molar   A tooth with a flattened surface.

Monosyllabic   Comprised of one syllable.

Phonetics   The science of speech sounds.

Polysyllabic   A word comprised of three or more syllables.

Pronunciation   The combination of articulation and enunciation.

Schwa   A central-middle and unstressed vowel.

Stress   The amount of intensity given to a sound, syllable, or word.

Transcribe   To write a word, phrase, or sentence phonetically.

Vowel   A speech sound in which there is a free, unobstructed flow of vibrating breath.

Wrenched Stress   Intentional misplacement of primary stress on a syllable; a device sometimes used in poetry.

Enunciation may be defined as the production of vowels and diphthongs. A **vowel** is a free and unobstructed flow of vibrating breath. A **diphthong** is a speech sound composed of two vowels coming together in the same syllable. Vowels and diphthongs are important in English because they not only provide the basis of the syllable but also give the language carrying power and beauty. Although the fricative /f/, for example, is a helpful sound, particularly if you want to say the word *friend* or *after,* few people would disagree that prolonging the /f/ sound is not very pleasant. On the other hand, prolonging the vowel in *calm* gives increased loudness and certainly a difference in auditory pleasure. Part of this response, however, is related to the word's meaning and **connotations**. For example, separate the meaning from the pronunciation in the word *confusion.* Again, the vowels give the sound of the word carrying power and a degree of pleasure, partly because of the combinations of consonants and vowels. The words *cellar door* are reputed to constitute one of the most pleasant sound combinations in English if the meaning is separated from the sound.

The major organ in vowel production is the tongue. Vowels are produced by altering both the position of and amount of tension in the tongue. Other active articulators are (1) the cheek and lip muscles, (2) the lower jaw (mandible), and (3) the tensed velum (since all vibrating air is resonated through the mouth in producing vowels and diphthongs). Compared with the precision necessary to articulate consonants, more latitude is allowable for vowels.

All vowels are voiced continuants. Although some vowels are produced in a similar manner, there are no cognate pairs. A different vowel is enunciated by shifting the position of the tongue, in some cases very slightly, and increasing or decreasing the amount of tension in the tongue. Prolong the vowels in the words *beet* and *bit* and feel the difference in tongue placement and amount of tension.

In **pronunciation** vowel adjustments require less articulatory movement than consonant sounds. Several vowel charts have been designed to illustrate these adjustments. In the accompanying chart, "High," "Middle," and "Low" refer to the position of the peak of the tongue's arch; "Front," "Central," and "Back" indicate where in the mouth (buccal cavity) the resonance is produced. You will notice that there are considerably more vowels than are included in the famous "*a, e, i, o, u,* and sometimes *y*" listing.

Each of the vowel sounds is **transcribed** into **phonetics** and accompanied by a key word containing that vowel. Since a word can often be pronounced in more than one way, there must be general agreement. Therefore, the key words must be pronounced as indicated in the text. There will not be a problem with many sounds, but remember that there are a number of correct pronunciations, and speakers from different parts of the country might have different pronunciations. A standard reference book for pronunciation is *A Pronouncing Dictionary of American English* by John S. Kenyon and Thomas A. Knott. The errors in the production of vowels and diphthongs (substitutions, additions, and distortions) are primarily due to regionalisms. This subject will be discussed in Chapter 11. Other errors will be detailed below.

In the exercises that appear in the sections below, there may be a variety of vowels that can be used for the underlined vowels. However, you will learn to

	Front	Central	Back
High	/i/ — see /ɪ/ — bit		/u/ — true /ʊ/ — put
Middle	/e/ — make /ɛ/ — met	/ɝ/ — her /ɜ/ — bird (New England/ British) /ɚ/ — after /ʌ/ — cut /ə/ — about	/o/ — go
Low	/æ/ — cat /a/ — half (New England/ British)		/ɔ/ — law /ɒ/ — hot (New England) /ɑ/ — father

differentiate vowel sounds more quickly by using the vowel under discussion rather than your **habitual** vowel sound. Remember that people in your area might use a variant pronunciation that is also acceptable.

In practice, always exaggerate the production and feeling of the sound. Get a sense of what the articulators are doing. When you habituate yourself to the sound, do not pull away too much from the exaggerated articulation.

FRONT VOWELS

/i/

Production

In the production of /i/ (as in *see*), the muscles of the tongue are tense. The tongue is slightly arched, and the front of the tongue is raised. The mouth is almost closed, and the lips are slightly tensed and spread. The vowel /i/ occurs only in stressed syllables.

EXERCISES

The first time you read the following exercises aloud, exaggerate the production of all of the sounds in the words, giving special attention to the vowels. Feel what is happening in the lip area as well as the tongue. Be careful! Do not pull away too much to gain the appropriate enunciation in later readings.

1. keen   release
   feed   leisure
   seal   pleasing
   feel   receive
   meal   machine
   mean   streamers
   creed   frequent
   read   teacher
   seen   eagles
   need   careen

2. The mean weasel had eaten three eagles under the tree.

3. The police agreed to please the people.

4. In the east the green leaves are falling.

5. Lee's deeds were appreciated by the team.

6. Frieda repeated her dream to Athena.

7. The geese were feeding on the beans.

8. We had seen the thief stuff the wheat in the beehive.

9. The screams were heard from the village green.

10. Phoebe made a scene at *Antigone*.

11. Free the bees in the hive.

The following selections are by W. S. Gilbert. It may seem that his works are overused in this text, but they happen to be among the best for developing good breath control and appropriate articulation.

12. My hopes will be blighted, I fear,
    My dear;
    In a month you'll be going to sea,
    Quite free,
    And all of my wishes
    You'll throw to the fishes
    As though they were never to be;
    Poor me!
    As though they were never to be.
    And I shall be left all alone
    To moan,
    And weep at your cruel deceit,
    Complete;
    While you'll be asserting

Your freedom by flirting
With every woman you meet,
You cheat—
With every woman you meet!

From RUDDIGORE   *W. S. Gilbert*

13. With base deceit
You worked upon our feelings!
Revenge is sweet,
And flavours all our dealings!
With courage rare
And resolution manly,
For death prepare,
Unhappy General Stanley.

From THE PIRATES OF PENZANCE   *W. S. Gilbert*

Over the ripening peach
Buzzes the bee.
Splash on the billowy beach
Tumbles the sea.
But the peach
And the beach
They are each Nothing to me!

From RUDDIGORE   *W. S. Gilbert*

/ɪ/

Production

In the production of /ɪ/ (as in *bit*), the muscles of the tongue are relaxed, which lowers the tongue slightly from the /i/ position, but the front of the tongue is slightly raised. The teeth are slightly farther apart compared with the production of /i/, and the sound is usually shorter in duration.

EXERCISES

The first time you read the following exercises aloud, exaggerate all of the sounds in the words, giving special attention to the vowels. Feel how this vowel differs from /i/.

1. Read aloud the words, alternating between the /ɪ/ and /i/ columns. The words enclosed in brackets are nonsense syllables and therefore written in phonetics. Sound them out! Pronounce them as they are transcribed. Make certain that you don't pull away too much when trying to develop appropriate pronunciation.

/ɪ/	/i/	/ɪ/	/i/
itch	each	mitten	meetin'
chill	[tʃil]	little	[litl̩]
dim	deem	river	reaver
kid	keyed	middle	[midl̩]
list	least	pity	pea tea
wish	[wiʃ]	filling	feeling
will	we'll	listen	lee son
mill	meal	whisper	whee spur
mit	meet	ripple	[ripl̩]
rid	read	children	[tʃildrən]

Read aloud the following sentences and selections.

2. Patricia was knitting little mittens for him.

3. "Miss Brill" is not a simple story.*

4. We got a bin of mixed biscuits for Christmas.

5. Rip Van Winkle is my favorite literary* character.

6. Silly Millie went fishing with Willie.

7. Thin vinegar is often used in salads.

8. Steve wished that Katy* would tickle Mister Greenjeans.

9. Vito picks thin chickens for his soup.

10. Gristle on liver is particularly* offensive.

11. The twins swam in flimsy* bathing suits.

12. But as for certain truth, no man has known it,
    Nor will he know it; neither of the gods,
    Nor yet of all the things of which I speak.
    And even if by chance he were to utter
    Finality, he would himself not know it:
    For all is but a woven web of guesses.

    Xenophanes

13. Perchance he for whom this Bell tolls, may be so ill, as that he
    knows not it tolls for him; And perchance I may thinke my self

---

*The vowel in the last syllable of these words (represented by the letter "y") is pronounced /ɪ/ (as in *bit*). In **dynamic speech** many /i/ vowels become /ɪ/, particularly in the final position.

so much better than I am, as that they who are about me, and see my state, may have caused it to toll for me, and I know not that.

From DEVOTIONS   *John Donne*

/e/

Production

In the production of /e/ (as in *make*), the front of the tongue is raised slightly toward the palate, the muscles of the tongue are tense, and the tongue is lowered slightly from the /ɪ/ position. The mouth is opened wider than for /ɪ/, and the lips are spread. When used in stressed syllables, the vowel /e/ often becomes the diphthong /eɪ/. The use of this diphthong is encouraged in professional speech even though the single vowel symbol is transcribed.

EXERCISES

In the following exercises, feel the increased tension in the tongue compared with the /ɪ/ position. The tongue is also slightly lowered. Exaggerate the pronunciation of the words. Make certain you do not pull away too much to produce the sounds appropriately.

1. Alternate reading aloud the words in the /e/ column with those in the /ɪ/ column and feel the adjustment. In addition, prolong the vowel.

/e/	/ɪ/	/e/	/ɪ/
bait	bit	satiate	[sɪʃijɪt]
rain	Rin	ungrateful	[əngrɪtfl̩]
mate	mit	famous	[fɪməs]
take	tick	ancient	[ɪnʃənt]
aim	[ɪm]	Hemingway	hemming[wɪ]
tray	[trɪ]	vacation	[vɪkɪʃən]
wade	[wɪd]	tornado	[tɔrnɪdo]
sale	sill	ailment	ill mint
wage	[wɪʤ]	display	[dɪsplɪ]
spade	[spɪd]	relation	[rɪlɪʃən]

Read aloud the following sentences and selections.

2. Mabel and Abe went on a vacation to Angel, Texas.

3. They gave a great deal of help to their neighbors during the rainstorm.

4. Katy put my name on the cake she baked for me.

5. With the aid of a cane Mavis can walk.

6. The weathervane indicated a rainy day.

7. Tracy raked the cranberries with a gray rake.

8. The mailman brought the mail very late today.

9. The maiden made a strange mistake on the paper.

10. Hazel would always remain faithful to the family name.

11. That lady was a candidate for mayor.

12. Why so pale and wan, fond lover?
    Prithee, why so pale?
    Will, when looking well can't move her,
    Looking ill prevail?
    Prithee, why so pale?

    From SONG   *Sir John Suckling*

13. If I can stop one heart from breaking,
    I shall not live in vain;

    From LIFE   *Emily Dickinson*

14. To-morrow, and to-morrow, and to-morrow
    Creeps in this petty pace from day to day
    To the last syllable of recorded time,
    And all our yesterdays have lighted fools
    The way to dusty death.

    From MACBETH   *William Shakespeare*

15. More strange than true. I never may believe
    These antique fables, nor these fairy toys.
    Lovers and madmen have such seething brains,
    Such shaping fantasies, that apprehend
    More than cool reason ever comprehends.

    From A MIDSUMMER NIGHT'S DREAM   *William Shakespeare*

/ɛ/

Production

In the production of /ɛ/ (as in *met*), the muscles of the tongue are relaxed, and the tip is behind the lower teeth and lower in the mouth than for /e/. The lips are slightly spread while the lower jaw drops slightly from the /e/ position.

Problems

One of the most common problems with this sound is the substitution of /ɪ/. Although this error is prevalent in the South, it is very common in all parts of the country. In the following word list, use negative practice and feel the error.

	Career	*Error*	*Career*
get[1]	[gɛt]	[gɪt]	[gɛt]
met	[mɛt]	[mɪt]	[mɛt]
forget	[forgɛt]	[fəgɪt]	[forgɛt]
better	[bɛtɚ]	[bɪtə]	[bɛtɚ]
relish	[rɛlɪʃ]	[rɪlɪʃ]	[rɛlɪʃ]
fetch	[fɛtʃ]	[fɪtʃ]	[fɛtʃ]
let	[lɛt]	[lɪt]	[lɛt]
next	[nɛkst]	[nɪkst]	[nɛkst]
very	[vɛrɪ]	[vɪrɪ]	[vɛrɪ]
chest	[tʃɛst]	[tʃɪst]	[tʃɛst]

EXERCISES

The first time you read the following exercises, exaggerate the production of all of the sounds, giving special attention to the vowels. Feel how the vowel /ɛ/ differs from /e/.

1. Alternate reading aloud the words in the /ɛ/ and /e/ columns. The words enclosed in brackets are nonsense words and therefore transcribed into phonetics. Sound them out. Make certain you do not pull away too much when trying to develop the appropriate pronunciation.

/ɛ/	/e/	/ɛ/	/e/
pen	pain	spectra	spake [trə]
sketch	[sketʃ]	America	[əmerəkə]
peck	[pek]	henpecked	[henpekt]
chef	[ʃef]	intention	[ɪntenʃən]
yell	Yale	utensils	[jutensəlz]

---

[1] Many speakers use the substandard "git" for "get."

check	[tʃek]	emphasis	aim [fəsɪs]
led	laid	breakfast	break [fəst]
hem	[hem]	wretched	Ray [tʃəd]
ten	[ten]	repentance	[rɪpentəns]
bed	[bed]²	penthouse	paint house

Read aloud the following sentences and selections.

2. It is a pleasure to remember that debt.

3. The keg was held by Ned and Fred.

4. *High Noon* is a Western epic that will be remembered forever.

5. Helen was selling the shells for a penny.

6. After eating the yellow melons, David and Adam felt helpless.

7. Rett and Ellen's eggs were delivered without much effort.

8. Steve pretended that he did not feel the intense pain.

9. Infamous Uncle Ned had a large welt on his leg when he arrived.

10. Heather always said that the well-bred horse was the best.

11. Did Ben beg his brother to give him the tent?

12. Now what is this, and what is that, and why does father leave his rest
    At such a time of night as this, so very incompletely dressed?
    Dear father is, and always was, the most methodical of men!
    It's his invariable rule to go to bed at half-past ten.
    What strange occurrence can it be that calls dear father from his rest
    At such a time of night as this, so very incompletely dressed?
    From THE PIRATES OF PENZANCE   *W. S. Gilbert*

13. And when Hadad heard in Egypt that David slept with his fathers, and that
    Joab the captain of the host was dead, Hadad said to Pharaoh, Let me depart,
    that I may go to mine own country.
    From 1 KINGS

14. And he said unto him that was over the vestry, Bring forth vestments for all
    the worshippers of Baal. And he brought them forth vestments.
    From 2 KINGS

---

²*Bade* is pronounced "bad."

15. The cellar smelled of dust and old moisture. The beams were fuzzed with
    cobwebs. There was only one light, a dim one in the corner. A little rivulet
    was running darkly down the wall and already had formed a footsquare pool
    on the floor.

    From THE STORM *McKnight Malmar*

16. Freddie the Frog would wed;
    He needed a frog in his bed.
    Every froggie said "No!"
    Every froggie said "Go!"
    So Fred wed a tadpole instead.

    FREDDIE THE FROG *Edward Lear*

/æ/

Production

In the production of /æ/ (as in *cat*), the muscles of the tongue are relaxed. The
front and back of the tongue are low, and the tip is behind the lower front teeth.
The mouth is opened wider than for /ɛ/.

Problems

The most common error in the production of this vowel is too much tension in
the tongue. This error is common in the speech of New Yorkers and Midwesterners, particularly Chicagoans. In phonetic transcriptions, a dot under a sound
indicates extreme tension. Use negative practice in reading aloud the following
word lists.

	Career	*New York/* *Chicago*	*Career*
mask	[mæsk]	[mæsk]	[mæsk]
glad	[glæd]	[glæd]	[glæd]
apple	[æpl̩]	[æpl̩]	[æpl̩]
trash	[træʃ]	[træʃ]	[træʃ]
gallon	[gælən]	[gælən]	[gælən]
pastoral	[pæstərl̩]	[pæstərl̩]	[pæstərl̩]
radical	[rædəkl̩]	[rædəkl̩]	[rædəkl̩]
calf	[kæf]	[kæf]	[kæf]
flash	[flæʃ]	[flæʃ]	[flæʃ]
clap	[klæp]	[klæp]	[klæp]

EXERCISES

The first time you read the following exercises aloud, exaggerate the production of all of the sounds in the words, giving special attention to the vowel. Feel how the vowel differs from /ɛ/.

1. Alternate reading aloud the words in the /æ/ and /ɛ/ columns. The words enclosed in brackets are nonsense words transcribed into phonetics. Sound them out, keeping the same **stress** as in the related /æ/ word. Make certain you don't pull away too much when trying to make the appropriate pronunciation a habit.

/æ/	/ɛ/	/æ/	/ɛ/
mask	[mɛsk]	balance	bell [ləns]
calf	[kɛf]	galaxy	[gɛləksɪ]
hash	[hɛʃ]	graduate	[grɛdʒuet]
glad	[glɛd]	gallon	[gɛlən]
stamp	[stɛmp]	pastoral	pest [ərəl]
apt	[ɛpt]	expansive	expensive
can	Ken	bombastic	bomb [bɛs] tick
telegram	[tɛləgrɛm]	sandman	send men
trash	[trɛʃ]	diagram	[daɪəgrɛm]

2. The following is a list of words that contrasts /æ/ with /e/ and /ɛ/, vowels that are frequently incorrectly used in conjunction with /ŋ/ (as in *ring*). In career speech the /æ/ is used. (However, /ɛ/ is used in words like *length*, *penguin*, and *strength*. The lower jaw is lower than in the production of the vowels /e/ or /ɛ/.

	Career	/e/ Error	/ɛ/ Error	Career
bank	[bæŋk]	[beŋk]	[bɛŋk]	[bæŋk]
thank	[θæŋk]	[θeŋk]	[θɛŋk]	[θæŋk]
hang	[hæŋ]	[heŋ]	[hɛŋ]	[hæŋ]
Frank	[fræŋk]	[freŋk]	[frɛŋk]	[fræŋk]
rang	[ræŋ]	[reŋ]	[rɛŋ]	[ræŋ]
spanking	[spæŋkɪŋ]	[speŋkɪŋ]	[spɛŋkɪŋ]	[spæŋkɪŋ]
flank	[flæŋk]	[fleŋk]	[flɛŋk]	[flæŋk]
sank	[sæŋk]	[seŋk]	[sɛŋk]	[sæŋk]
blank	[blæŋk]	[bleŋk]	[blɛŋk]	[blæŋk]
Hank	[hæŋk]	[heŋk]	[hɛŋk]	[hæŋk]

Read aloud the following sentences and selections.

3. Carole gave Dan a back scratcher.

4. Vangy battered the radical purse snatcher.

5. Dan asked Andrea if she saw the tan cat attack the dog.

6. "Candid Camera" is a very popular program.

7. Bob, the masked bandit grabbed half the calf and ran.

8. Cramming for examinations is a bad habit.

9. My Aunt Pat's attic is filled with antiques.

10. There is a grand piano for sale in Manchester.

11. Candied apples are traditional at Thanksgiving.

12. Harold has been called a rough taskmaster by his students.

Enunciate the vowel without the additional tension in the following exercises:

13. She began to drink the coffee. While she was drinking, holding the cup in both hands, she began to make the sound again. She made the sound into the cup and the coffee splashed out onto her hands and her dress.

    From THAT EVENING SUN   *William Faulkner*

14. Rats!
    They fought the dogs and killed the cats,
    And bit the babies in the cradles,
    And ate the cheeses out of the vats,
    And licked the soup from the cooks' own ladles,
    Split open the kegs of salted sprats,
    Made nests inside men's Sunday hats,
    And even spoiled the women's chats,
    By drowning their speaking
    With shrieking and squeaking
    In fifty different sharps and flats.

    From THE PIED PIPER OF HAMELIN   *Robert Browning*

15. There was an old Man of Madrás,
    Who rode on a cream-coloured ass;
    But the length of its ears, so promoted his fears,
    That it killed that Old Man of Madrás.

    Edward Lear

16. The grandeur of the dooms,
    We have imagined for the mighty dead.

    From ENDYMION   *John Keats*

/a/

The vowel /a/ (as in *half*) is primarily a New England sound, used when the letters "a" and "au" come before /s/, /n/, /θ/, and /f/. (Most speakers would pronounce the key word *half* with /æ/.) This sound is also prevalent in some parts of the Midwest, as well as around Rochester, New York, in words like *hot, Tom, cot,* and *Bob*. It is often used in the South in words like *night,* [nat], *fright* [frat], *fire* [far], *hire* [har], and *tire* [tar]. The phoneme /a/ is heard as the first sound in the diphthong /aɪ/, as in *I, cry,* and *might*.

It can be a useful sound for the performer to use in reading some poems by Robert Frost, O'Neill's *Desire under the Elms,* and other New England literature. It is a good sound to use for any communication occasion when there is a need to imitate a New Englander. Refer to the section on American dialects for additional characteristics of New England speech (p. 259). This sound can be unpleasant to the ear, especially when produced with too much tension, and is not recommended for career speech because it is regional as well as potentially abrasive.

Production

The muscles of the tongue are relaxed, and the front and back of the tongue are low in the mouth. The tongue lies midway between the positions used to produce /æ/ and /ɑ/ (as in *father*).

EXERCISES

The first time you read the following exercises aloud, exaggerate the production of all of the sounds in the words, giving special attention to the vowels. Feel how this vowel differs from /æ/.

1. Alternate reading aloud the words in the /a/ and /æ/ columns. Sound them out! Make certain you don't pull away too much when trying to habituate yourself to the appropriate pronunciation. Remember that most of these words are also pronounced with /æ/.

/a/	/æ/	/a/	/æ/
bath	bath	disaster	disaster
salve³	salve	bombastic	bombastic
fast	fast	laughter	laughter

---

³Notice that the letter "l" is silent.

aunt	aunt/ant	pasture	pasture
laugh	laugh	grasping	grasping
class	class	answer	answer
glass	glass	plasterer	plasterer
path	path	afterwards	afterwards
aft	aft	advantage	advantage
ask	ask	blaspheme	blaspheme

Read aloud the following sentences and selections.

2. There is an advantage to grant him his wish.

3. Take a chance and command the child to stay off the grass.

4. My aunt Doris thinks that the draft would be ghastly.

5. The cast gave Jack a set of brass candlesticks.

6. The photograph of Frances and Hank amazed the class.

7. They gasped when they heard I had returned from France already.

8. On behalf of my Uncle Ned, I thank you for the brass canister you were asked to bring.

9. Wilma pranced down the path like a real dancer.

10. Grant took a chance and glanced at Vange.

11. Joseph advanced into the alabaster bathroom.

12. The flowers that bloom in the spring,
    Tra la,
    Breathe promise of merry sunshine—
    As we merrily dance and we sing,
    Tra la,

    From THE MIKADO (as pronounced by a New Englander)   *W. S. Gilbert*

13. With brotherly readiness,
    For my fair sister's sake,
    At once I answer "Yes"—
    That task I undertake—
    My word I never break.
    I freely grant that boon,
    And I'll repeat my plight.
    From morn to afternoon—
    From afternoon to night.

    From THE YEOMEN OF THE GUARD (as pronounced by a New Englander
    [gad])   *W. S. Gilbert*

CENTRAL VOWELS

/ɜˑ/

Production

The vowel /ɜˑ/ (as in *her*) is used only in stressed syllables. It may occur in a **monosyllabic** word like *fur* or in a **polysyllabic** word like *usurping*. The muscles of the tongue are tense, the sides of the tongue are against the upper rear **molars,** and the tongue tip is free. The lips are slightly rounded.

EXERCISES

The first time you work with the following exercises, exaggerate the production of the words and sentences. Feel how this vowel is produced compared with other vowels. Make certain you don't pull away too much when trying to develop the appropriate pronunciation.

1. earth   verdict
   nerve   furnace
   stir   deserving
   heard   churlish
   term   disturb
   work   confirm
   curl   mercy
   surge   irksome
   err   cursing
   swerve   rehearse

2. Richard[4] Burton purchased some ermine furs.

3. Shirley was sure she would smirk at the sermon.

4. The verb occurs in the first verse of the poem.

5. Many girls are learning to assert themselves.

6. Reserve some time in the term for a long rehearsal.

---

[4]*Richard* contains an unstressed "er."

7. Herb the herbman prepares the meals for all the servants.

8. The nurse was irked by the less than perfect patient.

9. Research the records for Myrtle's birthday.

10. The cowboy's stirrup was made of sterling.

11. The blackbird was sitting on the perch.

12. O'er the season vernal,
Time may cast a shade;
Sunshine, if eternal,
Makes the roses fade!

    From TRIAL BY JURY   *W. S. Gilbert*

13. There was an Old Lady of Chertsey,
Who made a remarkable curtsey;
She twirled round and round, till she sunk underground,
Which distressed all the people of Chertsey.

    Edward Lear

14. For anything so overdone is from the purpose of playing, whose end, both
at the first and now, was and is to hold as 'twere the mirror up to Nature.

    From HAMLET   *William Shakespeare*

15. Beat! beat! drums!—blow! bugles! blow!
Through the windows—through doors—burst like a ruthless force
Into the solemn church, and scatter the congregation.

    From BEAT! BEAT! DRUMS   *Walt Whitman*

16. Workers earn it,
Spend thrifts burn it;

    From MONEY   *Richard Armour*

17. Aloof with hermit-eye I scan
The present work or present man.

    From ODE TO TRANQUILITY   *Samuel Coleridge*

18. The flowers appear on the earth; the time of the singing of birds is come,
and the voice of the turtle is heard in our land.

    From ECCLESIASTES

19. There was an old party of Lyme
Who married three wives at one time.
When asked: "Why the third?"
He replied: "One's absurd,
And bigamy, sir, is a crime."

/ɚ/

Production

The vowel /ɚ/ (as in *after*) sounds the same as /ɝ/ except in the degree of **stress**; /ɚ/ occurs only in *unstressed* or minimally stressed syllables. (Remember that an unstressed syllable is a misnomer, since a syllable must have some stress.) The production of /ɚ/ is almost identical to /ɝ/ except that the muscles of the tongue are more relaxed and the sound is shorter in duration. The sides of the tongue are pressed against the upper rear molars, and the tongue tip is free and slightly tense.

EXERCISES

The first time you read the following exercises aloud, exaggerate the production of all of the sounds in the words, giving special attention to the vowels.

1. The words in column I use the unstressed /ɚ/. (In isolated words, /ɚ/ only occurs in words of more than one syllable. A monosyllabic word may contain /ɚ/ in dynamic speech if the syllable is unstressed. Refer to exercises 2 and 10 below.) How would the words in column I sound if the syllables containing /ɚ/ were stressed? This is called shifted or **wrenched stress.** Such a pronunciation is transcribed into phonetics in column II. Compare and contrast the pronunciation of the words in both columns.

I	*II*
sister	[sɪstɝ]
brother	[brʌðɝ]
average*	[ævɝɪdʒ]
boundary*	[baʊndɝɪ]
comfortable†	[kʌmfɝtəbl̩]
southern	[sʌðɝn]
razor	[rezɝ]
camera*	[kæmɝə]
perhaps	[pɝhæps]
governor	[gʌvɝnɝ]

---

*If pronounced with three syllables.

†If pronounced with four syllables.

Read aloud the following sentences.

2. Louise lost her feathers in her dance number.

3. The state government has a great deal of power.

4. Mother cooked my favorite dinner—liver.

5. Arthur ordered butter for his lobster.

6. The banker put the picture of the thief on the posterboard.

7. Perhaps the chair was comfortable, but it looked uncomfortable to me.

8. History is my most interesting subject.

9. His father was studying to be an actor.

10. I wonder what the average grade was in her class?

11. The surveyors surveyed the land like masters.

12. Read aloud the following bisyllabic words containing both /ɝ/ and /ɚ/.

server [sɝvɚ]	merger [mɝdʒɚ]
murder [mɝdɚ]	worker [wɝkɚ]
stirrer [stɝɚ]	learner [lɝnɚ]
murmur [mɝmɚ]	burner [bɝnɚ]
Herbert [hɝbɚt]	

Read aloud the following sentences and selections.

13. Her nurse brought her a stirrer for her coffee.

14. Herbert loved raspberry sherbert.

15. Valerie's workers perverted the aims of the organization.

16. The Governor of New York talked about a merger with New Jersey.

17. The courtroom was filled with murmurs when the murderer learned of the juror's verdict.

18. I will sing of the mercies of the Lord for ever: with my mouth will I make known thy faithfulness to all generations.

From PSALM 89

19. I love him—I love him—with fervour unceasing

    I worship and madly adore;

    My blind adoration is always increasing,

    My loss I shall ever deplore.

    Oh, see what a blessing, what love and caressing

    I've lost, and remember it, pray,

    When you I'm addressing, are busy assessing

    The damages Edwin must pay!
    From TRIAL BY JURY   *W. S. Gilbert*

20. What perplexes the world is the disparity between the swiftness of the spirit,

    and the immense unwieldiness, sluggishness, inertia, permanence of

    matter.
    From THE MAGIC MOUNTAIN   *Thomas Mann*

21. Cold in the earth—and fifteen wild Decembers

    From those brown hills have melted into spring:

    Faithful, indeed, is the spirit that remembers

    After such years of change and suffering!
    From REMEMBRANCE   *Emily Brontë*

22. On the third day after they moved to the country he came walking back

    from the village carrying a basket of groceries and a twenty-four-yard coil

    of rope.
    Katherine Anne Porter

23. But the dance itself had been enjoyable. The best people were there, and

    Ivan Ilych has danced with Princess Trufonova, as sister of the distinguished founder of the Society "Bear My Burden."

From ANNA KARENINA   *Count Lyof Tolstoi*

/ɜ/

Production

The vowel /ɜ/ (as in *bird*) is used by some New England and Southern speakers. Like /ɝ/, the vowel /ɜ/ is used only in stressed syllables. The arch of the tongue is high, but the tip is relaxed and resting behind the lower front teeth. It is also a British sound used in stage speech.

All words containing /ɝ/ may be pronounced with /ɜ/ (as in *bird*). Both sounds occur only in stressed syllables. A speaker who uses /ɝ/ would not use /ɜ/ in conversational speech. For professional speech, the /ɝ/ is recommended, although /ɜ/ is preferred in British speech, as noted above.

For practice, refer to the exercises for the stressed /ɝ/. Using those word lists, compare and contrast the stressed /ɜ/ with /ɝ/.

/ʌ/

Production

The vowel /ʌ/ (as in *cut*) is also used only in stressed syllables, and it occurs in monosyllabic words (*but*) and words of more than one syllable (*butter, mother,* and *fluttering*). The muscles of the tongue are relaxed, and the central portion of the tongue is slightly raised. The tongue tip remains behind the lower teeth, and the lips are in a neutral position.

EXERCISES

The first time you read the following exercises aloud, exaggerate the production of all of the sounds in the words, giving special attention to the vowels. Make certain that you do not pull away too much when trying to develop the appropriate pronunciation.

1. just   mother
   love   double
   rush   money
   come   funding
   mutt   muttering

such   punish
some   underling
us   utterly
flood   hundred
young   judgment

2. The* young puppy dug in the* dirt.

3. A* skunk stood on a* stump. The* stump thunk the* skunk stunk.

4. "Shucks," muttered Sonny, "I can jump and touch the* ceiling."

5. Ed's truck was* just covered with repulsive words.

6. Louise told the* judge to make the* punishment fit the* crime.

7. Have you studied much about* the* humming bird?

8. Mother and Ludwig rushed to the* dumbwaiter for the* fudge.

9. The* hamburg was* on an ugly-looking bun covered with mustard. Humbug!

10. Hank grumbled that there was* some money in honey.

11. The* trucker's tires bumped the* potholes with hundreds of thuds.

12. Olympus is now in a terrible muddle,
    The deputy deities all are at fault;
    They splutter and splash like a pig in a puddle,
    And dickens a one of 'em's earning his salt,
    For Thespis as Jove is a terrible blunder,
    Too nervous and timid—too easy and weak—
    Whenever he's called on to lighten or thunder,
    The thought of it keeps him awake for a week!

    From THESPIS   *W. S. Gilbert*

13. Judge not, that ye be not judged.
    For with what judgement ye judge, ye shall be judged: and with
    what measure ye mete, it shall be measured to you again.
    And why beholdest thou the mote that is in thy brother's eye,
    but considerest not the beam that is in thine own eye?

    From ST. MATTHEW

14. All hail great Judge!
    To your bright rays

---

*These words are unstressed and therefore do not use /ʌ/.

We never grudge
Ecstatic praise.

From TRIAL BY JURY *W. S. Gilbert*

15. **Judge:**   For now I am a Judge!
    All: And a good Judge too.
    Judge: Yes, now I am a Judge!
    All: And a good Judge too!
    Judge: Though all my law is fudge,
       Yet, I'll never, never budge,
       But I'll live and die a Judge!
    All: And a good Judge too!

From TRIAL BY JURY *W. S. Gilbert*

16. Humpty Dumpty sat on a wall,
    Humpty Dumpty had a great fall;
    All the king's horses
    And all the king's men
    Couldn't put Humpty Dumpty together again.

17. Double, double, toil and trouble;
    Fire burn and cauldron bubble.

    From MACBETH *William Shakespeare*

18. For such as be blessed of him shall inherit the earth; and they that be cursed
    of him shall be cut off.

    From PSALM 37

19. It's a song of a merryman, moping mum,
    Whose soul was sad, and whose glance was glum,
    Who sipped no sup, and who craved no crumb,
    As he sighed for the love of a ladye.

    From THE YEOMEN OF THE GUARD *W. S. Gilbert*

/ə/

The vowel /ə/ (as in *about*) has its own name—the **schwa**. It is a neutral-sounding vowel that occurs only in unstressed syllables. There is the same relationship between /ʌ/ and /ə/ as between /ɝ/ and /ɚ/. The major difference between /ʌ/ and /ə/ is the degree of stress. The vowel /ʌ/ occurs only in stressed syllables, while the schwa is used in unstressed syllables. The schwa is the most common vowel in English.

Any unstressed vowel sound can turn into the schwa. Say the word "America" aloud as transcribed: [əmɛrɪkə]. Now increase the speed. You probably said [əmɛrəkə]. To the New Englander, it is quite acceptable to say [sɪstə] for [sɪstɚ], turning the unstressed /ɚ/ into the schwa. When you are not quite sure what vowel is being said, it is most likely the schwa. In New England and Southern speech, when the /ɜ/ is used, the unstressed /ɚ/ is replaced by the schwa ([mɜdə] for [mɜˈdɚ]).

Production

As in /ʌ/, the central portion of the tongue is raised slightly and the muscles of the tongue are relaxed. The tongue tip rests behind the lower teeth, and the lips are in a neutral position.

EXERCISES

The first time you read the following exercises aloud, exaggerate the production of all of the sounds in the words, giving special attention to the vowels. Remember that the major difference between /ʌ/ and /ə/ is the degree of stress.

1. The pronunciations of the words are transcribed properly in column I. In column II, the words are transcribed with shifted or wrenched stress. Read both columns, making certain that you accurately vocalize what is transcribed. Focus on the differences in stress. Make certain that you do not pull away too much when trying to develop the appropriate pronunciation.

	I	II
around	[əraʊnd]	[ʌraʊnd]
poetry	[poətrɪ]	[poʌtrɪ]
suppose	[səpoz]	[sʌpoz]
connect	[kənɛkt]	[kʌnɛkt]
banana	[bənænə]	[bʌnænə]
aloud	[əlaʊd]	[ʌlaʊd]
method	[mɛθəd]	[mɛθʌd]
apply	[əplaɪ]	[ʌplaɪ]
society	[səsaɪətɪ]	[sʌsaɪətɪ]
possibly	[pɑsəblɪ]	[pɑsʌblɪ]

Read aloud the following sentences. Pay close attention to the stress! [˘] indicates minimal stress. Note that a monosyllabic word can contain the schwa in connected speech when the syllable is unstressed.

2. Allen's family wăs frŏm California.

3. The idea ŏf going to Australia excited Minerva.

4. Have you ever been to ă traveling circus?

5. Here is ă book by thĕ famous author William Saroyan.

6. It is about time that performance wăs stressed in literature classes.

7. Harold could better understand thĕ dilemma facing thĕ group.

8. President Kennedy had strong views about Cuba.

9. Generally speaking, thĕ sophomore year at college is different frŏm high school.

10. Thĕ moment he saw Veronica he knew whăt to do. (Now read this sentence with an increased stress on "what." You would now use /ʌ/.)

11. He could recognize Sarah's voice ŏn thĕ telephone.

Many of the schwas used in the sentences above can be substituted with different vowels in the unstressed syllables. For example, in the word "dilemma," the first vowel could also be pronounced as /ɪ/.

Read aloud the following selections.

12. Ŏf all symposia,
    Thĕ best by half,
    Upon Olympus, here, await ŭs,
    We eat Ambrosia,
    And nectar quaff—
    It cheers bŭt don't inebriate ŭs.

    From THESPIS *W. S. Gilbert*

13. Sing ă song ŏf sixpence
    Ă pocket full ŏf rye,
    Four ănd twenty blackbirds,
    Baked in ă pie.
    When thĕ pie wăs opened,
    Thĕ birds began to sing,
    Wasn't that ă dainty dish
    To set before thĕ King?

14. God be thanked, thĕ meanest ŏf his creatures
    Boasts two soul-sides, one to face thĕ world with,
    One to show a woman when he loves her!

    From ONE WORD MORE *Robert Browning*

15. My garden will never make me fam<u>ou</u>s,
I'm ă h<u>o</u>rticultural ignoram<u>u</u>s.

   From HE DIGS, HE DUG, HE HAS D<u>UG</u>   *Ogden Nash*

Read aloud the following words, sentences, and selections, which contain /ʌ/ and /ə/.

16. husband   abutment above

   hubbub   cultivate onion

17. The cultivation of onions is a difficult task.

18. Animal husbandry is an interesting study.

19. The buildings abutted each other.

20. Ezra had fun playing with Irma and Thomas.

21. The vulture is a bird that is rarely up to charitable deeds.

22. He was used to both, to dreams and mistakes. How often in that other world, had he not dreamed that he was wildly shoveling up money from the street.

   I. L. Peretz

23. The camel's hump is an ugly lump

   Which well you may see at the Zoo;

   But uglier yet is the Hump you get

   From having little to do.

   From HOW THE CAMEL GOT HIS HUMP   *Rudyard Kipling*

24. I cried unto the Lord with my voice; with my voice unto the Lord did I make my supplication. I poured out my complaint before him; I showed before him my trouble.

   PSALM 142

The following reading emphasizes /ɝ/ and /ɚ/, and /ʌ/ and /ə/.

25. Plaintiff:

I love him—I love him—with fervour unceasing

I worship and madly adore;

My blind adoration is always increasing,

My loss I shall ever deplore.

Oh, see what a blessing, what love and caressing

I've lost, and remember it, pray,

When you I'm addressing, are busy assessing

The damages Edwin must pay!

Defendant:

I smoke like a furnace—I'm always in liquor

A ruffian—a bully—a sot;

I'm sure I should thrash her, perhaps I should kick her,

I am such a very bad lot!
I'm not prepossessing, as you may be guessing,

She couldn't endure me a day;

Recall my professing, when you are assessing

The damages Edwin must pay!

From TRIAL BY JURY   *W. S. Gilbert*

BACK VOWELS

/u/

Production

In the production of /u/ (as in *true*), the muscles of the tongue are slightly tense; the back of the tongue is high toward the palate, and the tip rests behind the lower front teeth. The lips are rounded and slightly protruded.

EXERCISES

The first time you read the following exercises aloud, exaggerate the production of all of the sounds in the words, giving special attention to the vowels. Make certain that you do not pull away too much when trying to make the appropriate pronunciation a habit.

1. zoo   balloon
   through   peruse
   fruit   voodoo
   June   blueberry
   roof   fruition
   school   spoonerism
   lose   kangaroo
   glue   wounded
   choose   recruit
   bruise   festoon

2. The troops in the platoon were crouching in a festoon of blooms.

3. Every noontime the boys loosen the balloons.

4. Daniel Boone had nothing to do with the hole in the canoe.

5. The recruits got tattooed in July.

6. The prudent woman told the truth about the cruel crew.

7. I assume* that his orders will be resumed* in June.

---

*Professional speech would feature the diphthong /ɪu/.

8. Choose the right glue for the roof.

9. The frost bruised the fruit trees, especially the blueberries.

10. The kangaroo was wounded by the foolish troops.

11. The train's caboose worked itself loose and went through the wall.

12. There was a young lady in blue,
    Who said, "Is it you?* Is it you?"*
    When they said, "Yes it is,"
    She replied only, "Whizz!"
    That ungracious young lady in blue.

    Edward Lear

13. There was an old lady who lived in a shoe,
    She had so many children she didn't know what to do.

14. They intend to send a wire
    To the moon—to the moon;
    And they'll set the Thames on fire
    Very soon—very soon.

    Anonymous

15. In Rangoon the heat of noon is just what the natives shun.

    From MAD DOGS AND ENGLISHMEN   *Noel Coward*

16. Oh, Georgia booze is mighty fine booze,
    The best yuh ever poured yuh.

    THE MOUNTAIN WHIPPOORWILL   *Stephen Vincent Benet*

17. Though she's twenty-one, it's true,
    I am barely twenty-two—
    False and foolish prophets you,
    Twenty years ago!

    From PRINCESS IDA   *W. S. Gilbert*

/ʊ/

Production

In the production of /ʊ/ (as in *put*), the muscles of the tongue are relaxed. The back of the tongue is high toward the palate, and the tip rests behind the lower front teeth. The lips are less rounded than for /u/.

---

*Use the diphthong /ju/.

EXERCISES

The first few times you read the following exercises aloud, exaggerate the production of all of the sounds in the words, giving special attention to the vowels. Feel how this vowel differs from /u/.

1. Alternate reading aloud the words in the /ʊ/ and /u/ columns. The words enclosed in brackets are nonsense words and therefore transcribed into phonetics. Sound them out. Make certain you do not pull away too much when trying to develop the appropriate pronunciation.

	/ʊ/	/u/		/ʊ/	/u/
wolf	[wʊlf]	[wulf]	cushion	[kʊʃən]	[kuʃən]
wood	[wʊd]	wooed	sugar	[ʃugɚ]	[ʃugɚ]
cooked	[kʊkt]	[kukt]	mistook	[mɪstʊk]	[mɪstuk]
pushed	[pʊʃt]	[puʃt]	Brooklyn	[brʊklən]	[bruklən]
bush	[bʊʃ]	[buʃ]	bulletin	[bʊlətən]	[bulətən]
butch	[bʊtʃ]	[butʃ]	neighborhood	[nebɚhʊd]	[nebɚhud]
pull	[pʊl]	pool	pulpit	[pʊlpɪt]	pool pit
stood	[stʊd]	stewed	bosom	[bʊzəm]	[buzəm]
could	[kʊd]	cooed	cookies	[kʊkiz]	[kukiz]
shook	[ʃʊk]	[ʃuk]	bushel	[bʊʃl]	[buʃl]

2. The cook took the sugar and put it in the pudding.

3. Reverend Woods read the bulletin from the pulpit.

4. Ferdinand the Bull pushed the flowers into[5] the bushes.

5. The neighborhood children were happy with their woolen pullovers.

6. Dot pulled the hood over the horse's head and checked his hoof.

7. Charlie stood in his woolies as long as he could.

8. Mrs. Fulton said she would always suffer from good looks.

9. The wooden keg was full of beer.

10. He shook the hook from the pushcart.

11. The wolf stole the pullet and forsook the farm.

---

[5] Since the word is minimally stressed and the sound precedes another consonant, professional speech uses the schwa rather than /ʊ/ or /u/. However, before another vowel sound, the /ʊ/ is preferred in professional speech (such as "to Atlanta" [tʊ ætlæntə]).

12. In May, when the sea-winds pierced our solitudes,
   I found the fresh Rhodora in the woods,
   Spreading its leaflets blooms in a damp nook,
   To please the desert and the sluggish brook.
   The purple petals, fallen in the pool,
   Make the black water with their beauty gay;
   Here might the red-bird come his plumes to cool,
   And court the flower that cheapens his array.

   Ralph Waldo Emerson

13. And he took about five thousand men, and set them to lie in ambush . . . on the west side of the city.

   From JOSHUA

/o/

Production

In the production of /o/ (as in *go*), the muscles of the tongue are tense. The back of the tongue is raised midway to the palate, and the tip rests behind the lower front teeth. The lips are rounded.

When used in stressed syllables, /o/ often becomes the diphthong /oʊ/. This is particularly true when the single vowel appears in the final position, as in the word *go,* or when used in stressed syllables. In professional speech, the use of this diphthong is encouraged. It is produced when the lips are relaxed after the production of /o/.

EXERCISES

The first time you read the following exercises aloud, exaggerate the production of all of the sounds in the words, giving special attention to the vowels. Feel how this vowel differs from /ʊ/.

1. Alternate reading aloud the words in the /o/ and /ʊ/ columns. The words enclosed in brackets are nonsense words and therefore transcribed in phonetics. Sound them out. Make certain that you do not pull away too much when trying to develop the appropriate pronunciation.

	/o/	/ʊ/		/o/	/ʊ/
scold	[skold]	[skʊld]	obey	[obeɪ]	[ʊbeɪ]
shown	[ʃon]	[ʃun]	soldier	[soldʒɚ]	[sʊldʒɚ]
boast	[bost]	[bʊst]	frozen	[frozn̩]	[frʊzn̩]

bowl	[bol]	bull	bureau	[bjʊro]	[bjurʊ]
grown	[gron]	[grʊn]	Ohio	[ohaɪjo]	[ʊhaɪju]
soul	[sol]	[sʊl]	Oklahoma	[okləhomə]	[ʊkləhumə]
goal	[gol]	[gʊl]	piano	[pɪæno]	[pɪænu]
woke	[wok]	[wʊk]	woeful	[wofʊl]	[wufʊl]
though	[ðo]	[ðu]	opium	[opɪəm]	[ʊpɪəm]
throw	[θro]	[θru]	Omaha	[oməhɔ]	[ʊməhɔ]

2. Joe was the only one at the bowling alley.

3. Go and bring me both folders from the desk.

4. The short stories by Poe are often odious and sorrowful.

5. Snow White sang "Heigh Ho" along with Dopey.

6. The opening of *Oklahoma* was loaded with celebrities.

7. Tony broke the woeful silence with a friendly "Hello."

8. Coal costs almost double what it did only ten years ago.

9. In poker the joker does not count.

10. Michele was catching toads and putting them into bowls of flowers.

11. The phony old man was rowing toward the other rowboat.

12. I grow old . . . I grow old . . .
    I shall wear the bottom of my trousers rolled.
    From THE LOVE SONG OF J. ALFRED PRUFROCK   *T. S. Eliot*

13. In vain to us you plead—
    Don't go!
    Your prayers we do not heed—
    Don't go!
    It's true we sigh,
    But don't suppose
    A tearful eye
    Forgiveness shows.
    Oh, no!
    From IOLANTHE   *W. S. Gilbert*

14. I, as the modest moon with crescent bow,
    Have always shown a light to nightly scandal,
    I must say I should like to go below,
    And find out if the game is worth the candle!
    From THESPIS   *W. S. Gilbert*

15. Sweet and low, sweet and low,
    Wind of the western sea,
    Low, low, breathe and blow,
    Wind of the western sea!
    Over the rolling waters go,
    Come from the dying moon, and blow,
    Blow him again to me.

    From THE PRINCESS   *Alfred Lord Tennyson*

16. Old King Cole
    Was a merry old soul,
    And a merry old soul was he,
    He called for his pipe,
    And he called for his bowl,
    And he called for his fiddlers three.

    Anonymous

17. Jupiter, Mars, and Apollo,
    Have quitted the dwellings of men;
    The other gods quickly will follow,
    And what will become of us then.
    Oh, pardon us, Jove and Apollo,
    Pardon us, Jupiter, Mars;
    Oh, see us in misery wallow,
    Cursing our terrible stars.

    From THESPIS   *W. S. Gilbert*

/ɔ/

Production

In the production of /ɔ/ (as in *law*), the muscles of the tongue are slightly tense. The back of the tongue is lower than for /o/, and the tip rests behind the lower front teeth. The lips are less rounded than in /o/.

EXERCISES

The first few times you read the following exercises aloud, exaggerate the production of all of the sounds in the words, giving special attention to the vowels. Feel how this vowel differs from /o/.

1. Alternate reading aloud the words in the /ɔ/ and /o/ columns. The words enclosed in brackets are nonsense words and therefore transcribed into pho-

netics. Sound them out. Make certain you do not pull away too much when trying to develop appropriate pronunciation. It is important to note that the following words can be pronounced using different vowels, but in learning this sound use /ɔ/.

	/ɔ/	/o/		/ɔ/	/o/
flaw	[flɔ]	flow	withdraw	[wɪðdrɔ]	[wɪðdro]
lawn	[lɔn]	loan	Australian	[ɔstreljən]	[ostreljən]
call	[kɔl]	coal	authentic	[ɔθɛntɪk]	[oθɛntɪk]
salt	[sɔlt]	[solt]	caucus	[kɔkəs]	coke us
wrong	[rɔŋ]	[roŋ]	caution	[kɔʃən]	co-shun
walk	[wɔk]	woke	because	[bɪkɔz]	[bɪkoz]
draw	[drɔ]	[dro]	automobile	[ɔtəmobil]	[otəmobil]
shawl	[ʃɔl]	shoal	auspicious	[ɔspɪʃəs]	[ospɪʃəs]
fawn	[fɔn]	phone	authority	[ɔθɔrətɪ]	[oθorətɪ]
sauce	[sɔs]	[sos]	Boston	[bɔstn̩]	[bostn̩]

2. There are many auspicious authors in Boston.

3. The Australian and the Austrian met because of chance.

4. Yvonne's Southern drawl called attention to her speech.

5. My boss thought that the longer song was better.

6. The automobile I bought had many flaws.

7. The newsman authenticated the awful details.

8. Some people caution putting salt on the fish.

9. Audrey insisted upon an audit.

10. The fawn was walking in the wrong direction.

11. Saul forgot he fought for the lost cause.

12. There is only one way to achieve happiness on this terrestrial ball,
And that is to have either a clear conscience, or none at all.
From INTER-OFFICE MEMORANDUM   *Ogden Nash*

13. I know not whether Laws be right,
Or whether Laws be wrong;
All that we know who lie in gaol
Is that the wall is strong;
And that each day is like a year,
A year whose days are long.
From THE BALLAD OF READING GAOL   *Oscar Wilde*

14. See-saw, Margery Daw,
    Jacky shall have a new master;
    Jacky must have but a penny a day,
    Because he can't work any faster.

    Anonymous

15. There are some things which cannot be learned quickly, and time, which is
    all we have, must be paid heavily for their acquiring. They are the very
    simplest things and because it takes a man's life to know them the little new
    that each man gets from life is very costly and the only heritage he has to
    leave.

    From DEATH IN THE AFTERNOON   *Ernest Hemingway*

16. He shall treat us with awe,
    If there isn't a flaw,
    Singing so merrily—Trial-la-law!
    Trial-la-law—Trial-la-law!
    Singing so merrily—Trial-la-law!

    From TRIAL BY JURY   *W. S. Gilbert*

/ɒ/

Most speakers would not say *hot* using this vowel. As a matter of fact, there is
no key word that would clarify the sound for all Americans. It is primarily an
Eastern and Southern sound, but it is used in both British speech and stage
speech, which is why it is considered acceptable in career speech. Continue to
use the sound if it is part of your speech. It is not important to use it, however,
unless your goal is professional acting or performance.

Production

The muscles of the tongue are relaxed; the back of the tongue is low, and the tip
of the tongue rests behind the lower front teeth. The mandible is lowered from
the /ɔ/ position. The lips are slightly rounded but not as rounded as in /ɔ/.

EXERCISES

The first few times you read aloud the following exercises, exaggerate the production of all of the sounds in the words, giving special attention to the vowels.
Feel how this vowel differs from /ɔ/.

1. Alternate reading aloud the words in the /ɒ/ and /ɔ/ columns. Sound them
   out. Make certain you do not pull away too much when trying to develop
   the appropriate pronunciation.

	/ɒ/	/ɔ/		/ɒ/	/ɔ/
lost	[lɒst]	[lɔst]	alot	[əlɒt]	[əlɔt]
cough	[kɒf]	[kɔf]	frosty	[frɒstɪ]	[frɔstɪ]
tossed	[tɒst]	[tɔst]	moral	[mɒrəl]	[mɔrəl]
frost	[frɒst]	[frɔst]	orange	[ɒrəndʒ]	[ɔrəndʒ]
soft	[sɒft]	[sɔft]	Oregon	[ɒrəgɒn]	[ɔrəgɔn]
scoff	[skɒf]	[skɔf]	office	[ɒfəs]	[ɔfəs]
broth	[brɒθ]	[brɔθ]	salty	[sɒltɪ]	[sɔltɪ]
cloth	[klɒθ]	[klɔθ]	Florence	[flɒrəns]	[flɔrəns]
crossed	[krɒst]	[krɔst]			

2. Frank's office windows were frosted.

3. Don't shut the hall closet.

4. He coughed when he lost his medicine.

5. Dorothy fostered a love for frosting.

6. He tossed the ball in the fog.

7. The cloth was filled with moth holes.

8. Does the cake have chocolate frosting?

9. But lo! at the door of our cottage,
   The knock of the Guest.
   From ELEGY FROM A COUNTRY DOORYARD   *Phyllis McGinley*

10. Hickory, dickory, dock,
    The mouse ran up the clock,
    The clock struck one,
    The mouse ran down,
    Hickory, dickory, dock.

11. "Who killed Cock Robin?"
    "I," said the sparrow,
    "With my bow and arrow,
    I killed Cock Robin."

12. You've got to get up, you've got to get up,
    You've got to get up this morning!
    From THIS IS THE ARMY   *Irving Berlin*

13. A Garden is a lovesome thing, God wot!
    Rose plot,
    Fringed pool. Ferned grot—
    The veriest school

Of Peace; and yet the fool
Contends that God is not—
Not God! in Gardens! when the eve is cool?
Nay, but I have a sign:
'Tis very sure God walks in mine.

MY GARDEN *Thomas Edward Brown*

/ɑ/

Production

In the production of /ɑ/ (as in *father*), the muscles of the tongue are relaxed; the back of the tongue is low; and the tip rests behind the lower front teeth. The mandible is dropped from the /ɒ/ position, and the mouth is wide open. This sound often precedes the semivowel /r/. See the section of New England regionalisms in Chapter 11 for a detailed discussion of this sound combination.

You may have noticed that in producing the back vowels from high to low, the lips become increasingly unrounded as the mouth opens more.

EXERCISES

The first few times you read aloud the following exercises, exaggerate the production of the sounds in the words, giving special attention to the vowels.

1. park   balmy*

   Psalms*   alarmed

   carve   darkened

   harm   Harvard

   Sarge   partner

   palm*   guardian

   cart   farmer

   charm   harvest

   calm*   articulation

   alms*   Arkansas

2. Arthur was originally from Arkansas.

---

*In these words, the letter "l" is silent.

3. The ardent students charged out the books in the archives.

4. Jacob Marley was Scrooge's smart partner.

5. They argued that they would not harm the cargo.

6. Farmers are known as the guardians of the harvest.

7. The Artful Dodger is a character from Charles Dickens.

8. The Sergeant-at-Arms sounded the alarm with little charm.

9. It is a hard task to read the Psalms with good articulation.

10. King Arthur's knights wore carved armor.

11. Park your proverbial car in Harvard Yard!

12. She won't believe my statement, and declares we must be parted,
    Because on a career of double-dealing I have started,
    Then gives her hand to one of these, and leaves me broken-hearted.

    From IOLANTHE   *W. S. Gilbert*

13. All that I know
    Of a certain star
    Is, it can throw
    (Like the angled spar)
    Now a dart of red,
    Now a dart of blue;
    Till my friends have said
    They would fain see, too,
    My star that dartles the red and the blue!

    From MY STAR   *Robert Browning*

14. The following word lists compare /ɒ/ and /ɑ/.

	/ɒ/	/ɑ/
Robert	[rɒbɚt]	[rɑbɚt]
Tom	[tɒm]	[tɑm]
grotto	[grɒto]	[grɑto]
probably	[prɒbəblɪ]	[prɑbəblɪ]
motto	[mɒto]	[mɑto]
locked	[lɒkt]	[lɑkt]
got	[gɒt]	[gɑt]
cot	[kɒt]	[kɑt]
doctor	[dɒktɚ]	[dɑktɚ]

DIPHTHONGS

A diphthong (notice the pronunciation: [dɪfθɔŋ]) is the combination of two vowels within the same syllable. One of the vowels has more emphasis because its duration is longer. Although any two vowels can constitute a diphthong, some are acceptable in professional speech and some are not. This section will introduce and discuss both kinds.

It was mentioned when the vowels /e/ and /o/ were introduced that many speakers commonly diphthongize these vowels, especially in stressed syllables, to /eɪ/ and /ou/, respectively. It is difficult to control the action of the tongue in the first vowel. Besides, in professional speech this process is generally allowed. The diphthongs in "go and stay" ([gou ænd steɪ]) are caused by the rhythm of the language and are difficult to isolate from the individual vowel.

The phonemic diphthongs that will be discussed in detail are /aɪ/, /au/, /ɔɪ/, /ju/, and /ɪu/.

/aɪ/

The diphthong /aɪ/ (as in *ice*) is sometimes transcribed as /ɑɪ/, which is a most acceptable allophone of the /aɪ/ diphthong. It might be a good idea for New Englanders to use /ɑɪ/ to help them eliminate any remnant of /a/ from their speech.

Production

In the production of /aɪ/, the first vowel requires a low tongue and a lowered jaw. The muscles of the tongue are relaxed, and the tip rests behind the lower front teeth. From that position the tongue moves to a high-front position. If the allophone is used, the first vowel is produced with a low-back tongue position /ɑ/ before moving into the /ɪ/.

Problems

Three errors are common in the production of /aɪ/. The first is to omit the /ɪ/ component completely, a trait that is quite common in some Southern and Eastern speech. In the following word list, use negative practice.

	/aɪ/	/a/	/aɪ/
fine	[faɪn]	[fan]	[faɪn]
blind	[blaɪnd]	[bland]	[blaɪnd]
final	[faɪnl̩]	[fanl̩]	[faɪnl̩]

tribe	[traɪb]	[trab]	[traɪb]
sight	[saɪt]	[sat]	[saɪt]
spite	[spaɪt]	[spat]	[spaɪt]
I'm	[aɪm]	[am]	[aɪm]

The second error is to use excessive tension on the /a/, which gives the sound a flat and very unpleasant quality. To correct this problem, use /ɑ/ (as in *father*) for the first vowel. Keep the tongue flat in the mouth and produce the sound with an open throat. After you feel the difference between the productions of the sounds /ɑɪ/ and /aɪ/, you may want to go back to using /a/ in /aɪ/ but retain a relaxed quality. If you choose /ɑɪ/, make certain that you do not exaggerate the production of the /ɑ/.

The third error is the New York pronunciation of the diphthong. Refer to Chapter 11 (p. 271) for an additional discussion of this problem and corrective exercises.

EXERCISES

Record the following list of words and sentences and focus on the production of /aɪ/.

1. eye   final
   pile   playwright
   mice   island
   spies   daylight
   wide   stylish
   right   finite
   twice   diary
   guide   certify
   high   license
   rise   biography

2. The bicycle arrived just in time.

3. I didn't realize the biography was by Myers.

4. The guide told us to turn right twice.

5. Iris got a diamond ring from Byron.

6. At the height of the lightning storm they arrived.

7. At night the tiger was hiding in the jungle.

8. The license certified that they could photograph the lions.

9. The ivory jewelry was mine.

10. The sky was clear and bright blue.

11. I'll not ask the guide to drive the Jeep.

12. The world stands out on either side
    No wider than the heart is wide.

    From RENASCENCE   *Edna St. Vincent Millay*

13. In Adam's fall
    We sinned all.

    My Book and Heart
    Must never part.

    Young Obadias,
    David, Josias,—
    All were pious.

    Peter denyed
    His Lord, and cryed.

    Young Timothy
    Learnt sin to fly.

    Xerxes did die,
    And so must I.

    Zaccheus he
    Did climb the tree
    Our Lord to see.

    From THE NEW ENGLAND PRIMER

14. "Who saw him die?"
    "I," said the Fly,
    "With my little eye,
    I saw him die."

    From WHO KILLED COCK ROBIN?

15. Along came a spider,
    And sat down beside her,
    And frightened Miss Muffet away.

16. Phoebus am I, with golden ray,
    The god of day, the god of day,
    When a shadowy night has held her sway,
    I make the goddess fly.
    'Tis mine the task to wake the world,
    In slumber curled, in slumber curled,

By me her charms are all unfurled,
The god of day and I!

From THESPIS   *W. S. Gilbert*

17. Oh, listen to the plaintiff's case:
    Observe the features of her face—
    The broken-hearted bride.
    Condole with her distress of mind:
    From bias free of every kind,
    This trial must be tried!

    From TRIAL BY JURY   *W. S. Gilbert*

18. Let fervent words and fervent thoughts be mine,
    That I may lead them to thy sacred shrine!

    From PRINCESS IDA   *W. S. Gilbert*

19. For storm or shine, pure peace is thine,
    Whate'er betide.

    From SATISFIED   *Mary Baker Eddy*

20. Whose wreathed friezes intertwine
    The viol, the violet, and the vine.

    From THE CITY IN THE SEA   *Edgar Allan Poe*

/aʊ/

Production

In the production of /aʊ/ (as in *house*), the first vowel requires a low tongue position and a lowered jaw. (For the preferred allophone, /ɑʊ/, the first vowel requires a low-back tongue position.) The muscles of the tongue are relaxed. The tongue tip starts at rest behind the lower front teeth; the tongue then moves to a high-back position, but the muscles stay relaxed. The lips are rounded.

Problems

In career speech, you should use the allophone /ɑʊ/ if you have any tension when producing /aʊ/. In fact, the allophone /ɑʊ/ will be used throughout the remainder of the text. However, if you chose /aʊ/ for yourself, the danger is tension in the production of /a/, as was the case with /aɪ/.

The most common error in the production of /aʊ/ is the substitution of /æ/ for the preferred vowel /ɑ/. What results is a very tense and unpleasant sound. The error is found in a number of dialects, which is why it appears here rather than in the section on regionalisms.

Produce /æ→u/ and /ɑ→u/ before making the correct sound /aʊ/. When you pronounce this diphthong properly, /u/ becomes /ʊ/. To get a sense of this error, record what is transcribed:

[æ→u]   [æ→u]   [æ→u]

The correction is

[ɑ→u]   [ɑ→u]   [ɑ→u]

Now say the following using negative practice.

	Correct	*Incorrect*	*Correct*
bound	[bɑʊnd]	[bæʊnd]	[bɑʊnd]
howl	[hɑʊl]	[hæʊl]	[hɑʊl]
now	[nɑʊ]	[næʊ]	[nɑʊ]
sour	[sɑʊr]	[sæʊr]	[sɑʊr]
vow	[vɑʊ]	[væʊ]	[vɑʊ]
count	[kɑʊnt]	[kæʊnt]	[kɑʊnt]
mouth	[mɑʊθ]	[mæʊθ]	[mɑʊθ]
wow	[wɑʊ]	[wæʊ]	[wɑʊ]
hour	[ɑʊr]	[æʊr]	[ɑʊr]

[hɑʊ nɑʊ brɑʊn kɑʊ]

[hɑʊ næʊ brɑʊn kæʊ]

[hæʊ nɑʊ bræʊn kɑʊ]

[hæʊ næʊ bræʊn kæʊ]

[hɑʊ nɑʊ brɑʊn kɑʊ]

Remember, do not pull away too much from the exaggeration when trying to habituate appropriate pronunciation.

EXERCISES

The first few times you work with these exercises, exaggerate the pronunciation of the words and phrases. Feel how the diphthong is produced. Make certain you don't pull away too much when trying to develop the appropriate pronunciation.

1. shout   housekeeper
   foul   ourselves
   bough   devout
   owl   tower
   south   counterfeit
   flour   Browning
   drown   mountainous
   crowd   outside
   bounce   boundary
   mouth   doubtful

2. How do you account for the amount of snow on the ground?

3. Shout at the crowd!

4. Howard thought it was about time to go around the house.

5. Browning and Housman are our favorite poets.

6. The brown cows are particularly foul smelling.

7. Now the flowers are blooming in the south.

8. The housekeeper came down the stairs with a frown on her face.

9. When she scowled and pouted I went outside.

10. The mountainous terrain made it doubtful that we could go south.

11. The chowder was filled with cauliflower and flounder.

12. Hark, the hour of ten is sounding:
    Hearts with anxious fears are bounding,
    Hall of Justice crowds surrounding,
    Breathing hope and fear—

    . . . .

    Oh, joy unbounded,
    With wealth surrounded,
    The knell is sounded
    Of grief and woe.

    From TRIAL BY JURY   *W. S. Gilbert*

13. We'll storm their bowers
    With scented showers
    Of fairest flowers
    That we can buy!

    From PRINCESS IDA   *W. S. Gilbert*

14. Up and down, and in and out,
    Here and there, and round about;
    Every chamber, every house,
    Every chink that holds a mouse.

    From THE YEOMEN OF THE GUARDS   *W. S. Gilbert*

15. He who doubts from what he sees,
    Will ne'er believe, do what you please,
    If the Sun and Moon should doubt,
    They'd immediately go out.

    From AUGURIES OF INNOCENCE   *William Blake*

16. My son, if thou be surety for thy friend, if thou hast stricken thy hand with
    a stranger, Thou art snared with the words of thy mouth, thou art taken with
    the words of thy mouth.

    From PROVERBS

17. A gourmet dining in St. Lou
    Found quite a large mouse in his stew.
    Said the waiter: "Don't shout
    And wave it about,
    Or the rest will be wanting one too."

    Anonymous

18. The owl looked down with his great round eyes
    At the lowering clouds and the darkening skies,
    "A good night for scouting," says he,
    "With never a sound I'll go prowling around.
    A mouse or two may be found on the ground
    Or a fat little bird in a tree."
    So down he flew from the old church tower,
    The mouse and the birdie crouch and cower,
    Back he flies in half an hour,
    "A very good supper," says he.

    Anonymous

19. I remember the whole beginning as a succession of flights and drops, a little
    seesaw of the right throbs and the wrong. After rising, in town, to meet his
    appeal, I had at all events a couple of very bad days—found myself doubtful
    again, felt indeed sure I had made a mistake. In this state of mind I spent
    the long hours of bumping in a swinging coach that carried me to the stop-
    ping place at which I was to be met by a vehicle from the house. This con-
    venience, I was told, had been ordered and I found, toward the close of the
    June afternoon, a commodious fly in waiting for me.

    From THE TURN OF THE SCREW   *Henry James*

/ɔɪ/

Production

In the production of /ɔɪ/ (as in *boy*), the first vowel requires the tongue to be in a low-back position with a lowered jaw. The muscles of the tongue are relaxed, and the tip rests behind the lower front teeth with the lips rounded. The tongue moves to a high-front position, the muscles of the tongue relaxed and the lips retracted.

EXERCISES

Exaggerate the production of the diphthong in addition to each sound in the words and sentences in the following exercises. Feel how the blending of the vowels is produced. Do not pull away too much from the exaggeration while developing the appropriate pronunciation.

1. foil   sirloin
   join   royalty
   boil   appointment
   voice   rejoice
   toy   embroil
   joist   boisterous
   choice   destroy
   soil   poignant
   oil   oyster
   noise   thyroid

2. Did you enjoy the choice of oysters on the menu?

3. Roy, avoid the sirloin steak in the oily restaurant.

4. The oil soiled the rug.

5. He had an adroit way of avoiding employment.

6. The noise of the boys made her avoid the den.

7. The people rejoiced when the royal family entered.

8. Don't destroy the ointment.

9. Although the soil was moist, it was too deep.

10. The boisterous crowd made him recoil in terror.

11. Don't disappoint your loyal fans.

12. When first my old, old love I knew,
    My bosom welled with joy;
    My riches at her feet I threw—
    I was a love-sick boy!
    No terms seemed too extravagant
    Upon her to employ—
    I used to mope, and sigh, and pant,
    Just like a love-sick boy!
    Tink-a-Tank—Tink-a-Tank.

    But joy incessant palls the sense;
    And love, unchanged, will cloy,
    And she became a bore intense
    Unto her love-sick boy!
    With fitful glimmer burnt my flame,
    And I grew cold and coy,
    At last, one morning, I became
    Another's love-sick boy.
    Tink-a-Tank—Tink-a-Tank.

    From TRIAL BY JURY   *W. S. Gilbert*

13. There was a fellow from Roiling
    Whose temper was quick to come boiling;
    He'd leap and he'd hum as he banged on his drum,
    That boiling old Fellow from Roiling.

    Edward Lear

14. Music to hear, why hear'st thou music sadly?
    Sweets with sweets war not, joy delights in joy.
    Why lovest thou that which thou receivest no gladly,
    Or else receivest with pleasure thine annoy?

    From SONNET   *William Shakespeare*

15. If somebody there chanced to be
    Who loved me in a manner true,
    My heart would point him out to me,
    And I would point him out to you.
    But here it says of those who point,
    Their manners must be out of joint—
    You "may" not point—
    You "must" not point—
    It's manners out of joint, to point!

    From RUDDIGORE   *W. S. Gilbert*

/ju/

Production

In the production of this diphthong, the tongue begins in a high-front position and ends in a high-back position. The muscles of the tongue are tense, and the diphthong ends with lip rounding. The /ju/ diphthong is often found in the initial position in words of more than one syllable.

EXERCISES

It is important, in order to differentiate between /ju/ and the diphthong /ɪu/, to exaggerate the articulation. Do not pull away from this exaggeration too much when you develop the appropriate pronunciation.

1. hue   unison
    few   university
    Ute   eulogy
    huge   unit
    mute   uniform
    Hugh   unusual
    beaut   puberty
                 humility
                 mutation
                 usurp

2. Few institutions are without constitutions.

3. Tune into Tuesday's news.

4. The lute player's enthusiasm was infectious.

5. Unitarians' eulogies are usually short.

6. Hugh renewed his interest in nuclear fission.

7. The nuisance was caused by the weak test tubes.

8. The tutor's duties were established by the university officials.

9. Eulalia's teaching imbued the students with confidence.

10. Humility is a human characteristic.

11. He was duly amused by the duplication of the huge manuscript.

12. No woman would ever be quite accurate about her age. It looks so calculating.

    From THE IMPORTANCE OF BEING EARNEST *Oscar Wilde*

13. Ignorance of the law excuses no man; not that all men know the law, but because 'tis an excuse every man will plead, and no man can tell how to refute him.

    From TABLE TALK *John Selden*

/ɪu/

Production

This is an alternative diphthong to /ju/. As a matter of fact, it is preferred to /ju/ in professional speech in many situations. It is produced like /ju/ except that the muscles of the tongue are relaxed somewhat. In some words, such as *tune,* the singular vowel /u/ or the diphthong may be used. In career speech, the diphthong /ɪu/ is preferred. If /ju/ is used, the pronunciation may become labored and seem showy. The diphthong /ɪu/ contains very little of the gliding movement produced by the semivowel /j/.

EXERCISES

1. Produce the three pronunciations transcribed for the following words.

	/u/	/ju/	/ɪu/
new	[nu]	[nju]	[nɪu]
Tuesday	[tuzde]	[tjuzde]	[tɪuzde]
dew	[du]	[dju]	[dɪu]
nude	[nud]	[njud]	[nɪud]
tune	[tun]	[tjun]	[tɪun]
astute	[æstut]	[æstjut]	[æstɪut]
neuter	[nutɚ]	[njutɚ]	[nɪutɚ]

   Compare the /ɪu/ diphthong with /ju/ in the following sentences.

2. Few institutions are without constitutions.

3. Tune in Tuesday's news.

4. The lute player's enthusiasm was infectious.

5. Unitarians' eulogies are usually short.

6. H_ugh ren_ewed his interest in n_uclear fission.

7. Make a distinction between /u/ and /ɪu/ in the following word pairs.

stoop—stupid	[stup]—[stɪupɪd]
noon–new	[nun]—[nɪu]
two—tune	[tu]—[tɪun]
do—dew	[du]—[dɪu]
moo—mew	[mu]—[mɪu]
pooh—pew	[pu]—[pɪu]
who—hew	[hu]—[hɪu]
tooter—tutor	[tutɚ]—[tɪutɚ]

8

PRONUNCIATION

GLOSSARY

Anaptyxis   A linguistic error in which a vowel, usually the schwa, is placed between two consonants, adding an extra syllable (for example, [laɪtənɪŋ] for [laɪtnɪŋ]).

Assimilation   The influence of one sound upon another.

Bilabial   Pertaining to the two lips.

Continuant   A classification of sound in which there is a free flow of breath through the articulatory mold; except for the plosives, all sounds are continuants.

Dentalization   The erroneous use of the teeth in the production of sounds.

Diadochokinesis   The ability to produce difficult sound combinations with rapidity and precision.

Explosion   The release of impounded breath in the production of a plosive.

Haplology   A linguistic error in which a repeated sound or syllable is omitted (for example, [laɪbɛrɪ] for [laɪbrɛrɪ]).

Implosion   The coming together of the articulators with the buildup of breath but without the release of the impounded breath in the production of a plosive.

Linguistics   The study of human speech.

Metathesis   A linguistic error in which sounds are reversed in the pronunciation of a word (for example, "prespiration" for "perspiration").

Restressing   The changing of a vowel due to a change in stress; frequently a schwa turns into /ʌ/ instead of retaining the original vowel (for example, in its restressed form, *was* becomes [wʌz] instead of [wɑz] or [wɒz]).

Spoonerism   The transposition of sounds in different words.

In dynamic or conversational speech, there are three processes. First, it is necessary to produce the sound at the larynx (discussed in Chapters 2, 3, and 4). Second, the sound must be resonated into various speech sounds (Chapters 6 and 7). Third, the speech sounds must combine into syllables that are transformed into words (Chapter 8), which are eventually used to form vital or fluid speech (Chapters 11, 12, and 13).

The combination of articulation and enunciation creates pronunciation. It has been said that a word is a picture to the ear, with the vowel as the painting and the consonant as the frame. One is of little use without the other. This chapter deals with pronunciation—combining consonants and vowels into words that are uttered correctly and that work together to create dynamic speech.

STRESS

Although a discussion of stress could have been included earlier in the text, it appears here because stress is a relatively sophisticated concept, requiring a developed ear. Intelligence has little relevance in the ability to use stress correctly. Its use has been the downfall of many voice and speech students. Without some training, stress can cause great frustration.

There are two main types of stress in the English language. Primary stress is indicated by the placement of [ˊ] over the vowel in the syllable receiving the strongest emphasis. Minimal or weak stress is represented by [ˇ] appearing over the vowel in the syllable containing less stress. Sometimes weak or minimal stress is called "unstressed." This is a misnomer, since any spoken syllable must receive some stress. However, many teachers still use the term *unstressed,* and certainly everyone understands what is meant.

Every spoken word contains some kind of stress. If a word of one syllable is uttered aloud by itself, it receives primary stress, because it cannot be heard in relation to another syllable. Thus, in the sentence

Í ám á bíg trée.

the primary stress marks indicate either that there is a significant pause after each word or that the speaker is an oak or a robot. If the adjective were *little* instead of *big,* a decision would have to be made regarding the degree of stress.

In English there are several other systems for stress. There is the four-stress system, in which [´] signifies primary stress, [ˆ] signifies secondary stress, [`] signifies tertiary stress, and [˘] signifies minimal or weak stress. In a three-stress system, [´] represents primary, [`] represents secondary, and [˘] represents minimal stress.

The syllable that contains the primary stress (and there is usually only one primary stress in a word or phrase) is also the loudest syllable. Read the following sentences as marked. The parenthetical matter indicates the situation, which will determine the proper stress.

(You brought me the pencils, paper, and ink but . . .)
    Whêre àre thĕ bóoks?

(I did not ask you, What are the books; I want to know . . .)
    Whére àre thĕ boôks?

(I give up . . .)
    Whêre áre thĕ boòks?

And so stress is related not only to the loudness of the surrounding syllables but also to the underlying meaning. Using the four-stress system, say the following phrases aloud as transcribed.

1. *Thĕ Côrn Ìs Gréen*

2. Ĭ mèt ă greˆat gírl.

3. Thĕ tîme ĭs nów.

4. *Gône with thĕ Wínd*

5. Whàt ĭs thĕ meˆaning ŏf thát phrâse?

6. Dò yoû bĕliêve ĭn thĕ stárs?

7. Hoòráh fŏr thĕ lîttlĕ màn!

8. Gô ănd càtch ă fâllĭng stár.

9. Thàt wăs nót vêrў smârt.

10. Î knòw. Lèt's âll gò skíˆng!

What changes of meaning are there in the following sentences?

1. The President lives in the Whíte Hoûse.
   Did you like the whíte hoùse?

2. She is a líghthoùse keˆepĕr.
   She is a lîght hóusekeˆepĕr.

3. These are hôthòuse flówĕrs.
   This is a hôt hóuse.

4. He is a boŏkkeêpĕr.
   Marian the librarian called herself a boŏk keêpĕr.

   Throughout this text we have noted that the criteria for your standard of speech are determined by the demands made by your career. The appropriateness is further determined by your personality, the audience, and the speech occasion. As you move along in this chapter, you will be dealing with some sophisticated speech principles. Do not minimize their importance. Many of the principles presented here make the difference between a professional speaker and a nonprofessional.

RESTRESSING

Certain words usually contain minimal stress in conversational speech because they are less important than other words in the same phrase or sentence. These words very often contain the unstressed schwa, /ə/. If, to clarify meaning, these words are given additional stress, the original vowel should be used. In the previous chapter, it was stated that any unstressed vowel can become a schwa. However, if this **restressing** occurs, which often happens in professional speech, the speaker should use the original vowel. Say the following words aloud.

	Unstressed Form	*Restressed Form*	*Professional Form*
because	[bɪkəz]	[bɪkʌz]	[bɪkɔz]
was	[wəz]	[wʌz]	[wɑz], [wɒz]
of	[əv]	[ʌv]	[ɑv], [ɒv]
for	[fɚ]	[fɝ]	[fɔr]
from	[frəm]	[frʌm]	[frɑm], [frɒm]
can	[kən], [kn̩]	[kʌn]	[kæn]

"WRONG WORDS"

In the following words, learn and use the proper meaning. The subject is brought up here because these words are often mispronounced as well as misused.

uninterested [ənɪntrəstəd] (adj.): not paying attention;
   indifferent, not interested

disinterested [dɪsɪntrəstəd] (adj.): impartial; unbiased

elusive [ɪlɪusəv] (adj.): tending to escape from grasp; baffling

illusive [ɪlɪusəv] (adj.): unreal; deceiving

(As you will note, *elusive* and *illusive* are pronounced the same and contain the diphthong /ɪu/ in professional speech.)

alumna [əlʌmnə] (n., sing.): female graduate

alumnae [əlʌmni] (n., pl.): female graduates

alumnus [əlʌmnʊs] (n., sing.): male graduate

alumni [əlʌmnaɪ] (n., pl.): male or male and female graduates

except [ɪksɛpt] (v.): to take out; to omit

accept [æksɛpt] (v.): to receive with consent; to approve

affect [əfɛkt] (v.): to act upon; to produce an effect upon; to influence

effect [ɪfɛkt] (v.): to bring about; to accomplish; to produce

illusion [ɪlɪuʒən] (n.): misleading image; state of being deceived

delusion[dɪlɪuʒən] (n.): a false belief

allusion [əlɪuʒən] (n.): an implied or indirect reference; a figure of speech

sensual [sɛnʃuəl] (adj.): devoted or preoccupied with the senses or appetites; deficient in moral, spiritual, or intellectual interests

sensuous [sɛnʃuəs] (adj.): impressions or imagery pertaining to the senses

altar [ɔltɚ] (n.): raised and enclosed structure

alter [ɔltɚ] (v.): to make different; to change

(Notice that both words are pronounced the same.)

continual [kəntɪnjuəl] (adj.): implies a close prolonged succession or recurrence

continuous [kəntɪnjuəs] (adj.): implies an uninterrupted flow or spatial extension

perpetual [pɚpɛtjuəl] (adj.): pertaining to unfailing repetition or lasting duration

perennial [pɚɛnɪəl] (adj.): pertaining to an enduring existence, often through constant renewal

ASSIMILATION

This subject has been treated as a basic principle in the production of speech sounds. This part of the text will deal more extensively with the positive as well as negative influences of assimilation. As defined earlier, **assimilation** is the influence of one sound upon another. Ordinarily, in producing sounds, words, and dynamic speech, the mouth tends to the simplest and easiest articulation. The results may be acceptable or unacceptable pronunciation.

In the words below, the last sound becomes /s/ or /z/, or /t/ or /d/, depending upon the preceding sound. If a surd precedes the last sound, /s/ or /t/ is used because they, too, are surds. Conversely, if the next-to-last sound is a sonant, the /z/ or /d/ is used.

It is easier for the articulatory mechanism to stay voiced or unvoiced than to switch on and off. This principle does not apply in all cases, however. Exaggerate the production of the words below before pulling away in order to develop the appropriate articulation.

EXERCISES

In the following lists of words, pay close attention to the unvoiced and then the voiced endings.

Unvoiced-Unvoiced Endings

flakes [fleks]	omits [omɪts]	lips [lɪps]
tops [tɑps]	shakes [ʃeks]	shirks [ʃɝks]
grasped [græspt]	thinks [θɪŋks]	floats [flots]
digits [dɪdʒɪts]	baths [bæθs]	maps [mæps]
shrinks [ʃrɪŋks]	cheeps [tʃips]	laughs [læfs]
planks [plæŋks]	loafs [lofs]	sticks [stɪks]
licks [lɪks]	coughs [kɔfs]	works [wɝks]
flips [flɪps]	soaps [sops]	habits [hæbɪts]
coats [kots]	smarts [smɑrts]	cakes [keks]
kicks [kɪks]	flits [flɪts]	kites [kaɪts]

Voiced-Voiced Endings   ～symbol for ðə

raved [revd] ～ symbol for ðə	paths [pæðz]	deeds [didz]
clothes [kloðz]	thrills [θrɪlz]	tongues [tʌŋz]

snows [snoz]   thieves [θivz]   cabs [kæbz]

diphthongs [dɪfθɔŋz] berries [bɛriz]   schemed [skimd]

adjectives [ædʤɛktɪvz] creams [krimz]   wigs [wɪgz]

judged [ʤʌʤd]   winds [wɪndz]   hanged [hæŋd]

bowls [bolz]   riddles [rɪdl̩z]   copies [kɔpiz]

washes [wɔʃəz]   runners [rʌnɚz]   tools [tulz]

adverbs [ædvɚbz]   closed [klozd]   butters [bʌtɚz]

lungs [lʌŋz]   graves [grevz]   dreamed [drimd]

Omission of /t/ and /d/

A nonprofessional speaker often omits the /t/ and /d/ phonemes. In the following word list, exaggerate the production of these words so that you feel the articulation of the /t/ and /d/. Use negative practice. Do not pull away too much in trying to habituate the appropriate articulation.

EXERCISES

	Career	*Error*	*Career*
interval	[ɪntɚvl̩]	[ɪnɚvl̩]	[ɪntɚvl̩]
interface	[ɪntɚfes]	[ɪnɚfes]	[ɪntɚfes]
interlace	[ɪntɚles]	[ɪnɚles]	[ɪntɚles]
enter	[ɛntɚ]	[ɛnɚ]	[ɛntɚ]
cantaloupe	[kæntəlop]	[kænəlop]	[kæntəlop]
intermix	[ɪntɚmɪks]	[ɪnɚmɪks]	[ɪntɚmɪks]
interlunar	[ɪntɚlɪunɚ]	[ɪnɚlɪunɚ]	[ɪntɚlɪunɚ]
renter	[rɛntɚ]	[rɛnɚ]	[rɛntɚ]
interlude	[ɪntɚlɪud]	[ɪnɚlɪud]	[ɪntɚlɪud]
antic	[æntɪk]	[ænɪk]	[æntɪk]
enterprise	[ɛntɚpraɪz]	[ɛnɚpraɪz]	[ɛntɚpraɪz]
frantic	[fræntɪk]	[frænɪk]	[fræntɪk]
intermingle	[ɪntɚmɪŋgl̩]	[ɪnɚmɪŋgl̩]	[ɪntɚmɪŋgl̩]
interjection	[ɪntɚʤɛkʃən]	[ɪnɚʤɛkʃən]	[ɪntɚʤɛkʃən]
intersperse	[ɪntɚspɝs]	[ɪnɚspɝs]	[ɪntɚspɝs]
holding	[holdɪŋ]	[holɪŋ]	[holdɪŋ]
underling	[ʌndɚlɪŋ]	[ʌnɚlɪŋ]	[ʌndɚlɪŋ]

underneath	[əndɚniθ]	[ənɚniθ]	[əndɚniθ]
wonder	[wʌndɚ]	[wʌnɚ]	[wʌndɚ]
blond	[blɔnd]	[blɔn]	[blɔnd]
hand	[hænd]	[hæn]	[hænd]
spend	[spɛnd]	[spɛn]	[spɛnd]

Substitution of /d/ for /t/

In many words, a /t/ phoneme is changed to a /d/ phoneme because of assimilation. To produce the voiceless phoneme /t/, the vocal mechanism must shut off the vibration. When the /t/ is placed between two voiced sounds, the vocal mechanism tends to substitute the phonating /d/ for the voiceless /t/, as in [lɪdl̩] for *little*. Remember that we are basically lazy animals. Professional speech requires attention to this error.

EXERCISES

The following list is exemplary rather than extensive. Make your own list. Doing so will aid in your hearing and kinetic reinforcement. Use negative practice. Note that this error is very common in the pronunciation of numbers. Read the words as they are transcribed in order to hear and feel the differences.

	Career	*Error*	*Career*
otter	[ɑtɚ]	[ɑdɚ]	[ɑtɚ]
fraternity	[frətɝnətɪ]	[frətɝnədɪ]	[frətɝnətɪ]
accreditation	[əkrɛdəteʃən]	[əkrɛdədeʃən]	[əkrɛdəteʃən]
entirety	[ɛntaɪrtɪ]	[ɛntaɪrdɪ]	[ɛntaɪrtɪ]
creditor	[krɛdətɚ]	[krɛdədɚ]	[krɛdətɚ]
dirty	[dɝtɪ]	[dɝdɪ]	[dɝtɪ]
ninety	[naɪntɪ]	[naɪndɪ]	[naɪntɪ]
eighty	[etɪ]	[edɪ]	[etɪ]
seventy	[sɛvəntɪ]	[sɛvəndɪ]	[sɛvəntɪ]
sixty[1]	[sɪkstɪ]	[sɪksdɪ]	[sɪkstɪ]

[1] Can you feel that the /t/ is easier to produce in this word than the others? This is because the /t/ continues the surd adjustment begun with the /k/ phoneme. However, there must be vibration of the vocal folds in the production of the last sound in that word, the vowel /ɪ/.

EXPLOSION AND IMPLOSION

A plosive sound may be imploded (unaspirated) or exploded (aspirated). In explosion, breath is built up behind the articulators and then released in a puff of air. The amount of air released (**explosion**) depends on the placement of the plosive in the word. Place a piece of paper in front of your mouth and say the word *pan;* now say the word *span.* Does the movement of the paper show less aspiration in *span* than in *pan?*

In **implosion,** the articulators come together and, as in explosion, pressure is built up, but the articulators do not release the puff of air into that sound. Instead, the air is absorbed into the next sound. Although this is a sophisticated process, it is an important one for the communication specialist. A few examples should help to clarify the distinction between implosion and explosion. In this text, the mark indicating explosion is ['], and it is placed to the right of the plosive: /pʻ/, /bʻ/, and /kʻ/. Implosion is designated by ['] as in /p'/, /b'/, /k'/.

Read the following sentence as indicated by the transcriptions. Focus your attention on the underlined portions.

I don't know.   [aɪ dono]   (omission of /t/)

            [aɪ dontʻno]   (exploded /t/)

            [aɪ dont'no]   (imploded /t/)

Which pronunciation is preferred in career speech? If you use the first one, you are an animal answering to the name of Moose. The third pronunciation is preferred. If all plosives are exploded in speech, the impression created is one of pedantic prissiness. This is the quality of speech encouraged by history teachers forced to direct the high school play. How many times have you heard, "Pronounce all of the consonants distinctly and clearly"? In following this suggestion, often all of the plosive sounds are exploded.

Plosives are always exploded when they are either the initial sound in a word or the final sound with no word immediately following.

EXERCISE

In pronouncing the following words, all of the plosives should be exploded. Feel what the articulators are doing.

cup   [kʻʌpʻ]

gift   [gʻɪftʻ]

took [tʻʊkʻ]

Kent   [kˈɛntˈ]

brunch   [bˈrʌntʃˈ]

bridge   [bˈrɪʤˈ]

peep   [pˈipˈ]

cheap   [tʃˈipˈ]

coast   [kˈostˈ]

toast   [tˈostˈ]

In an imploded plosive, the articulators come together and pressure builds up behind the articulators, but the breath is released into the next sound.

EXERCISES

In the group of words below, pronunciation using explosion is followed by a pronunciation using implosion. The implosion occurs immediately before a syllabic consonant.

	Explosion	*Implosion*
Latin	[lætˈn̩]	[læt'n̩]
mitten	[mɪtˈn̩]	[mɪt'n̩]
middle	[mɪdˈl̩]	[mɪd'l̩]
Hutton	[hʌtˈn̩]	[hʌt'n̩]
muddle	[mʌdˈl̩]	[mʌd'l̩]

As you pronounce the following phrases, exaggerate the explosion and implosion so that you feel what is happening in sound production.

	Explosion	*Implosion*
don't know	[dontˈ no]	[dont' no]
won't go	[wontˈ go]	[wont' go]
quick temper	[kwɪkˈ tɛmpɚ]	[kwɪk' tɛmpɚ]
book store	[bʊkˈ stɔr]	[bʊk' stɔr]
Cape clam	[kepˈ klæm]	[kep' klæm]
Spot Pond	[spɑtˈ pɑnd]	[spɑt' pɑnd]
right hand	[raɪtˈ hænd]	[raɪt' hænd]
put it	[pʊtˈ ɪt]	[pʊt' ɪt]
talk fast	[tɔkˈ fæst]	[tɔk' fæst]
sank quickly	[sæŋkˈ kˈwɪkˈlɪ]	[sæŋk' kˈwɪkˈlɪ]

When one plosive is followed by another, the first is imploded and the second is exploded. Say the following words twice. The first time explode all of the plosives. The second time, use implosion followed by explosion; this latter pronunciation should be used in career speech.

EXERCISE

	Explosion Only	*Implosion and Explosion*
looked	[lʊkˈtˈ]	[lʊkʾtˈ]
asked	[æskˈtˈ]	[æskʾtˈ]
husked	[hʌskˈtˈ]	[hʌskʾtˈ]
basked	[bæskˈtˈ]	[bæskʾtˈ]
robbed	[rɑbˈdˈ]	[rɑbʾdˈ]
gaped	[gepˈtˈ]	[gepʾtˈ]
grasped	[græspˈtˈ]	[græspʾtˈ]

When a word ends with a plosive sound and the next word begins with another plosive (the same or different), the first plosive is imploded and the second is exploded. The duration of the implosion creates the two separate sounds.

EXERCISES

In the following words, first explode the final plosive in the first word; then implode the final plosive in the first word and hold the implosion long enough to feel and hear the production.

	Explosion Only	*Implosion and Explosion*
act two	[ækˈtˈ tˈu]	[ækʾtˈ tˈu]
ripe berries	[raɪpˈ bˈɛriz]	[raɪpʾ bˈɛriz]
red pajamas	[rɛdˈ pˈədʒˈaməz]	[rɛdʾ pˈədʒˈaməz]
rhubarb pie	[rubˈɑrbˈ pˈaɪ]	[rubˈɑrbʾ pˈaɪ]
black cat	[blækˈ kˈætˈ]	[blækʾ kˈætˈ]
cooked dinner	[kʊkˈtˈ dˈɪnɚ]	[kʊkˈtʾ dˈɪnɚ]

In the lists below, say the phrases three times as indicated and feel the explosion and implosion in the plosives. The first time use straight explosion. The second time exaggerate the length of the implosion; the third time give the implosion the proper amount of time. Note that the modifying mark [:] after a sound signifies that the sound is prolonged. (Although the sound of a plosive cannot be prolonged, its buildup of pressure can.)

	Explosion Only	*Prolonged Implosion and Explosion*	*Proper Implosion and Explosion*
act two	[æk't' t'u]	[æk't': t'u]	[æk't' t'u]
ripe berries	[raɪp' b'ɛriz]	[raɪp': b'ɛriz]	[raɪp' b'ɛriz]
red pajamas	[rɛd' p'ədʒ'aməz]	[rɛd': p'ədʒ'aməz]	[rɛd' p'ədʒ'aməz]
rhubarb pie	[rub'arb' p'aɪ]	[rub'arb': p'aɪ]	[rub'arb' p'aɪ]
black cat	[blæk' k'æt]	[blæk': k'æt]	[blæk': k'æt]
cooked dinner	[kʊk't' d'ɪnɚ]	[kʊk': t': d'ɪnɚ]	[kʊk't' d'ɪnɚ]

A very common error is the omission of medial plosives. Sometimes these incorrect pronunciations create unintended but legitimate words, such as "paining" for *painting*.

EXERCISES

Using negative practice, pronounce the following words and phrases.

	Career	*Error*	*Career*
rental	[rɛntl̩]	[rɛnl̩]	[rɛntl̩]
problem	[prabləm]	[praləm]	[prabləm]
mental	[mɛntl̩]	[mɛnl̩]	[mɛntl̩]
painting	[pentɪŋ]	[penɪŋ]	[pentɪŋ]
gentle	[dʒɛntl̩]	[dʒɛnl̩]	[dʒɛntl̩]
Bedford	[bɛdfɚd]	[bɛfəd]	[bɛdfɚd]
probably	[prabəblɪ]	[pralɪ]	[prabəblɪ]
dental	[dɛntl̩]	[dɛnl̩]	[dɛntl̩]
chanting	[tʃæntɪŋ]	[tʃænɪŋ]	[tʃæntɪŋ]
splinter	[splɪntɚ]	[splɪnɚ]	[splɪntɚ]
breakfast	[brɛkfəst]	[brɛfəst]	[brɛkfəst]
Medford	[mɛdfɚd]	[mɛfəd]	[mɛdfɚd]
That's a problem.	[ðæts ə prabləm]	[ðæts ə praləm]	[ðæts ə prabləm]
a mental trick	[ə mɛntl̩ trɪk]	[ə mɛnl̩ trɪk]	[ə mɛntl̩ trɪk]

painting a house	[pentɪŋ ə haʊs]	[penɪŋ ə haʊs]	[pentɪŋ ə haʊs]
Gently does it.	[dʒɛntlɪ dʌz ɪt]	[dʒɛnlɪ dʌz ɪt]	[dʒɛntlɪ dʌz ɪt]
probably true	[prɑbəblɪ tru]	[prɑlɪ tru]	[prɑbəblɪ tru]
a dental plan	[ə dɛntl̩ plæn]	[ə dɛnl̩ plæn]	[ə dɛntl̩ plæn]

/nd/ and /md/ Clusters

In connected speech, the combinations /nd/ and /md/ are often produced carelessly. Sometimes the plosives should be imploded and aren't, and sometimes they should be exploded but aren't. In the following phrases and sentences, make certain that the plosive is imploded before you proceed to the next word. The flow of the **continuant** before the plosive must be interrupted. Many of the clusters can also be pronounced with exploded plosives.

the end of the story	[ðɪ ɛnd' əv ðə stɔrɪ]
The hand aches.	[ðə hænd' eks]
Find me the way!	[faɪnd' mɪ ðə weɪ]
Don't hound me!	[dont' haʊnd' mɪ]
Beth blamed the boy.	[bɛθ blemd' ðə bɔɪ]
Ned claimed the box.	[nɛd' klemd' ðə bɑks]
Ralph informed the troops.	[rælf ɪnfɔrmd' ðə trups]

/ts/ and /dz/ Clusters

The /ts/ and /dz/ combinations are frequently mispronounced. The /t/ and /d/ are often omitted, or the combination is sloppily produced.

EXERCISES

Overarticulate the following word list. Do not pull away too much when you practice. Feel the tongue in contact with the alveolar ridge to make closure in the production of /t/ and /d/. The tongue tip then drops, and the escaping air is forced through the narrow groove down the front of the tongue in the production of /s/ and /z/.

/ts/	/dz/
goats [gots]	goads [godz]
invites [ɪnvaɪts]	loads [lodz]
totes [tots]	toads [todz]
coats [kots]	codes [kodz]

rights [raɪts̲]   rides [raɪd̲z]
cats [kæts̲]   cads [kæd̲z]
votes [vots̲]   plaids [plæd̲z]
mates [mets̲]   maids [med̲z]
spots [spɑts̲]   spuds [spʌd̲z]
huts [hʌts̲]   suds [sʌd̲z]

/sts/ Clusters

This is a difficult combination that takes practice to make habitual. However, in career speech it is one of the most important combinations in the language. Its correct pronunciation reflects a speaker of precision and care. Anyone interested in a communications career must master this combination.

The most common error is to omit the imploded /t/ plosive and make one long /s/ phoneme.

EXERCISES

Exaggerate the articulation of the following word list. If you have difficulty inserting the plosive, separate the cluster /sts/ into /s/ and /ts/. Go back to the /ts/ word list just above and feel what is happening in the production of the cluster. Remember that the modifying mark [:] prolongs the production of the phoneme.

hosts   [hos:ts]   blasts   [blæs:ts]
priests   [pris:ts]   boasts   [bos:ts]
coasts   [kos:ts]   masts   [mæs:ts]
frosts   [frɔs:ts]   tastes   [tes:ts]
casts   [kæs:ts]   thrusts   [θrʌs:ts]
wrists   [rɪs:ts]   insists   [ɪnsɪs:ts]
lasts   [læs:ts]   fists   [fɪs:ts]
posts   [pos:ts]   assists   [əsɪs:ts]

In the following tongue twisters, work first to exaggerate the proper production of the sounds. When you have that under control, quicken the pace. When you have succeeded in producing the difficult sound combinations with rapidity and clarity, you are exemplifying **diadochokinesis.** As you can see, you are also exhibiting it when you pronounce the word successfully!

Amidst the mists and coldest frosts,
With barest wrists and stoutest boasts,
He thrusts his fists against the posts,
And still insists he sees the ghosts.

A Swiss wrist wrestler's watch lasts longer when it rests on the wrestlers' wrists rather than their fists.

/θs/ and /ðz/ Clusters

Say the following words and phrases aloud using negative practice. The untrained speaker tends to omit the fricative before the /s/ and /z/ phonemes. Exaggerate the production of the sound and feel the placement of the articulators. When you try to develop the proper pronunciation, make certain that you do not pull away too much from overarticulation.

	Career	*Error*	*Career*
fourths	[fɔrθs]	[fɔrs] (force)	[fɔrθs]
fifths	[fɪfθs]	[fɪfs]	[fɪfθs]
lengths	[lɛŋθs]	[lɛŋs]	[lɛŋθs]
sixths	[sɪksθs]	[sɪks] (six)	[sɪksθs]
depths	[dɛpθs]	[dɛps]	[dɛpθs]
breaths	[brɛθs]	[brɛs]	[brɛθs]
breathes	[briðz]	[briz] (breeze)	[briðz]
writhes	[raɪðz]	[raɪz] (rise)	[raɪðz]
tithes	[taɪðz]	[taɪz] (ties)	[taɪðz]
clothes	[kloðz]	[kloz] (close)	[kloðz]
teethes	[tiðz]	[tiz] (tease)	[tiðz]

	Career	*Error*	*Career*
lengths of cord	[lɛŋθs əv kɔrd]	[lɛŋs əv kɔrd]	[lɛŋθs əv kɔrd]
breathes some air	[briðz səm er]	[briz səm er]	[briðz səm er]
washes the clothes	[wɔʃɪz ðə kloðz]	[wɔʃɪz ðə kloz]	[wɔʃɪz ðə kloðz]
writhes with pain	[raɪðz wɪð pen]	[raɪz wɪð pen]	[raɪðz wɪð pen]
breathes diaphragmatically	[briðz daɪəfrægmætɪklɪ]	[briz daɪəfrægmætɪklɪ]	[briðz daɪəfrægmætɪklɪ]

When you think you are ready, recite one of Carl Sandburg's definitions of poetry with speed and continuity:

Poetry is the synthesis of hyacinths and biscuits.

Omission of /l/

In the following words, the /l/ phoneme is correctly omitted even though some professional communicators say it. Consult your dictionary.

EXERCISES

Use negative practice in saying the following words. Exaggerate the production of the sounds so you can focus on the feel of the placement. This is also a good exercise for people learning English as a second language.

	Career	*Error*	*Career*
salmon	[sæmən]	[sælmən]	[sæmən]
half	[hæf]	[hælf]	[hæf]
walk	[wɔk]	[wɔlk]	[wɔk]
calf	[kæf]	[kælf]	[kæf]
palm	[pɑm]	[pɑlm]	[pɑm]
behalf	[bɪhæf]	[bɪhælf]	[bɪhæf]
Psalms	[sɑmz]	[sɑlmz]	[sɑmz]
balk	[bɔk]	[bɔlk]	[bɔk]
almond	[ɑmənd]	[ɑlmənd]	[ɑmənd]
calm	[kɑm]	[kɑlm]	[kɑm]
chalk	[tʃɔk]	[tʃɔlk]	[tʃɔk]
embalm	[ɛmbɑm]	[ɛmbɑlm]	[ɛmbɑm]

On the other hand, sometimes the /l/ phoneme is omitted when it should be articulated. Practice the words below.

	Career	*Error*	*Career*
milk	[mɪlk]	[mɪuk]	[mɪlk]
welcome	[wɛlkəm]	[wɛukəm]	[wɛlkəm]
railroad	[relrod]	[reurod]	[relrod]
million	[mɪljən]	[mɪujən]	[mɪljən]
William	[wɪljəm]	[wɪjəm]	[wɪljəm]

Substitution of /ŋ/ for /n/

The problem of substituting /ŋ/ for /n/ arises when /n/ precedes the plosives /k/ or /g/. Because /ŋ/ has a similar articulatory adjustment to /k/ and /g/, it is easier to anticipate the plosives by changing the /n/ to /ŋ/.

EXERCISE

Read the following words aloud and employ negative practice. Exaggerate the production of the words and feel what the articulators are doing. Do not pull away too much.

	Career	*Error*	*Career*
income	[ɪnkəm]	[ɪŋkəm]	[ɪŋkəm]
incongruous	[ɪnkɑngruəs]	[ɪŋkɑŋgruəs]	[ɪŋkɑngruəs]
incantation	[ɪnkænteʃən]	[ɪŋkænteʃən]	[ɪŋkænteʃən]
incapable	[ɪnkepəbl̩]	[ɪŋkepəbl̩]	[ɪŋkepəbl̩]
in case	[ɪnkes]	[ɪŋkes]	[ɪŋkes]
incoming	[ɪnkʌmɪŋ]	[ɪŋkʌmɪŋ]	[ɪŋkʌmɪŋ]
inclose	[ɪnkloz]	[ɪŋkloz]	[ɪŋkloz]
incomplete	[ɪnkəmplit]	[ɪŋkəmplit]	[ɪŋkəmplit]
increase	[ɪnkris]	[ɪŋkris]	[ɪŋkris]
incorrect	[ɪnkərɛkt]	[ɪŋkərɛkt]	[ɪŋkərɛkt]
incredible	[ɪnkrɛdəbl̩]	[ɪŋkrɛdəbl̩]	[ɪŋkrɛdəbl̩]
innkeeper	[ɪnkipɚ]	[ɪŋkipɚ]	[ɪnkipɚ]
ingrain	[ɪngren]	[ɪŋgren]	[ɪŋgren]
ingrate	[ɪngret]	[ɪŋgret]	[ɪŋgret]
ingoing	[ɪngoɪŋ]	[ɪŋgoɪŋ]	[ɪŋgoɪŋ]
ingredient	[ɪngridɪənt]	[ɪŋgridɪənt]	[ɪŋgridɪənt]

Substitution of /m̩/ for /nf/ and /nv/

You will remember that the symbol /m̩/ indicates that the phoneme /m/ is **dentalized,** that is, produced with the upper teeth touching the lower lip rather than its usual **bilabial** production. When either /nf/ or /nv/ follows /m/, the /m/ is often dentalized because of assimilation. For instance, it is easier to articulate /m̩f/ than /nf/ in the word *confine,* and whatever is easier is usually the route of the untrained speaker.

EXERCISES

In the following words, make certain that you take the time to produce the /n/ before moving to the fricative /f/ or /v/. Exaggerate the pronunciation using negative practice. During habituation, make certain that you do not pull away too much from the exaggerated articulation.

	Career	*Error*	*Career*
confine	[kənfaɪn]	[kəɱfaɪn]	[kənfaɪn]
confection	[kənfɛkʃən]	[kəɱfɛkʃən]	[kənfɛkʃən]
confederate	[kənfɛdɚət]	[kəɱfɛdɚət]	[kənfɛdɚət]
confess	[kənfɛs]	[kəɱfɛs]	[kənfɛs]
confer	[kənfɝ]	[kəɱfɝ]	[kənfɝ]
confirm	[kənfɝm]	[kəɱfɝm]	[kənfɝm]
confuse	[kənfɪuz]	[kəɱfɪuz]	[kənfɪuz]
convert	[kənvɝt]	[kəɱvɝt]	[kənvɝt]
converge	[kənvɝdʒ]	[kəɱvɝdʒ]	[kənvɝdʒ]
convey	[kənveɪ]	[kəɱveɪ]	[kənveɪ]
convince	[kənvɪns]	[kəɱvɪns]	[kənvɪns]
infirm	[ɪnfɝm]	[ɪɱfɝm]	[ɪnfɝm]
infection	[ɪnfɛkʃən]	[ɪɱfɛkʃən]	[ɪnfɛkʃən]
inference	[ɪnfɚəns]	[ɪɱfɚəns]	[ɪnfɚəns]
infidel	[ɪnfədl̩]	[ɪɱfədl̩]	[ɪnfədl̩]
infinitive	[ɪnfɪnətɪv]	[ɪɱfɪnətɪv]	[ɪnfɪnətɪv]
inflate	[ɪnflet]	[ɪɱflet]	[ɪnflet]
infringe	[ɪnfrɪndʒ]	[ɪɱfrɪndʒ]	[ɪnfrɪndʒ]
influence	[ɪnfluəns]	[ɪɱfluəns]	[ɪnfluəns]
informal	[ɪnfɔrməl]	[ɪɱfɔrməl]	[ɪnfɔrməl]
unfit	[ʌnfɪt]	[ʌɱfɪt]	[ʌnfɪt]
unfold	[ʌnfold]	[ʌɱfold]	[ʌnfold]
unflinch	[ʌnflɪntʃ]	[ʌɱflɪntʃ]	[ʌnflɪntʃ]
unfeeling	[ʌnfilɪŋ]	[ʌɱfilɪŋ]	[ʌnfilɪŋ;

Dentalization of /p/ and /b/

In the following exercise use negative practice. When making the correction, do not allow the upper teeth to touch the lower lip on the bilabial plosive before articulating the fricatives /f/ and /v/, as in the words "stop fast" [stɑp fæst]. Give the plosive sounds their full bilabial adjustment. Hold the imploded plosive longer than usual so that you will feel the bilabial adjustment. Remember [:] after a sound indicates prolongation.

	Career	*Error*	*Career*
step first	[stɛp: fɝst]	[stɛp̪: fɝst]	[stɛp: fɝst]
top value	[tɑp: vælju]	[tɑp̪: vælju]	[tɑp: vælju]

obvious	[ɑb:vɪəs]	[ɑb:vɪəs]	[ɑb:vɪəs]
stop Frank	[stɑp: fræŋk]	[stɑp: fræŋk]	[stɑp: fræŋk]
mob violence	[mɑb: vaɪələns]	[mɑb: vaɪələns]	[mɑb: vaɪələns]
rob Verne	[rɑb: vɝn]	[rɑb: vɝn]	[rɑb: vɝn]
Fab vendors	[fæb: vɛndɚz]	[fæb: vɛndɚz]	[fæb: vɛndnz]
troup fatigue	[trup: fətig]	[trup: fətig]	[trup: fətig]

SYLLABLE OMISSION AND ADDITION

There are a number of words whose pronunciations have been altered through the omission of a syllable. Obviously, enough speakers have made the change in pronunciation that the changes are reflected in the dictionary. The following list of words is divided into "Career" and "Conversational." *Conversation* is defined as "informal." Thus, actors might present themselves with professional speech but use conversational speech when in character. Professional speakers would obviously use the career pronunciation. You are encouraged, however, to maintain flexibility in communication in your career.

	Career	*Conversational*
sophomore	[sɑfəmɔr] or [sɑfm̩ɔr]	[sɑfmɔr]
traveling	[trævəlɪŋ] or [trævl̩ɪŋ]	[trævlɪŋ]
camera	[kæmərə]	[kæmrə]
veteran	[vɛtərən]	[vɛtrən]
battery	[bætərɪ]	[bætrɪ]
federal	[fɛdərəl]	[fɛdrəl]
victory	[vɪktərɪ]	[vɪktrɪ]
family	[fæməlɪ]	[fæmlɪ]
boundary	[baʊndərɪ]	[baʊndrɪ]
bakery	[bekərɪ]	[bekrɪ]
grocery	[grosərɪ]	[grosrɪ]
delivery	[dɪlɪvərɪ]	[dɪlɪvrɪ]
different	[dɪfərənt]	[dɪfrənt]
history	[hɪstərɪ]	[hɪstrɪ]
salary	[sælərɪ]	[sælrɪ]
temperamental	[tɛmpərəmɛntəl]	[tɛmprəmɛntəl]

liberal	[lɪbərəl]	[lɪbrəl]
celery	[sɛlərɪ]	[sɛlrɪ]
memory	[mɛmərɪ]	[mɛmrɪ]

ANAPTYXIS

Sometimes speakers add syllables where none exist. This is an error in **linguistics** called **anaptyxis**.

EXERCISE

Use negative practice on the following list of frequently mispronounced words and add new words to the list.

	Career	*Error*	*Career*
lightning	[laɪtnɪŋ]	[laɪtənɪŋ]	[laɪtnɪŋ]
sparkling	[spɑrklɪŋ]	[spɑrkəlɪŋ]	[spɑrklɪŋ]
athletic	[æθlɛtɪk]	[æθəlɛtɪk]	[æθlɛtɪk]
laundry	[lɔndrɪ]	[lɔndɚɪ]	[lɔndrɪ]
troubling	[trʌblɪŋ]	[trʌbəlɪŋ]	[trʌblɪŋ]
heartrending	[hɑrtrɛndɪŋ]	[hɑrtrɛndɚɪŋ]	[hɑrtrɛndɪŋ]
evening	[ivnɪŋ]	[ivənɪŋ]	[ivnɪŋ]
bubbling	[bʌblɪŋ]	[bʌbəlɪŋ]	[bʌblɪŋ]
ticklish	[tɪklɪʃ]	[tɪkəlɪʃ]	[tɪklɪʃ]
grievous	[grivəs]	[griviəs]	[grivəs]
business	[bɪznɪs]	[bɪzənɪs]	[bɪznɪs]
chuckling	[tʃʌklɪŋ]	[tʃʌkəlɪŋ]	[tʃʌklɪŋ]
please	[pliz]	[pəliz]	[pliz]

THE SNEEZING ERROR

One of the most common errors made by the untrained (and too many trained) speakers is assimilation when the pronoun *you* (or its variations) follows a plosive, particularly /t/ and /d/. The resulting sound often imitates the sneeze (ətʃu). This error is exemplified in the following:

Question: [ʤitjɛt]

Answer: [noʤu]

The translation of this is:

Question: [dɪdju it jɛt]
                     Did you eat yet?

Answer: [no dɪd ju]
                     No, did you?

You must correct this error. Only the basest of beasts continue to make these barbaric utterances—and they don't use them professionally! In correcting this error, attention must first be given to the imploded plosive. Then you must move into the /j/ and often the diphthong [ju].

EXERCISES

In the following exercises, hold the indicated imploded plosive for a full second before moving into the [ju] diphthong. This will help you focus on the proper articulatory adjustment. Then give appropriate timing to the plosives.

	Practice	*Correct*
Did you?	[dɪd: ju]	[dɪd ju]
Won't you?	[wont: ju]	[wont ju]
He didn't cast you.	[hɪ dɪdn̩t kæst: ju]	[hɪ dɪdn̩t kæst ju]
Couldn't you do it?	[kʊdn̩t: ju du ɪt]	[kʊdn̩t ju dṳ ɪt]
It's the cat you mean.	[ɪts ðə kæt: ju min]	[ɪts ðə kæt ju min]
Let the baby pat you.	[lɛt ðə bebɪ pæt: ju]	[lɛt ðə bebɪ pæt ju]
the pad you bought	[ðə pæd: ju bɔt]	[ðə pæd ju bɔt]

Use negative practice in the following exercise. Exaggerate the articulation of the error as well as the correct pronunciation. Make certain that you do not pull away too much from the overarticulation when you speak correctly.

	Career	*Error*	*Career*
Don't you?	[dont ju]	[dontʃu] (Gesundheit!)	[dont ju]
Won't you?	[wont ju]	[wontʃu]	[wont ju]

Did you?	[dɪd ju]	[dɪdʒu]	[dɪd ju]
Can't you?	[kænt ju]	[kæntʃu]	[kænt ju]
trust you	[trʌst ju]	[trʌstʃu]	[trʌst ju]
but you	[bʌt ju]	[bʌtʃu]	[bʌt ju]
Would you?	[wʊd ju]	[wʊdʒu]	[wʊd ju]
Bite your nails.	[baɪt jɔr nelz]	[baɪtʃɚ nelz]	[baɪt jɔr nelz]
Lift your leg.	[lɪft jɔr lɛg]	[lɪftʃɚ lɛg]	[lɪft jɔr lɛg]
Hold your temper.	[hold jɔr tɛmpɚ]	[holdʒɚ tɛmpɚ]	[hold jɔr tɛmpɚ]
Could you?	[kʊd ju]	[kʊdʒu]	[kʊd ju]
What's your name?	[ʌʌts jɔr nem]	[ʌʌtʃɚ nem]	[ʌʌts jɔr nem]
Change your mind.	[tʃendʒ jɔr maɪnd]	[tʃendʒɚ maɪnd]	[tʃendʒ jɔr maɪnd]

with you

witch ju

meryl strep

SAME SPELLING, DIFFERENT PRONUNCIATION

Several words are spelled the same way but pronounced differently, according to their part of speech. The difference is primarily in the stressed syllable. Professional communicators must know these differences even though secondary pronunciations appear in dictionaries. Reflect the best possible standard and join the campaign to keep your language as pure as possible.

EXERCISE

Read the following list of words, paying close attention to the shifts in stress.

	Noun	*Verb*	*Adjective*
permit	[ˈpɝmɪt]	[pɚˈmɪt]	
discharge	[ˈdɪstʃɑrdʒ]	[dɪsˈtʃɑrdʒ]	
object	[ˈɑbdʒɛkt]	[əbˈdʒɛkt]	
pervert	[ˈpɝvɚt]	[pɚˈvɝt]	
conduct	[ˈkɑndəkt]	[kənˈdʌkt]	
convict	[ˈkɑnvɪkt]	[kənˈvɪkt]	
conflict	[ˈkɑnflɪkt]	[kənˈflɪkt]	
convert	[ˈkɑnvɚt]	[kənˈvɝt]	

insult	['ɪnsəlt]	[ɪn'sʌlt]	
overflow	['ovɚflou]	[ovɚ'flou]	
frequent		[frɪ'kwɛnt]	['frikwənt]
intimate		['ɪntəmet]	['ɪntəmət]

METATHESIS AND HAPLOLOGY

Two common errors in pronunciation are metathesis and haplology. **Metathesis** is the reversal of sounds within the same word. Recently politicians have been talking about the possibility of a [njukjulɚ] (instead of a [njuklɪɚ]) war. This slip of the tongue is often highlighted on radio and television "blooper" shows. This error is similar to a **spoonerism,** in which sounds in different words are transposed (as in "getting your mords wixed").

The second error, **haplology,** is the omission of a repeated sound or syllable ([hæpɔlədʒɪ] for [hæplɔlədʒɪ]).

EXERCISES

As you read the following word lists aloud, use negative practice. Exaggerate the correct and incorrect pronunciations. When developing the correct pronunciation, use a mirror and do not pull away too much from the overdone articulation. Let the visual image determine to what degree you add or minimize articulation.

METATHESIS

	Career	*Error*	*Career*
cavalry	[kævəlrɪ]	[kælvərɪ]	[kævəlrɪ]
Calvary	[kælvərɪ]	[kævəlrɪ]	[kælvərɪ]
relevant	[rɛləvənt]	[rɛvələnt]	[rɛləvənt]
hospital	[haspɪtl]	[hapsɪtl]	[haspɪtl]
I asked her	[aɪ æskt hɚ]	[aɪ ækst hɚ][1]	[aɪ æskt hɚ]
spaghetti	[spəgɛtɪ]	[pɪsgɛtɪ]	[spəgɛtɪ]
asterisk	[æstərɪsk]	[æstərɪks]	[æstərɪsk]
introduction	[ɪntrədʌkʃən]	[ɪntɚdʌkʃən]	[ɪntrədʌkʃən]

---

[1] [ænd nau aɪm ɪn prɪzn̩]

perspire	[pɚ·spaɪr]	[prəspaɪr]	[pɚ·spaɪr]
apron	[eprən]	[epɚ·n]	[eprən]
perspiration	[pɚ·spərɛʃən]	[prɛspərɛʃən]	[pɚ·spərɛʃən]
hundred	[hʌndrəd]	[hʌndɚ·d]	[hʌndrəd]
professor	[prəfɛsɚ·]	[pɚ·fɛsɚ·]	[prəfɛsɚ·]
children	[tʃɪldrən]	[tʃɪldɚ·n]	[tʃɪldrən]
prescribe	[prəskraɪb]	[pɚ·skraɪb]	[prəskraɪb]
perform	[pɚ·fɔrm]	[prəfɔrm]	[pɚ·fɔrm]

HAPLOLOGY

	Career	*Error*	*Career*
Atlanta	[ætlæntə]	[ælæntə]	[ætlæntə]
		[ætlænə]	
antecedent	[æntəsidn̩t]	[ænəsidn̩t]	[æntəsidn̩t]
dentistry	[dɛntɪstrɪ]	[dɛnɪstrɪ]	[dɛntɪstrɪ]
interact	[ɪntɚ·ækt]	[ɪnɚ·ækt]	[ɪntɚ·ækt]
interject	[ɪntɚ·dʒɛkt]	[ɪnɚ·dʒɛkt]	[ɪntɚ·dʒɛkt]
entertain	[ɛntɚ·ten]	[ɛnɚ·ten]	[ɛntɚ·ten]
twenty	[twɛntɪ]	[twɛnɪ]	[twɛntɪ]
interesting	[ɪntərɪstɪŋ]	[ɪnɚ·ɪstɪŋ]	[ɪntərɪstɪŋ]
interdepartmental	[ɪntɚ·dɪpɑrtmɛntl̩]	[ɪnɚ·dɪpɑrtmɛnl̩][2]	[ɪntɚ·dɪpɑrtmɛntl̩]
antidote	[æntədot]	[ænədot]	[æntədot]
governor	[gʌvɚ·nɚ·]	[gʌvnɚ·]	[gʌvɚ·nɚ·]
February	[fɛbruɛrɪ]	[fɛbjuɛrɪ]	[fɛbruɛrɪ]
library	[laɪbrɛrɪ]	[laɪbɛrɪ]	[laɪbrɛrɪ]
secretary	[sɛkrətɛrɪ]	[sɛkətɛrɪ]	[sɛkrətɛrɪ]
particularly	[pɑrtɪkjulərlɪ]	[pɑrtɪkjulɪ]	[pɑrtɪkjulərlɪ]
arctic	[ɑrktɪk]	[ɑrtɪk]	[ɑrktɪk]
substitute	[sʌbstətɪut]	[sʌbsətɪut]	[sʌbstətɪut]
tentative	[tɛntətɪv]	[tɛnətɪv]	[tɛntətɪv]

---

[2]Notice only one /t/ remains.

9

VOCAL
DYNAMICS

GLOSSARY

Inflection   The changes of stress, tempo, and pitch and the use of pauses to support, enhance, reflect, and amplify meaning.

Pace   A form of speech emphasis in which changes of verbal speed are used for contrast and highlight.

Pause   A form of speech emphasis in which there is an absence of speech before or after an utterance.

Prosody   "The art or science of patterning in poetry";[1] prosody includes patterns of meter and images as well as other repetitions.

Slide   A movement through steps; in inflection, sliding occurs through changes in voice quality and projection as well as pitch.

Step   The interval between two adjoining pitches.

Stress   A form of speech emphasis in which attention is given to words important to meaning. This form of emphasis has been called *force*. In broadcasting, this form of emphasis is called "punching."

---

[1] Wallace Bacon, *The Art of Interpretation,* 3rd ed. (New York: Holt, Rinehart and Winston, 1979), p. 548.

The basic tools of voice and speech have been discussed in previous chapters. Open throat, good diaphragmatic control, and good pronunciation are relatively useless in and of themselves. They must be applied to the communication of some message to an audience (even if the audience is yourself). Otherwise, there is no speech or meaningful message imparted.

However, having good tools does not insure successful communication. The tools of a Shakespearean scholar, for example, would certainly include content. But if the audience is bored by the delivery, this content has little value. How many of us have had a professor (or two!) who clearly knew the subject matter but was unable to communicate this knowledge to an audience?

Obviously, for truly effective communication, there must be a melding of materials with delivery. One of the most important components of delivery is the choices available to the speaker for underscoring and amplifying meaning. How can certain words and ideas be colored to clarify the meaning and attitude of the speaker? These techniques, which are learned behaviors rather than innate, can insure that the speaker will not be monotonous (that is, will not use the same pitch and intensity).

There are a number of reasons why a speaker is monotonous. The most important is a lack of variety in thought and emotion. Therefore, it is fundamental for a speaker to understand the content of his or her communication thoroughly. Washington Irving stated that "at sea, everything that breaks the monotony of the surrounding expanse attracts attention."[2] The study of **prosody** tells us that the meter in a poem may not be as significant to meaning as the foot that breaks the pattern. Our eyes and ears are more alert when a pattern is broken. For a detailed discussion of variety in poetry, refer to the book *Oral Interpretation* by Charlotte Lee and Timothy Gura.

In the early 1880s, Charles Wesley Emerson identified four forms of speech emphasis that are useful in contemporary speech and help give a speaker vocal dynamics. These forms are stress, pace or tempo, slide, and pause.[3]

In an earlier chapter, we mentioned the difficulty in separating the factors of voice (quality, pitch, rate, and volume). These factors work together to form a whole voice. Similarly, the forms of speech emphasis should not be separated in the communication process. Indeed, they too are parts relating to the whole and work together to energize the entire speech performance. To learn to communicate effectively, however, the forms of speech emphasis must be isolated, identified, and discussed. When these elements are combined and used to express the intended meaning, appropriate inflection is achieved. **Inflection** is defined as the variations of vocal techniques that support, enhance, reflect, and amplify meaning.

---

[2] Washington Irving, *The Sketch Book* (New York: United States Book Company, 1819), p. 13.

[3] Charles Wesley Emerson, *The Evolution of Expression* (Boston: Emerson College Press, 1881), p. 26.

STRESS

A natural evolution takes place when you begin studying stress or force and proceed through tempo, slide, and pause. **Stress** or force is one of the most basic and primitive forms of speech emphasis. In this emphasis, the speaker selects the most important words and images and simply stresses them, usually through increased volume but sometimes through decreased volume. The danger with using only one of these forms exclusively throughout a message, performance, reading, or sermon is that the communication becomes colorless. Like any art form, attention is drawn to the meaning through the use of variations.

Ordinarily, the words that receive attention are the words that give a thought clarity and dynamism: nouns, verbs, adverbs, and adjectives. Usually pronouns, connectives, and prepositions are not stressed. Of course, there are exceptions to this. As a matter of fact, television policies vary to the degree that often, each has its own style of delivery. It is important to get your immediate meaning across. For example, ask your roommate to put the wastebasket on the desk so that you will not forget to empty it. If your roomie places it under the desk, you respond, "I said to put it *on* the desk." In this case stressing a preposition is important to the meaning. Ordinarily, of course, the preposition *on* would not receive a great deal of stress.

EXERCISES FOR STRESS

1. In this poem, color words are underscored according to one person's interpretation. You may have a few additions or deletions according to your understanding. Read the poem and record yourself, stressing the underscored words. As you listen to the playback, make certain that you were accurate.

Come live with me and be my love,
And we will all the pleasures prove,
That hills and valleys, dales, and fields,
And all the craggy mountains yields.

There we will sit upon the rocks,
And see the shepherds feed their flocks,
By shallow rivers to whose falls
Melodious birds sing madrigals.

And I will make thee beds of roses
With a thousand fragrant posies,
A cap of flowers, and a kirtle
Embroidered all with leaves of myrtle;

A Gown made of the finest wool
Which from our pretty lambs we pull;

Fur lined slippers for the cold,
With buckles of the purest gold;

A belt of straw and ivy buds,
With coral clasps and amber studs:
And if these pleasures may thee move,
Come live with me and be my love.

The shepherds' swains shall dance and sing
For thy delight each May morning:
If these delights thy mind may move,
Then live with me and be my love.

THE PASSIONATE SHEPHERD TO HIS LOVE   *Christopher Marlowe*

In exercises 2 and 3 underline the important words according to your interpretation. Then record your reading according to what you have underlined.

2. If all the world and love were young,
   And truth in every shepherd's tongue,
   These pretty pleasures might me move,
   To live with thee, and be thy love.

   Time drives the flocks from field to fold,
   When rivers rage, and rocks grow cold,
   And Philomel becometh dumb,
   The rest complains of cares to come.

   The flowers do fade, and wanton fields,
   The wayward winter reckoning yields,
   A honey tongue, a heart of gall,
   Is fancy's spring, but sorrow's fall.

   Thy gowns, thy shoes, thy beds of roses,
   Thy cap, thy kirtle, and thy posies,
   Soon break, soon wither, soon forgotten:
   In folly ripe, in reason rotten.

   Thy belt of straw and ivy buds,
   Thy coral clasps and amber studs,
   All these in me no means can move,
   To come to thee, and be thy love.

   But could youth last, and love still breed,
   Had joys no date, nor age no need,
   Then these delights my mind might move,
   To live with thee and be thy love.

   THE NYMPH'S REPLY TO THE SHEPHERD   *Sir Walter Raleigh*

3. And the Lord spake unto Moses and unto Aaron, saying: This is the ordinance
   of the law which the Lord hath commanded, saying, Speak unto the children

of Israel, that they bring thee a red heifer without spot, wherein is no blemish, and upon which never came yoke.

From EXODUS

4. Force and stress can become extremely irritating when overused. This is the favorite form of speech emphasis for a number of neophyte television and radio news announcers. Using negative practice, read aloud and tape the following news report. Exaggerate the use of force and stress. Listen to yourself! Play the tape and realize how "stress-full" you sounded. Then reread the report using stress more selectively. Know when and why you use it.

GOOD MORNING. I'M _____ AND THIS IS NEWSBRIEF. AT THE TOP OF THE HOUR FORMER HOUSE MAJORITY WHIP _____ HAS BEEN ACQUITTED OF CONSPIRACY AND EXTORTION CHARGES. THE JURY FOUND _____ HAD BEEN ENTRAPPED BY AN UNDERCOVER FBI AGENT. THE FIRST TRIAL ENDED IN A HUNG JURY LAST FALL. _____ HAD NO COMMENT AS TO WHETHER HE WOULD RETURN TO PUBLIC LIFE.

AND THE REPORT IS IN ON THE FUTURE OF THE MX MISSILES. THE U.S. SENATE VOTED IN ONE POINT FIVE BILLION DOLLARS FOR THE PRODUCTION OF TWENTY-ONE WEAPONS. THE MISSILES MUST PASS ANOTHER SENATE VOTE LATER THIS WEEK AS WELL AS IN THE HOUSE OF REPRESENTATIVES. INDIANA REPUBLICAN SENATOR _____ SAYS HE VOTED FOR THE MISSILES AS A BARGAINING CHIP AT THE GENEVA TALKS.

In the following exercises, use as much force or stress as you can in your first reading without distorting the meaning as determined by the color words.

5. But oh! shipmates! on the starboard hand of every woe, there is a sure delight; and higher the top of that delight, than the bottom of the woe is deep. Is not the main-truck higher than the kelson is low? Delight is to him—a far, far upward, and inward delight—who against the proud gods and commodores of this earth, ever stands forth his own inexorable self. . . .

And eternal delight and deliciousness will be his, who coming to lay him down, can say with his final breath—O Father!—chiefly known to me by Thy rod—mortal or immortal, here I die. I have striven to be Thine, more than to be the world's, or mine own. Yet this is nothing; I leave eternity to Thee; for what is man that he should live out the lifetime of his God? . . .

The Nantucketer, out of sight of land, furls his sails and lays him to his rest, while under his very pillow rush herds of walruses and whales. . . .

Give me a condor's quill! Give me Vesuvius' crater for an inkstand! . . . To produce a mighty book, you must choose a mighty theme.

From MOBY DICK *Herman Melville*

The country needs and, unless I mistake its temper, the country demands bold, persistent experimentation. It is common sense to take a method and try it: If it fails, admit it frankly and try another. But above all, try something.

Franklin Delano Roosevelt

PACE OR TEMPO

From stress we proceed to a change in tempo or pace. **Pace** in speech is akin to emotion. The tempo of a voice is often an outward manifestation of what is happening emotionally inside. Therefore, it is extremely important to control your tempo so that it reflects what is desired. For example, a person's pace usually speeds up as pressure or emotional intensity increases. A slower pace is equated with serenity, which may or may not be so.

Frequently the importance of a message is reflected in the pace used. Usually the important parts of a message are delivered slowly; less important parts are usually delivered more quickly. However, sometimes the opposite technique is used. For example, a comedian may deliver the punch line with rapid-fire speech and then slow up the pace while the audience responds to the joke. This is a delivery technique that Bob Hope often uses. Thus, a change in tempo can frequently underscore meaning or indicate a change in thought. In addition, an increase in tempo and volume, like music, often builds to a climax followed by a decrescendo.

Various effects can be achieved through changing the pace. Sometimes, as in the opening of Robert Frost's "The Death of the Hired Man," a mood of contemplation can be emphasized by using a relatively slow pace. In this example, the slow pace also works with the tone color (use of sounds) to create an atmosphere of contemplation. After the musing mood has been established, the poet continues in lines 3 and 4:

She ran on tip-toe down the darkened passage
To meet him in the doorway with the news.

The mood changes from meditation to action, a fact amplified by the poet's use of plosive sounds and run-on lines. By using these devices and increasing the tempo, you can effectively suggest Mary's movements in an oral performance.

EXERCISES FOR TEMPO

1. The opening lines from Alfred Lord Tennyson's "Ulysses" are contemplative in mood. Read them aloud, using a slow pace to emphasize Ulysses' discontent and dissatisfaction with life. Lines 6 through 11 build in emotional ten-

sion to the epigram "I am become a name"; this climactic moment can be clarified for an audience by an increase in tempo, along with other forms of speech emphasis.

It little profits that an idle king,
By this still hearth, among these barren crags,
Matched with an aged wife, I mete and dole
Unequal laws unto a savage race,
That hoard, and sleep, and feed, and know not me.
I cannot rest from travel; I will drink
Life to the lees. All times I have enjoyed
Greatly, have suffered greatly, both with those
That loved me, and alone; on shore, and when
Through scudding drifts the rainy Hyades[4] ['haɪədiz]
Vext the dim sea: I am become a name.

2. Record the following selection and determine the varieties of pace according to the meaning and imagery presented by the poet. Listen to the recording as objectively as you can. Did you make the most out of the pacing that the poet gave you?

Into the street the Piper stept,
Smiling first a little smile,
As if he knew what magic slept
In his quiet pipe the while;
Then, like a musical adept,
To blow the pipe his lips he wrinkled,
And green and blue his sharp eyes twinkled
Like a candle-flame where salt is sprinkled
And ere three shrill notes the pipe uttered,
You heard as if an army muttered;
And the muttering grew to a grumbling;
And the grumbling grew to a mighty rumbling;
And out of the houses the rats came tumbling.
Great rats, small rats, lean rats, brawny rats,
Brown rats, black rats, gray rats, tawny rats.
Grave old plodders, gay young friskers,
Fathers, mothers, uncles, cousins,
Cocking tails and pricking whiskers,
Families by tens and dozens,
Brothers, sisters, husbands, wives—
Followed the Piper for their lives.

---

[4]*Hyades* is a cluster of stars believed by the ancients to indicate rainy weather when they rose with the sun.

From step to step he piped advancing,
And step for step he followed dancing,
Until they came to the river Weser [vezɚ],
Wherein all plunged and perished!

From THE PIED PIPER OF HAMELIN   *Robert Browning*

SLIDE

A **slide** is a form of speech emphasis in which pitch always changes; often vocal quality and volume change as well. The use of this vocal technique is dictated by the speaker's intended meaning.

The interval between two adjoining pitches is called a **step.** The term *slide* is particularly vivid because of its implicit visual imagery. A slide provides vocal movement and energy. This movement is realized when the intended meaning is conveyed. For example, say the following "pitch graphic" as it appears on the page:

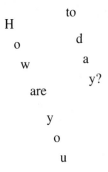

When spoken as written, this sentence carries little meaning, even though changes in pitch are designated. There is no thought behind these changes in pitch. It is a sentence said by an android or robot.

When appropriate, thoughtful inflection is used, there is usually not only a change in pitch but also a change in the quality and projection of the voice. Record and exaggerate the following pitch graph:

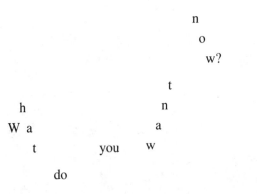

If you have produced the sentence as written, there will be a change of pitch on the words "What," "want," and "now." Can you detect a difference in the quality and projection of the voice in addition to the more obvious change in pitch? These changes in pitch as dictated by the meaning are slides. This sliding effect between words (and frequently within a word) is a more sophisticated form of emphasis than either stress or tempo.

The use of the slide can be illustrated easily if you read a child's story to an imaginary kindergarten class. The slides become exaggerated. (However, most kindergarten students do not like this technique, because they feel as if the reader were talking down to them. Nevertheless, this exaggeration will clarify the slide.)

The question-and-answer technique is useful in familiarizing oneself with the slide. Read the following sentence aloud:

The sky is blue.

Now ask yourself, "What color is the sky?"

```
                              u
The   sky          bl  u
           is          ue.
```

On the last word, you use a slide. Listen to it again.

EXERCISES FOR THE SLIDE

In the following exercises ask a question that has to be answered by the under-scored words. Record your answer and listen carefully to what you have said. If there was a change of pitch (and perhaps of quality and projection), you probably slid! If not, repeat your answer and exaggerate the slide. Example: Quietly (how?) put your papers (what?) on the table (where?).

1. Go, sir, gallop, and don't forget that the world was made in six days. You can ask me for anything you like, except time.

   Napoleon Bonaparte

2. Three years she grew in sun and shower,
   Then Nature said, "A lovelier flower
   On earth was never sown.
   This Child I to myself will take;
   She shall be mine, and I will make
   A Lady of my own."

   From LUCY   *William Wordsworth*

3. Near this spot are deposited the remains of one who possesses Beauty without
Vanity, Strength without Insolence, Courage without Ferocity, and all the
Virtues of Man, without his Vices. This Praise, which would be unmeaning
Flattery if inscribed over human ashes, is but a just tribute to the Memory of
Boatswain, a Dog.

INSCRIPTION ON THE MONUMENT OF A NEWFOUNDLAND DOG   *Lord Byron*

4. Hatred comes from the heart; contempt from the head;
and neither feeling is quite within our control.

From STUDIES IN PESSIMISM   *Arthur Schopenhauer*

5. Therefore to this dog will I,
Tenderly not scornfully,
Render praise and favor:
With my hand upon his head,
Is my benediction said
Therefore and for ever.

From TO FLUSH, MY DOG   *Elizabeth Barrett Browning*

In the following exercises, concentrate on the slide. The meaning that you want
to communicate will determine which words you slide on. The first few times
you read the selections aloud, practice exaggerated slide. Then pull away to
what you think is appropriate, but do not pull away too much. Using a mirror,
observe what is happening to your face while exhibiting exaggerated and appropriate slides.

6. If I speak in the tongues of men and of angels, but have not love, I am a noisy
gong or a clanging cymbal. And if I have prophetic powers, and understand
all mysteries and all knowledge, and if I have all faith, so as to remove mountains, but have not love, I am nothing. If I give away all I have, and if I deliver
my body to be burned, but have not love, I gain nothing.

From I CORINTHIANS

7. I've got a letter, parson, from my son away out west,
And my old heart's as heavy as an anvil in my breast,
To think the boy whose future I had once so proudly planned
Should wander from the path of right and come to such an end!
I told him when he left us, only three short years ago,
He'd find himself a-plowing in a mightly crooked row.

His letters come so seldom that I somehow sort of knowed
That Billy was a-trampling on a mightly rocky road.
He wrote from out in Denver, and the story's very short;
I just can't tell his mother; it'd crush her poor old heart.
And so I reckoned, parson, you might break the news to her—
Bill's in the legislature, but he doesn't know what for.

Anonymous

8. Lady Bracknell (a Victorian aristocrat):

Mr. Worthing, I confess I feel somewhat bewildered by what you have just told me. To be born, or at any rate bred, in a handbag, whether it had handles or not, seems to me to display a contempt for the ordinary decencies of family life that reminds one of the worst excesses of the French Revolution. And I presume you know what that unfortunate movement led to? As for the particular locality in which the hand-bag was found, a cloak-room at a railway station might serve to conceal a social indiscretion—has probably, indeed, been used for that purpose before—but it could hardly be regarded as an assured basis for a recognized position in good society. You can hardly imagine that I and Lord Bracknell would dream of allowing our only daughter—a girl brought up with the utmost care—to marry into a cloakroom and form an alliance with a parcel? Good morning, Mr. Worthing!

From THE IMPORTANCE OF BEING ERNEST   *Oscar Wilde*

PAUSE

A **pause** is the absence of speech before or after an utterance. It is a temporary stop in verbalization but with a continuation of thought—it is not a break in the continuity of the thought. The pause is an integral part of meaning. A true pause is the "loud" silence that intensifies a communication. During this silence the thought is maintained until the vocalization resumes. This bridge of thought is usually emphasized through facial expressions (particularly the eyes) and tension in the body.

A pause may be likened to an electric arc (Figure 9.1). There are two wires, one of which is plugged into a live socket. The other wire is uncharged. This second wire is slowly brought toward the charged wire. Eventually an arc of electricity springs from the live wire to the other when the charge is great enough.

FIGURE 9.1   CURRENT ARCING FROM LIVE WIRE TO ADJACENT, POWERLESS WIRE

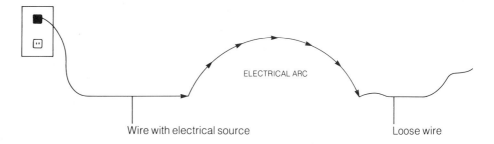

Wire with electrical source

ELECTRICAL ARC

Loose wire

A similar situation occurs with the use of the pause (Figure 9.2). If the thought before the pause is sufficiently energized, the thought will be maintained and intensified until it is verbally completed. The pause is "the servant of the thought."

The pause is the most artistic form of speech emphasis. There are three types of pauses: (1) reflection, (2) anticipation, and (3) implication. The pause of reflection causes the listener to think back on something that has been said. This technique is often employed by comics. Frequently the expression on the face is an indication or "tip off" that something significant has been said. The response of the audience comes after a couple of beats.

The pause of anticipation is used when the audience anticipates something that is about to be said. Again, a comic uses this form of pause very frequently. Sometimes the audience itself completes the thought.

The third type of pause (and perhaps the most meaningful) is the pause of implication, in which the pause implies something more than has been said. For example, Aunt Maude and Uncle Ned had been invited to a party on Friday night. Aunt Maude did not attend. She met Uncle Ned on Saturday morning and he said, "Maude, you missed [pause of implication] quite a party last night." This pause was probably accompanied by some form of nonverbal communication, perhaps a nod of the head or widened eyes.

It is very important to underscore that all of the forms of speech emphasis (stress, pace, slide, and pause) work together to create an appropriate whole. Using all of the inflective forms gives the speaker variety, energy, and above all clarity. No one form of emphasis should be used to the exclusion of the others. Obviously, the material presented will help to determine which forms of emphasis to use.

EXERCISES FOR EMPHASIS

Tape the following exercises using the separate forms of emphasis. This is a very difficult challenge. Apply stress (punching) the first time. Then read it with changes of pace. Then add inflection, and finally pause. This procedure will be very mechanical and in many cases humorous, but the purpose is to isolate and highlight the separate forms. Then read the exercise with a mixture of all four forms of emphasis. Remember that an overused technique diminishes its effec-

FIGURE 9.2   PAUSE PROVIDING ENERGIZED MEANING BETWEEN TWO WORDS

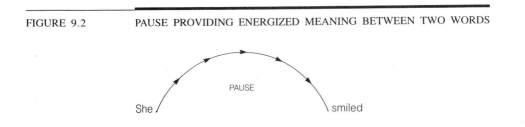

tiveness. Determine your own choices according to the meaning you desire to convey to your audience.

1. "Hallelujah" was the only observation
   That escaped Lieutenant-Colonel Mary Jane,
   When she tumbled off the platform in the station,
   And was cut in little pieces by the train.
   Mary Jane, the train is through yer:
   Hallelujah, hallelujah!
   We will gather up the fragments that remain.

   HALLELUJAH   *A. E. Housman*

2. When Sir Joshua Reynolds died
   All nature was degraded;
   The King dropped a tear into the Queen's ear,
   And all his pictures faded.

   SIR JOSHUA REYNOLDS   *William Blake*

3. Hermit hoar, in solemn cell,
   Wearing out life's evening gray,
   Smite thy bosom, Sage, and tell,
   What is bliss? And which the way?

   Thus I spoke; and speaking sigh'd;
   Scarce repress'd the starting tear;
   When the hoary sage reply'd:
   "Come, my lad, and drink some beer."

   HERMIT HOAR . . .   *Anonymous*

4. *Constable Dogberry* (to First Watchman): You are thought here to be the most senseless and fit man for the constable of the watch, therefore bear you the lantern. This is your charge: you shall comprehend all vagrom men; you are to bid any man stand, in the prince's name.
   Watchman: How, if a'well not stand?
   Dogberry: Why, then, take no note of him, but let him go; and presently call the rest of the watch together, and thank God you are rid of a knave. . . . You shall also make no noise in the streets; for, for the watch to babble and to talk is most intolerable and not to be endured.
   Second Watchman: We will rather sleep than talk; we know what belongs to a watch.
   Dogberry: . . . Well, you are to call at all the alehouses, and bid those that are drunk get them to bed.
   Watchman: How if they will not?
   Dogberry: Why, then, let them alone till they are sober; if they make you not then the better answer, you may say they are not the men you took them for.

   From MUCH ADO ABOUT NOTHING   *William Shakespeare*

EXERCISES FOR VOCAL DYNAMICS

In the following exercises, the forms of speech emphasis should be determined by the meaning. Read the exercises aloud and tape them. You are encouraged to exaggerate your use of the forms at first. However, when you pull away from the exaggeration, make certain that you retain appropriate vocal dynamics.

1. Sally Salter, she was a young teacher who taught,
   And her friend, Charley Church, was a preacher, who praught;
   Though his enemies called him a screecher, who scraught.

   His heart, when he saw her, kept sinking, and sunk;
   And his eye, meeting hers, began winking and wunk;
   While she, in her turn, fell to thinking, and thunk.

   He hastened to woo her, and sweetly he wooed,
   For his love grew until to a mountain it grewed,
   And what he was longing to do, then he doed.

   In secret he wanted to speak, and he spoke,
   To seek with his lips what his heart long had soke;
   So he managed to let the truth leak, and it loke.

   He asked her to ride to the church, and they rode;
   They so sweetly did glide, that they both thought they glode,
   And they came to the place to be tied, and were tode.

   Then homeward he said let us drive, and they drove,
   And soon as they wished to arrive, they arrove;
   For whatever he couldn't contrive, she controve.

   The kiss he was dying to steal, then he stole;
   At the feet where he wanted to kneel, then he knole;
   And he said, "I feel better than ever I fole."

   So they to each other kept clinging, and clung,
   While Time his swift circuit was winging, and wung;
   And this was the thing he was bringing and brung:

   The man Sally wanted to catch, and had caught—
   That she wanted from others to snatch, and had snaught—
   Was the one she now liked to scratch, and she scraught.

   And Charley's warm love began freezing, and froze,
   While he took to teasing, and cruelly toze
   The girl he had wished to be squeezing, and squoze.

   "Wretch!" he cried, when she threatened to leave him, and left,
   "How could you deceive, as you have deceft?"
   And she answered, "I promised to cleave, and I've cleft."

   Anonymous

2. Make a joyful noise unto the Lord, all ye lands. Serve the Lord with gladness: come before his presence with singing. Know ye that the Lord he is God: it is he that hath made us, and not we ourselves; we are his people, and the sheep of his pasture. Enter into his gates with thanksgiving and into his courts with praise: be thankful unto him, and bless his name. For the Lord is good; his mercy endureth to all generations.

   PSALM 100

3. For obvious reasons there is generally little time for a news anchor to make much use of the pause. For radio and television reporting, all forms of emphases are constrained by time. An increase in speed allows for the use of slide, however. Do not use stress, or the "punch" approach, to the exclusion of the other forms. In the following copy, make certain that you incorporate tempo and slide into your presentation along with stress.

   A COALITION OF EDUCATORS, COMMUNITY LEADERS, AND CITY OFFICIALS THROUGHOUT THE STATE SAY LEGISLATORS SHOULD FOCUS ON EARLY EDUCATION PROGRAMS RATHER THAN PAY RAISES TO TEACHERS TO IMPROVE EDUCATION.

   THE COALITION MADE THEIR SUGGESTIONS YESTERDAY IN A LETTER TO THE LEGISLATOR'S EDUCATION COMMITTEE.

   THE LEGISLATOR'S COMMITTEE IS EXPECTED TO RELEASE NEXT MONTH ITS VERSION OF SEVERAL BILLS TO OVERHAUL PUBLIC EDUCATION IN THE STATE.

   THE NEXT SUMMIT TALKS MAY BE POSTPONED FOR A WHILE.

   THE SOVIETS WANT TO HOLD OFF ON THE TALKS UNTIL SEPTEMBER.

   THE RUSSIANS SAY THEY WILL WAIT UNTIL AFTER THE SOVIET LEADER'S MEETING WITH THE U.N. TO DISCUSS PEACE INITIATIVES.

   WEATHER-WISE IT IS 38 DEGREES AND CLOUDY OUTSIDE OUR STUDIOS.

   THERE WILL BE CONTINUED SUNSHINE THROUGHOUT THE DAY AS THE CLOUDS MOVE OUT OF VIEW.

   TONIGHT THE TEMPERATURES WILL DROP BACK INTO THE HIGH TWENTIES WHICH WILL MAKE IT A BIT NIPPY.

   AND IN SPORTS, IT WILL BE SAMMY MUMFORD ON THE MOUND FOR THE ANGELS AND JOE FOSS FOR THE YANKEES AS THE TEAMS OPEN UP A 10-GAME HOMESTAND TONIGHT.

   WE'LL HAVE HIGHLIGHTS OF THE GAME TONIGHT ON THE ELEVEN O'CLOCK NEWS.

THIS IS _____ FOR "HEADLINES." MORE NEWS AT SIX. HAVE A
GOOD DAY.

4. Oscar Wilde wrote the following poem for his sister Isola, whose childhood
   death profoundly influenced the poet. The title means "may she rest in peace."

   Tread lightly, she is near,
   Under the snow,
   Speak gently, she can hear
   The daisies grow.

   All her bright golden hair
   Tarnished with rust,
   She that was young and fair
   Fallen to dust.

   Lily-like, white as snow,
   She hardly knew
   She was a woman, so
   Sweetly she grew.

   Coffin-board, heavy stone,
   Lie on her breast,
   I vex my heart alone,
   She is at rest.

   Peace, Peace, she cannot hear
   Lyre or sonnet
   All my life's buried here,
   Heap earth upon it.

   REQUIESCAT   *Oscar Wilde*

5. O God! methinks it were a happy life,
   To be no better than a homely swain;
   To sit upon a hill, as I do now,
   To carve out dials quaintly, point by point,
   Thereby to see the minutes how they run,
   How many makes the hour full complete;
   How many hours bring about the day;
   How many days will finish up the year;
   How many years a mortal man may live.
   When this is known, then to divide the times:—
   So many hours must I tend my flock;
   So many hours must I take my rest;
   So many hours must I contemplate;
   So many hours must I sport myself;
   So many days my ewes have been with young;

So many weeks ere the poor fools will yean;[5]
So many months ere I shall shear the fleece:
So minutes, hours, days, months and years,
Past over to the end they were created,
Would bring white hairs unto a quiet grave.
Ah, what a life were this! how sweet! how lovely!

From HENRY VI, PART 3 *William Shakespeare*

6. The following selection is a challenge. Without sacrificing the rhythmic patter
   or breath control, incorporate stress, tempo, and slide.

My eyes are fully open to my awful situation
I shall go at once to Roderic and make him an oration.
I shall tell him I've recovered my forgotten moral senses,
And I don't care twopence-halfpenny for any consequences.
Now I do not want to perish by the sword or by the dagger,
But a martyr may indulge a little pardonable swagger,
And a word or two of compliment my vanity would flatter,
But I've got to die to-morrow, so it really doesn't matter!

If I were not a little mad and generally silly
I should give you my advice upon the subject, willy-nilly;
I should show you in a moment how to grapple with the question,
And you'd really be astonished at the force of my suggestion.
On the subject I shall write you a most valuable letter,
Full of excellent suggestions when I feel a little better,
But at present I'm afraid I am as mad as any hatter,
So I'll keep 'em to myself, for my opinion doesn't matter!

If I had been so lucky as to have a steady brother
Who could talk to me as we are talking now to one another—
Who could give me good advice when he discovered I was erring
(Which is just the very favour which on you I am conferring),
My story would have made a rather interesting idyll,
And I might have lied and died a very decent indiwiddle.
This particularly rapid, unintelligible patter
Isn't generally heard, and if it is it doesn't matter!

From RUDDIGORE *W. S. Gilbert*

7. In the following poem, make certain that you decide on a meaning for the
   made-up words. Lewis Carroll called them "portmanteau words"; for example, "slithy" melds the words *slimy* and *lithe*. Create a character/narrator
   and a fictive world or environment.

---

[5] *Yean* means "to give birth."

'Twas brillig, and the slithy toves
Did gyre and gimble in the wabe;
All mimsy were the borogoves,
And the mome raths outgrabe.

"Beware the Jabberwock, my son!
The jaws that bite, the claws that catch!
Beware the Jubjub bird, and shun
The frumious Bandersnatch!"

He took his vorpal sword in hand:
Long time the manxome foe he sought—
So rested he by the Tumtum tree,
And stood awhile in thought.

And, as in uffish thought he stood,
The Jabberwock, with eyes of flame,
Came whiffling through the tulgey wood,
And burbled as it came!

One, two! One, two! And through and through
The vorpal blade went snicker-snack!
He left it dead, and with its head
He went galumphing back.

"And hast thou slain the Jabberwock?
Come to my arms, my beamish boy!
O frabjous day! Callooh! Callay!"
He chortled in his joy.

'Twas brillig, and the slithy toves
Did gyre and gimble in the wabe;
All mimsy were the borogoves,
And the mome raths outgrabe.

JABBERWOCKY   *Lewis Carroll*

8. The following is a commercial. Try out your island accent!

| :60 | Trinidad Carnival |
| | Young Urban Professionals |

Slow Music—	I know, you're going through your fifth cold of the
"Phase Dance" by	winter season. Your nine-to-five job is getting you
Pat Metheny	down. The groundhog brought you disappointing
	news. And you've got those Valentine Blues.

Segue to "Carnival"	Forget about it men . . .
by Sergio Mendes	Take a break!!!
	Come to Trinidad, the island in the sun that is full of
	fun for everyone.

Join us for Carnival, where the party never stops.
Carnival is color!
Carnival is vibrant!
Carnival is Life!
Experience the authentic sound of steel band and
calypso.
Experience three days of continuous dancing in the
streets.
Bask in the potpourri that is Trinidad Carnival.
You have not lived until you experience Trinidad
Carnival.

9. Only a wise man knows what things really mean. Wisdom makes him smile
and makes his frowns disappear. Do what the king says, and don't make any
rash promises to God. The king can do anything he likes, so depart his presence; don't stay in such a dangerous place. The king acts with authority, and
no one can challenge what he does. As long as you obey his commands, you
are safe, and a wise man knows how and when to do it. There is a right time
and a right way to do everything, but we know so little! None of us knows
what is going to happen, and there is no one to tell us. No one can keep
himself from dying or put off the day of his death. That is a battle we cannot
escape; we cannot cheat our way out.

From ECCLESIASTES

10

KINESICS

GLOSSARY

Autistic Mannerism   Unconscious muscular movements usually caused by nervousness.

Countenance   The face, including the eyes.

Gesture   Upper body movement, including use of the arms and hands.

Homophenous Sounds   Sounds that look alike on the lips (for example, *pan, man,* and *mat*)

Homophonous Words   Words that sound alike (for example, *vain, vane,* and *vein*)

Kinesics   The study of movement of the body.

Labiodental   Pertaining to the lips and teeth.

Linguaalveolar   Pertaining to the tongue and alveolar ridge.

Linguadental   Pertaining to the tongue and teeth.

Paralanguage   Language other than vocalized speech.

Speechreading   The technique of understanding verbal communication primarily through vision.

Thus far, this text has dealt with the incorporation of the voice and speech into the communication process. There is another important component in communication, a nonverbal one called kinesics, a kind of action language. You may be familiar with the phrase "kinesthetic sense image," referring to the awareness of muscular movement. **Kinesics** is the study of bodily movement. Bodily movement in this text will mean gesture, countenance (the use of the face), and posture. We will not attempt to discuss other nonverbal cues, which are numerous. We have chosen the above-mentioned topics because of their practicality and relevance to professional communication.

As in the study of the factors involved in sound and voice, it is difficult to separate the various components of kinesics, because they all work together to form the entire communication experience. However, for discussion and clarification, we will deal with them individually.

GESTURE

Gesture as the term is used here refers to the underscoring or amplification of words through the speaker's upper body movements, including movements of the arms and hands. It should be stressed at the outset that gestures, like other positive nonverbal components, should result naturally from the desire to get the message across. Gestures should not be taught.

Some individuals use **autistic mannerisms**, which interfere with the communication process. These mannerisms should be pointed out to a speaker and eliminated. The speaker should begin by eliminating all gestures. Before you can concentrate on what is right for you, you must rid yourself of those gestures that stand in the way of good communication. Because of the stress involved in speaking, people are usually not composed enough to control their gestures and their message. During delivery, however, total concentration must be on getting the message across. The accompanying amplification of that message, whether through vocal technique or body movement, ought to be developed.

Gestures that are prescribed are usually false because they are imposed from the outside. In time, however, freeing gestures can be developed and become natural. As in developing voice and speech, one should be loathe to say, "But that's not me!" You don't know who you are gesticulatively until you have investigated the possibilities. The major point is to eliminate those gesticulations that do not add to your message and use those that are appropriate and supportive.

Although specific gestures should not be taught, you should be encouraged to explore all possibilities through exercises. Here we are promoting physical freedom rather than prescribed gestures. If the speaker is open to the content of his or her message and has processed the message intellectually and emotionally, the physical response ought to be truthful. Inhibiting a physical response through nervousness, a lack of control of the content, or some other fault does a great disservice to the communication experience as well as to the speaker.

There is a place for the mechanical gesture. The place is not, however, an actual performance but exercises or rehearsals before the communication event. Students who are controlled by fear tend to restrict their physical movement. It is sometimes helpful to force yourself to make a particular gesture with the arm and hand. For example, in the sentence "I will not do it!", stress the "not" with a pointed index finger on your dominant hand. Make certain that the tension that is in the message gets into the muscles of that finger. That gesture must be viewed as an extension of you. If the wrist is weak, the listener will get a confused message. Rework that sentence until your gesture feels comfortable. If necessary, try using your fist rather than the pointed finger. Perhaps that expresses your feeling more successfully. Thus, even though the gesture has been imposed mechanically, it has been made to work effectively for you. Besides, any mimetic gesture must be processed through the speaker's own perceptions.

An autistic gesture reflects the speaker's nervousness about the oral performance. Most of us have autistic mannerisms that reveal our "self." The teacher who tosses and catches a piece of chalk during a lecture reveals self. As students we get caught up not in taking notes, but in hoping that the teacher will drop the chalk, which will shatter into a million pieces! What about the speaker who twists his wedding ring throughout a presentation? Does that mean that he is unhappily married? Of course not!

However, before you can correct these types of mannerisms, you have to know what they are. As an exercise, videotape an informative speech about yourself. Discuss your hobbies or what you hope to be doing professionally in ten years. Do not use notes or a lectern. During the playback, note those gestures that distract from your intended message. We all have these idiosyncratic mannerisms. Among the most common are shifting the weight from one foot to the other, brushing hair out of the eyes, clearing the throat, and the dreaded interjection "ah."

Every speaker faces the problem of dealing with nonverbal symbols. Sometimes they are in the form of **paralanguage**, such as the vocalized pause, nervous giggling, or the use of silences. With some speakers this physical process is more difficult than dealing with either the intellectual or emotional factors involved in speaking. One of the great dangers in teaching gesture is that the speaker may be so concerned with the body that the physical responses become self-conscious and out of proportion, thus interfering with the message.

Too often, when gesture is taught directly, the speaker is too concerned with bodily actions and becomes self-conscious; as a result, the physical response is out of proportion. When a speaker must think of gesturing on a particular word, the most important part of getting a message across to an audience, *concentration,* is broken. If a speaker is encouraged to em-"body" the message, the mind, emotions, and body must work together. The speaker's body should significantly amplify the thought. It has been stated that "gestures are used to illustrate, to emphasize, to point, to explain, or to interrupt; therefore, they cannot be isolated from the verbal components of speech. The understanding of most spoken messages is dependent upon the observation of both verbal and nonverbal codifications, and any isolation of oratorical or conversational gesture is out of the question."[1]

Although a physical activity does not always accompany a verbal communication, any gesture that is used must bear some relationship to the verbal language. A simple shrug of the shoulders might say, "Who cares?", "I don't know," or "So what!" You should use those gestures that will underscore and clarify meaning.

"WHEN-YOU-SAY-IT-DON'T-DO-IT" PRINCIPLE

One of the dangers in concentrating on gesture is to use too many, many of which are the wrong kind. Don't use gestures to support an obvious verbal message. For example, how many times have you heard a politician or a cleric say, "There are three reasons for this. One [accompanied by one finger, of course], two [you guessed it!], and three [yup!]." Be grateful that there were not eleven reasons! What would the speaker have done then? A more extreme example would be singing the song "Tea for Two" while sipping from an imaginary cup on the word "tea" and holding up two fingers on the word "two." Try the "do-it-and-say-it" principle!

These kinds of actions are quite humorous. Their use is an effective technique when laughter is the desired response. Be very careful, however, to use this technique with discrimination and for the proper effect.

EXERCISES FOR GESTURE

Read the following selections in a full-length mirror using the "do-it-and-say-it" principle. Underscore the word with a descriptive gesture. Keep in mind that these exercises are forms of negative practice. Make certain that you understand why the accompanying gesture is wrong! A comic effect is not the intent, although it will be the result. Then read the exercises with appropriate gesture. Reinforce the thoughts physically, but do *not* "do it and say it."

1. **Hjalmar:**   It's Father's old shot-gun. It doesn't shoot any more; something's gone wrong with the lock. But it's quite fun to have it, all the same, because we can take it to pieces and clean it every now

---

[1] Jurgen Ruesch and Weldon Kees, *Nonverbal Communication: Notes on the Visual Perception of Human Relations* (Berkeley: University of California Press, 1970), p. 37.

and then, and grease it and put it together again. Of course, it's mostly Father who plays with that sort of thing.

Hedvig: Now you can see the wild duck properly.

Gregers: I was just looking at it. She seems to me to drag one wing a little.

Hjalmar: Well, that's not very surprising; she's been wounded.

Gregers: And she's a little lame in one foot, too.

From THE WILD DUCK *Henrik Ibsen*

2. By the cigars they smoke, and the composers they love, ye shall know the texture of men's souls.

From INDIAN SUMMER *John Galsworthy*

3. The poet is like the prince of the clouds who haunts the tempest and laughs at the man with the bow; exiled on the ground amid the hue and cry, his giant's wings prevent him from walking.

From FLEURS DU MAL *Charles Baudelaire*

4. Othello:

It is the cause, it is the cause, my soul,—
Let me not name it to you, you chaste stars!—
It is the cause.—Yet I'll not shed her blood;
Nor scar that whiter skin of hers than snow,
And smooth as monumental alabaster.
Yet she must die, else she'll betray more men.
Put out the light, and then put out the light.

From OTHELLO *William Shakespeare*

5. Notice how the use of gestures in the following selection are supportive and effective in clarifying the despicable nature of the character. In this case comedy is desired.

Volpone:

Ah, Mosca, you clever puppy, what a fool you are, how little you have learned of me! Do you really think you have to let the ducats fly in order to have everything? No, you fool! Let them rest quietly, side by side. Then, people will come of their own accord to offer you everything. Get this through your head: the magic of gold is so great that its smell alone can make men drunk. They only need to sniff it, and they come creeping here on their bellies; they only need to smell it, and they fall into your hands like moths in a flame. I do nothing but say I am rich—they bow their backs in reverence. Then I make a pretense at mortal illness. Ah, then the water drips off their tongues, and they begin to dance for my money. And how they love me: Friend Volpone! Best beloved friend! How they flatter me! How they serve me! How they rub against my shins and wag their tails! I'd like to trample the life out of these cobras, these vipers, but they dance to the tune of my pipe.

From VOLPONE *Ben Jonson*

COUNTENANCE

Countenance actions are movements of the head and face, particularly the eyes, "the orbs of the soul." It is through the use of the eyes that the proper relationship is set up between the speaker and the audience.

Making direct eye contact with the audience is perhaps the best advice, even though people talking to each other actually look at each other only about 35 percent of the time, according to some psychologists. But remember that the speech occasion is not conversation. It is your responsibility to make contact at some level with everyone in your audience. It is also one of the most difficult things for the beginning speaker to achieve. The tendency is to look almost anywhere except into the eyes of the listeners—you don't want them to discover that you are uncomfortable and nervous. With your momentary neurosis you are unable to realize that you relate your tensions to an audience by *not* looking at them.

Older textbooks have advised speakers not to look directly into the eyes of the audience. The writers say, "Look over their heads!" Poppycock! One of the reasons for looking into the eyes of an audience member is to read the feedback. This is perhaps the most important technique to be learned. Direct eye contact may cover a multitude of sins. On the other hand, the speaker should not be glued to the eyes of the listeners. That kind of intensity should be avoided as well. There are appropriate times for a speaker's gaze to wander. Observe a conversation between two friends. Do they constantly stare at each other? No! However, their eyes probably do make frequent connections. What techniques do you use when you do not want to listen to someone? You do not make direct eye contact. Perhaps you take a quick glance at your wristwatch or smile at someone else who is passing by. The point is that direct eye contact indicates an interest on the parts of both the speaker and listener.

Historically, a great deal of attention has been given to the power in the look of an eye. In grade B movies, a look is often used to hypnotize and gain control over another. Some popular adages state "if looks could kill" and "a person who does not look directly into your eyes when speaking should not be trusted." In the Spanish and American Indian cultures, there is the *ojo de dios,* or the eye of god, which protects against evil. In Robert Browning's dramatic monologue, "The Laboratory," the female character, after she has been given the poison to kill her rival, states:

What a drop! She's not little, no minion like me!
That's why she ensnared him: this will never free
The soul from those masculine eyes,—say, "no!"
To that pulse's magnificent come-and-go.
For only last night, as they whispered, I brought
My own eyes to bear on her so, that I thought
Could I keep them one half minute fixed, she would fall
Shrivelled; she fell not; yet this does it all!

Direct eye contact is an important technique when dictated by the material. In a performance, if an imagined listener is receiving the contact, you should not look into the eyes of the actual audience. Elizabeth Barrett Browning's "How Do I Love Thee" would not be read to the fellow in the third row. He might feel a little uncomfortable.

Facial expression, or countenance, reinforced by gesture should work together to create a total message that amplifies the intellectual meaning. Facial expression is often used to cue an audience for a desired response. For example, a speaker would not smile if an atmosphere of gloom were desired. Conversely, a somber expression is not the best cue to create a comedic environment. For our purposes the movements of the arms, hands, and head (with particular emphasis on facial expression) work together to perform "an additional function in that it is interpreted as a meta-communicative instruction accompanying verbal messages."[2]

People with hearing problems must develop the skill of reading nonverbal cues given by a speaker. This skill is also very helpful for speakers who are not hearing impaired, even though they do not have to rely exclusively on these visual components of the message.

A person with a serious hearing loss must gain more from the visual component. He or she relies more on **speechreading**, a term that has supplanted *lipreading*. Experts in the field of communication disorders recognize that there is more speechreading than a total focus on the lips. Since the impaired person is unable to hear the sounds produced, "the cues provided by the general situation are very helpful. Facial expression, gestures, and reactions are frequently more expressive than the words that are uttered."[3]

Speechreading techniques can be extremely helpful to the person with normal hearing as well as those with hearing impairment. Why shouldn't the hearing community benefit from techniques used by the hearing impaired?

Everyone interested in speechreading soon becomes aware of the role played by **homophenous sounds**, sounds that look alike on the lips as they are pronounced. The following sets of English consonants are considered homophenous sounds.[4]

Group	Consonants
I	/p/, /b/, /m/
II	/f/, /v/

---

[2] Ruesch and Kees, p. 64.

[3] Miriam D. Pauls, "Speechreading," in *Hearing and Deafness,* rev. ed., Hallowell Davis and S. Richard Silverman ed., (New York: Holt, Rinehart and Winston, 1964), p. 356.

[4] This classification of homophenous sounds was suggested by John J. O'Neill and Herbert J. Oyer, *Visual Communication for the Hard of Hearing* (Englewood Cliffs, N.J.: Prentice-Hall, 1961), p. 46.

III	/ʍ/, /w/, /r/
IV	/tʃ/, /ʤ/
	/ʃ/, /ʒ/
V	/t/, /d/, /l/, /n/, /s/, /z/, /θ/, /ð/
VI	/k/, /g/, /ŋ/, /h/

The acoustic components in these sounds are either unvoiced, voiced, or nasal. In Group I the three consonants are bilabial; since the hard-of-hearing or deaf person cannot perceive the acoustic components, the three sounds appear to be the same. Both of the consonant sounds in Group II are fricative **labio- dentals** (sounds articulated with the lower lip and upper teeth); the acoustic components vary in terms of the action of the vocal folds. In Group III, /ʍ/ and /w/ are bilabials and differ in the action of the vocal folds even though there is more observable cheek movement with /ʍ/. Although the tongue plays an important part in the production of the semivowel /r/, the primary visual cue is the movement of the two lips. Group IV consists of two sets of cognate pairs /tʃ/ and /ʤ/, and /ʃ/ and /ʒ/. In Group V all of the sounds are considered **linguaalveolar** (articulated with the tip of tongue against the hard ridge behind the upper teeth) except for the last set of cognates, /θ/ and /ð/. The articulatory adjustment for these sounds is **linguadental** (articulated with the tip of tongue touching the upper teeth). However, because of assimilation, Group V sounds can be mistaken for other sounds in dynamic speech. Group VI includes the cognate plosives /k/ and /g/, the nasal /ŋ/, and the fricative /h/.

It is very difficult for the person with impaired hearing to differentiate sounds made in the back of the throat, because they are not easily seen. Remember that people with a significant hearing loss must rely almost exclusively on speechreading for communication, since they cannot hear or frequently see the difference between the flow of breath and action of the vocal folds. The hearing individual can easily appreciate the problems of the hearing impaired when they face these homophenous sounds in dynamic speech. The difficulties are compounded when the same vowel is used with these homophenous sounds.

Homophonous words, on the other hand, sound exactly alike, such as *ate* and *eight; vale* and *veil;* and *vein, vane,* and *vain.* Homophenous words are those that use homophenous consonants, which look alike on the lips, with the same vowel or diphthong. Examples are *fault* and *vault; tan, Dan,* and *Nan;* and *chin* and *shin.* Kenneth Walter Berger has dramatized the problems with homophenous words in the following sentence: "I sat down and wrote a letter to my mother."[5] The homophonous words are in parentheses:

---

[5] Kenneth Walter Berger, *Speechreading: Principles and Methods* (Baltimore: National Educational Press, 1972), p. 101.

High	sad	doubt	add	rode	a	letter	do	by	mother.
I	sand	down	an	(road)	hey		new	(buy)	
	sat	noun	and	wrote	(hay)		(knew)	my	
		tout	ant	(rote)			to	pie	
		town	(aunt)				(too)		
			at				(two)		
			had						
			hand						
			hat						

Say this sentence aloud (without voice and with minimal facial expression) to a person with normal hearing and you might appreciate the difficulties facing the deafened person.

Exercises using speechreading principles but designed for the normal hearing community are extremely helpful in developing freedom in using the body for gesturing. In using exercises composed of homophenous words, it becomes necessary to communicate with the body as well as with the voice and speech. Consequently, such exercises increase body awareness.

EXERCISES USING HOMOPHENOUS SOUNDS

1. The following is a list of homophenous words. Although the consonants are different, all of the words contain the same vowel, /æ/:

man

pan

ban

mat

pat

bat

mad

pad

bad

Before an audience, articulate each of the words in order but do not vocalize. Do not use your countenance, especially the eyes. Since the words look alike on the lips, the listener should experience a "healthy" confusion. Repeat the exercise but skip around the list. The confusion should increase.

2. The homophenous words in exercise 1 are used in the following sentences.

He is the <u>man</u> who did it!

Watch out! The <u>pan</u> is hot!

Have you ever tried <u>Ban</u> deodorant?

The bathroom <u>mat</u> is still wet.

Be careful! Don't <u>pat</u> the dog. It might bite you!

I could have belted him with a baseball <u>bat</u>.

Don't be <u>mad</u> at me.

Come up to my <u>pad</u> when the class is over.

My brother was a very <u>bad</u> boy.

Select one of the sentences above to present to classmates without vocalization. The first time, be careful that you do not use any kinesic clues in your delivery.

3. Repeat each of the sentences in exercise 2 with nonverbal amplifications, but do not exaggerate the use of gesture. Deliver the sentences in a conversational, natural manner. After you can do this effectively and accurately, maintain the same degree of kinesic behavior while you vocalize the sentences.

4. Take a short stanza from a poem, speech, short story, or monologue and present it before an audience without vocalizing. Rely exclusively on the nonverbal components to convey the meaning or at least the emotion inherent in the segment. Do not exaggerate your gestures. Maintain a natural, conversational manner.

ADDITIONAL HOMOPHENOUS WORDS AND SENTENCES

The following combinations of sounds constitute additional homophenous words and sentences.

1. Initial position: palatal sounds /tʃ/, /dʒ/, /ʃ/, /ʒ/, /j/
   Final position: bilabial sounds /p/, /b/, /m/
   Medial vowel: /æ/

chap—What is that chap's name?

Jap(anese)—The Japanese are very musical people.

yap—All his dog does is yap, yap, yap.

jab—He gave Tom a quick jab to the head and another jab to the stomach.

jam—My mother makes the best strawberry jam in the world!

sham—I found the whole contest a big sham.

2. Initial position: labiodental sounds /f/, /v/
   Final position: linguaalveolar sounds /t/, /d/, /n/
   Medial vowel: /æ/

   fat—Boy, am I getting fat!

   vat—Put the vat of milk on the table, please.

   fad—Long hair was just a passing fad.

   fan—It's so hot. Where is the fan?

   van—I think the moving van will be a big help.

3. Initial position: linguaalveolar sounds /l/, /s/, /z/, /t/, /d/, /n/
   Final position: bilabial sounds /m/, /p/, /b/
   Medial vowel: /æ/
   (Homophonous words are in parentheses.)

   tam—Why do you like to wear a tam?

   tap—What is that tap-tap-tapping on my window pane?

   tab—It is your turn to pay the tab.

   dam—Boulder Dam is incredibly huge!

   (damn)—I really don't give a damn.

   dab—Put a little dab of blue in the paint.

   nap—I'm very tired. I think that I'll take a little nap.

   (knap)—We can climb that knap without any trouble. But this knapsack is mighty heavy!

   nab—Don't let the police nab you for speeding.

   lamb—I don't like lamb chops.

   (lam)—Hey, Mugsy, we better take it on the lam.

   lap—Get off my lap. You're too heavy.

   lab—Meet me in the lab in an hour.

Sam—Who doesn't love Uncle <u>Sam</u>?

sap—The blasted <u>sap</u> is all over my hands and clothes.

4. Initial position: linguavelar sounds /k/, /g/; glottal /h/
   Final position: linguaalveolarpalatal sound /tʃ/; linguapalatal sound /ʃ/
   Medial vowel: /æ/

catch—You'd better <u>catch</u> the ball before it breaks the window!

hatch—Batten down the <u>hatch</u>!

cash—Why didn't you <u>cash</u> the check?

gash—He had a two-inch <u>gash</u> in his leg.

hash—My favorite meal is corned beef <u>hash</u>.

5. Initial position: linguavelar sounds /k/, /g/; glottal /h/
   Final position: linguaalveolar sounds /t/, /d/, /n/, /l/, /s/, /z/
   Medial vowel: /æ/

cat—I wouldn't have a <u>cat</u> in my house!

gat—Hey, Tony, put the <u>gat</u> away.

hat—What a beautiful <u>hat</u> you're wearing, Michele!

cad—Marvin, you're a rat and a <u>cad</u>!

has—Does Martha have the flu? Yes, she <u>has</u> it.

gad—Oh, Chuck and Tracy are just <u>gad</u>abouts!

Remember the major purpose of homophenous word drills with and without vocalization is to encourage you to develop a flexible, meaningful physical response during the speech process.

BODY STANCE

The final aspect of bodily movement in communication is the stance of the body. This is important because many points are not made as the result of too little attention to this factor. Stance is closely related to posture.

Make certain that in performance you stand with the weight evenly distributed on both feet. The tendency is to bend one knee because it looks more casual. The danger is that under the tension of the situation, you will constantly shift your weight from one leg to the other. That is the surest way of revealing your tension to the audience.

The attitude of the speaker is also transmitted through stance. A timid, ill-prepared image is conveyed by slouched shoulders, hanging arms, and lowered head and eyes. This is the "judge-me-severely-because-I-am-unworthy-to-be-in-front-of-you-wasting-your-valuable-time" syndrome. Spare all audiences from these poor wretches!

On the other hand, there is the speaker who stands erectly with chest out, looking down his nose and communicating such an arrogant "you're so incredibly lucky to have an opportunity of seeing and hearing me that I could scream" attitude that the audience wants to see the person self-destruct. Both of these stances represent negative extremes.

Stand tall (but not too tall!) with shoulders back (but not too far back!), weight on both legs, and your head in a comfortable position so that you can see the audience easily.

Also, be neither a pacer nor a meandering nomad. If you take a step, it ought to be because you want to get closer to some member of the audience. Do not move just for the sake of moving. That is what it will look like. Any movement should come as a result of a desire to communicate a message. That is what prompts the movement—the desire to communicate a message to that audience, at that time, and in that place. No other message, time, place, or audience will do! That is what gives the performance dynamism and vitality!

Many of the selections in this text have been chosen with body movement in mind. Therefore, choose some selections from other chapters and apply the principles of kinesics to them as you read them aloud.

C H A P T E R

11

THE FOUR MAJOR DIALECTS OF AMERICAN ENGLISH

GLOSSARY

Allophone   A variation of a phoneme.

Dialect   The general pronunciation practiced by people in a particular region who speak the same language.

Sound Addition   Anaptyxis.

Sound Distortion   The distortion of a sound (for example, the excessive nasalization of /æ/ in [mæ̃n].

Sound Omission   The omission of a sound (for example, [sɔfkliz] for *Sophocles*).

Sound Substitution   The use of one sound for another (for example, [wæbɪt] for *rabbit*).

Suprasegmental Features   Those aspects of speech that concern more than individual phonemes, such as duration, stress, and juncture.

Triphthong   Three vowels coming together within the same syllable, an unacceptable pronunciation in professional speech.

A **dialect** is the general pronunciation practiced by people in a particular region who speak the same language. Within and outside the continental United States, there are a number of dialects. The American English in Hawaii, for example, is highly influenced by Oriental languages. As you study dialects, remember that some speakers will have a stronger dialect than others.

Obviously, a text on voice and articulation must limit its discussion to the most common dialects. The four dialects of American English that will be presented here are New England, New York City, Southern, and General American, which is the prevailing dialect in the Midwest, West, and Northwest.

There are many reasons why dialects develop. The most important, perhaps, is the influence of another language used by previous generations. A couple whose primary language is Italian is likely to speak English with an accent. Consequently, their children, although born in America, will be influenced by their parents' speech.

The early settlers in New England were primarily British. Accordingly, New England speech contains strong elements of British speech along with its own concoctions. British characteristics are also present in Southern speech, which includes additional Southern characteristics. Within a dialect, there are standard and substandard pronunciations.

Whether you are a "regional culturist" (a person who wishes to retain the best standards of speech within a particular region) or someone who does not want regional elements in your speech, it is important to know the voice and speech characteristics of different geographic locations. For example, there are many kinds of radio stations: hard rock, classical, country, gospel, and so on. If you are interested in becoming an on-air personality, you will want to know the recommended style of speech for the type of station you want to work for. Program requirements within a market will usually dictate appropriate speech or dialect.

You want your speech to be flexible, able to adapt to different styles and environments. Maintain your Down East or Southern speech if it is helpful and natural or required for the people with whom you interact—your listening or viewing audience, students, members of the congregation, or clients.

Used on the national level is the speech of the professional communicator; this is heard on television and radio, in motion pictures, and on the stage, as well as in other forums. However, many of these professionals have speech that does not reflect the standards of a trained speaker. In some cases their speech is even defective. Since we tend to imitate the speech of personalities we admire, it would be beneficial for everyone to mimic someone with a professional standard. It is important to realize that the speech of professional speakers substantially affects the average listener.

The material on dialects in this chapter is far from complete. It is by no means exhaustive, nor does it deal with dialectical variations. Your teacher will determine the dialectical standards for your class. The purpose of the chapter is simply to introduce you to the most obvious characteristics of the four major dialects of American English. The discussions and drills are helpful if you want to control or eliminate a dialect or to adopt a dialect for professional reasons.

The following modifying marks will be used in this and the following chapter to furnish additional information regarding the production of the sounds.

1. [:] appearing after the sound indicates that the sound is prolonged.

2. [ʔ] appearing before a sound indicates that the sound is glottalized. The breath is stopped with increased subglottal pressure and then the glottis is relaxed, allowing the breath to escape freely. The glottal stop is often used in place of the plosive /t/ (for example, [bɑʔl] for [bɑtl] *bottle*). This sound occurs frequently in the Cockney and Scottish dialects.

3. [~] placed over a sound indicates that the sound is produced with nasality. This modifying mark frequently appears with the vowel /æ/ and indicates excessive assimilation nasality. It is also quite evident in French.

4. ['] placed before a syllable indicates a primary accent on that syllable. [ˌ] placed before a syllable indicates secondary stress on that syllable. Obviously, these marks are only used with bisyllabic and polysyllabic words. (Examples are [ɪ'vækjuˌet] for *evacuate* and ['sɪmpləˌfaɪ] for *simplify*.)

5. [̩] placed beneath a vowel indicates greater tension than usual.

6. [̯] under a consonant signifies that the sound is dentalized (the blade of the tongue against the alveolar ridge with the tip touching the upper teeth). Other sounds can also be dentalized.

7. /ɾ/ indicates a single trill of the tongue tip on the consonant /r/.

8. /ř/ indicates a multiple trill on the tongue tip on the consonant /r/. (Imitate the stereotypical English duchess and roll that /r/!)

9. /ɻ/ indicates an /r/ where the tip of the tongue is curled too far back toward the palate (example: some midwesterners might say [ɻʌn] for [rʌn]).

10. [⊥] indicates that the tongue position is higher than usual.

In most of the exercises, the dialectical substitution of sound will appear above the appropriate letters. Each dialectic characteristic will be presented one at a time, and only sounds that are discussed will be included in the examples.

NEW ENGLAND

The speech of New Englanders is heavily influenced by their forefathers, the British. However, the New Englander not only uses **sound addition** and **sound**

omission but often creates an abrasive vocal quality most unlike the speech of the original English. In addition New England speech makes several **sound substitutions**.

Omission of /r/ and Substitution of /a/ for /ɑ/

One of the most distinguishing characteristics of New England speech is the omission of the semivowel /r/ and the substitution of the vowel /a/ (as in *ask*) for /ɑ/ (as in *father*).

Using negative practice, read the following word list as indicated by the column headings. If your speech is a New England dialect, record the following exercises as presented and *then reverse the procedure*. For example, in the following drill the New England pronunciation appears between the career pronunciations. Rerecord the exercise using New England, career, and then New England pronunciations. This will sensitize you to the correct and incorrect sounds.

	Career	New England	Career
park	[pɑrk]	[pak]	[pɑrk]
Harvard	[hɑrvɚd]	[havəd]	[hɑrvɚd]
sharp	[ʃɑrp]	[ʃap]	[ʃɑrp]
farm	[fɑrm]	[fam]	[fɑrm]
far	[fɑr]	[fa]	[fɑr]
army	[ɑrmɪ]	[amɪ]	[ɑrmɪ]
harm	[hɑrm]	[ham]	[hɑrm]
harp	[hɑrp]	[hap]	[hɑrp]
cart	[kɑrt]	[kat]	[kɑrt]
Arthur	[ɑrθɚ]	[aθə]	[ɑrθɚ]
partridge	[pɑrtrɪʤ]	[patrɪʤ]	[pɑrtrɪʤ]
marvelous	[mɑrvələs]	[mavələs]	[mɑrvələs]
garter	[gɑrtɚ]	[gatə]	[gɑrtɚ]
harmonize	[hɑrmənaɪz]	[hamənaɪz]	[hɑrmənaɪz]
arson	[ɑrsən]	[asən]	[ɑrsən]
pardon	[pɑrdn̩]	[padn̩]	[pɑrdn̩]

In trying to correct this regionalism, very frequently the New Englander adds the consonant /r/ but keeps the vowel /a/. This is not sufficient; the vowel must also be changed to /ɑ/.

Read the following word lists aloud.

	New England	/a/ Plus /r/	Career Speech
park	[pak]	[park]	[pɑrk]
Harvard	[havəd]	[harvəd]	[hɑrvɚd]
sharp	[ʃap]	[ʃarp]	[ʃɑrp]
farm	[fam]	[farm]	[fɑrm]
far	[fa]	[far]	[fɑr]
army	[amɪ]	[armɪ]	[ɑrmɪ]
harm	[ham]	[harm]	[hɑrm]
harp	[hap]	[harp]	[hɑrp]
cart	[kat]	[kart]	[kɑrt]
Arthur	[aθə]	[arθə]	[ɑrθɚ]
partridge	[patrɪʤ]	[partrɪʤ]	[pɑrtrɪʤ]
marvelous	[mavələs]	[marvələs]	[mɑrvələs]
garter	[gatə]	[gartɚ]	[gɑrtɚ]
harmonize	[hamənaɪz]	[harmənaɪz]	[hɑrmənaɪz]
arson	[asən]	[arsən]	[ɑrsən]
pardon	[padn̩]	[pardn̩]	[pɑrdn̩]

Use of /ɒ/

Refer to the discussion on the production of the sound /ɒ/ with the accompanying representative words and sentences (Chapter 7). In some areas of New England, this sound is distorted by opening the mouth too wide and using excessive lip action.

Addition of /r/ or /ɚ/

Frequently the New Englander adds /r/ to the end of a word ending with the letter "w" or after /ɔ/ (as in *law*). Also, the New Englander often changes /ɔ/ to /ɒ/ or /a/. This is particularly true when the word ending with /ɔ/ is followed by another word beginning with a vowel or diphthong. For example, in the sentence "The winter thaw is beginning," the New Englander is likely to say "The winter [θɒr] is beginning."

Read the following phrases and sentences aloud several times using negative practice. Do not hesitate to overdo the pronunciation of the words so that you can feel the addition as well as the omission of the /r/.

"He didn't draw it today."
Career: [hɪ dɪdn̩t drɔ ɪt tədeɪ]
New Engand: [hɪ dɪdn̩t drɒr ɪt tədeɪ]
Career: [hɪ dɪdn̩t drɔ ɪt tədeɪ]

"Steve was injured by the clawing tiger."
Career: [stiv wəz ɪnʤɚd baɪ ðə klɔɪŋ taɪgɚ]
New England: [stiv wɒz ɪnʤəd baɪ ðə klɒrɪŋ taɪgə]
Career: [stiv wəz ɪnʤɚd baɪ ðə klɔɪŋ taɪgɚ]

"Antigone had a flaw in her character."
Career: [æntɪgənɪ hæd ə flɔ ɪn hɚ kærəktɚ]
New England: [æntɪgənɪ hæd ə flɒr ɪn hɚ kærəktə]
Career: [æntɪgənɪ hæd ə flɔ ɪn hɚ kærəktɚ]

"A cawing bird can be very aggravating."
Career: [ə kɔɪŋ bɝd kæn bɪ vɛrɪ ægrəvetɪŋ]
New England: [ə kɒrɪŋ bɝd kæn bɪ vɛrɪ ægrəvetɪŋ]
Career: [ə kɔɪŋ bɝd kæn bɪ vɛrɪ ægrəvetɪŋ]

"If you get tired, draw up a chair."
Career: [ɪf ju gɛt taɪrd drɔ ʌp ə tʃɛr]
New England: [ɪf ju gɛt taɪəd drɒr ʌp ə tʃɛr]
Career: [ɪf ju gɛt taɪrd drɔ ʌp ə tʃɛr]

"Draw a picture."
Career: [drɔ ə pɪktʃɚ]
New England: [drɒr ə pɪktʃə]
Career: [drɔ ə pɪktʃɚ]

Substitution of /ɚ/ for /ə/

Another very recognizable and imitable New England speech characteristic is the substitution of the /ɚ/ for the schwa when it is the last sound of a word. President John F. Kennedy often used this sound.

Read the following word list using negative practice. Do not hesitate to exaggerate the pronunciation. This will help you to feel the production.

	Career	*New England*	*Career*
Asia	[eʒə]	[eʒɚ]	[eʒə]
pneumonia	[nɪumonjə]	[nɪumonjɚ]	[nɪumonjə]
idea	[aɪdiə]	[aɪdiɚ]	[aɪdiə]
stamina	[stæmɪnə]	[stæmɪnɚ]	[stæmɪnə]
umbrella	[əmbrɛlə]	[əmbrɛlɚ]	[əmbrɛlə]
euphoria	[jufɔrɪjə]	[jufɔrɪjɚ]	[jufɔrɪjə]
regalia	[rɪgeɪljə]	[rɪgeɪljɚ]	[rɪgeɪljə]

sofa	[sofə]	[sofɚ]	[sofə]
Alabama	[æləbæmə]	[æləbǽmɚ]	[æləbæmə]
Cuba	[kjubə]	[kjubɚ]	[kjubə]

Substitution of /ɜ/ for /ɝ/

This distinguishing characteristic is slowly disappearing in New England. Some residents of parts of Maine, New Hampshire, Vermont, and Cape Cod still retain it and pass it to their children.

For exercises, refer to the discussion of /ɜ/ on p. 169.

Substitution of /ə/ for /ɚ/

This substitution is also characteristic of London speech. Read the following word list using negative practice. Exaggerate the pronunciation so that you feel the production.

	Career	New England	Career
sister	[sɪstɚ]	[sɪstə]	[sɪstɚ]
brother	[brʌðɚ]	[brʌðə]	[brʌðɚ]
mother	[mʌðɚ]	[mʌðə]	[mʌðɚ]
father	[fɑðɚ]	[fɑðə]	[fɑðɚ]
actor	[æktɚ]	[æktə]	[æktɚ]
keeper	[kipɚ]	[kipə]	[kipɚ]
talker	[tɔkɚ]	[tɒkə]	[tɔkɚ]
walker	[wɔkɚ]	[wɒkə]	[wɔkɚ]
minister	[mɪnəstɚ]	[mɪnəstə]	[mɪnəstɚ]
mister	[mɪstɚ]	[mɪstə]	[mɪstɚ]

Substitution of /a/ for /æ/

This substitution is typical of New England speech. Record the following words using negative practice.

	Career	New England	Career
half	[hæf]	[haf]	[hæf]
bath	[bæθ]	[baθ]	[bæθ]
last	[læst]	[last]	[læst]

aunt	[ænt]	[ant]	[ænt]
ant	[ænt]	[ãnt]¹	[ænt]
fast	[fæst]	[fast]	[fæst]
cast	[kæst]	[kast]	[kæst]
passed	[pæst]	[past]	[pæst]
flask	[flæsk]	[flask]	[flæsk]
calf	[kæf]	[kaf]	[kæf]

Excessive Assimilation Nasality

New England speech often exhibits excessive assimilation nasality, although this characteristic is by no means limited to New England speech. You will remember that the modifying mark for nasality, [~], is placed over the affected phoneme. Refer to the drills on excessive assimilation nasality on pp. 79–81.

EXERCISES FOR NEW ENGLAND AND CAREER SPEECH

Read the following sentences carefully and exaggerate the pronunciation. Feel what the articulators are doing in the production of the sounds.

1. "Asia and Africa are large continents."

   Career: [eʒə ænd æfrɪkə ɑr lɑrʤ kɑntənənts]
   New England: [eʒɚ æ̃nd æfrɪkɚ a laʤ kɒntn̩ənts]
   Career: [eʒə ænd æfrɪkə ɑr lɑrʤ kɑntənənts]

2. "Martha had the idea of bringing the umbrella to the beach."

   Career: [mɑrθə hæd ðɪ aɪdiə əv brɪŋɪŋ ðɪ əmbrɛlə tə ðə bitʃ]
   New England: [maθɚ hæd ðɪ aɪdiɚ əv brɪŋɪŋ ðɪ əmbrɛlɚ tə ðə bitʃ]
   Career: [mɑrθə hæd ðɪ aɪdiə əv brɪŋɪŋ ðɪ əmbrɛlə tə ðə bitʃ]

3. "Harvey must have had a lot of stamina to wear all that underwater regalia."

   Career: [hɑrvɪ mʌst həv hæd ə lɑt əv stæmɪnə tə wer ɔl ðæt ʌndɚwɔtɚ rəgeljə]
   New England: [havɪ mʌst həv hæd ə lɒt əv stæ̃mɪnɚ tə weə ɒl ðæt ʌndəwɒtə rəgeljɚ]

---

¹The New Englander distinguishes between *aunt* and *ant*. (She resents being called an insect!) In addition, the New Englander tends to nasalize the vowel in *ant*. You will notice that in career speech, the relative and the insect are pronounced the same—and without nasality on /æ/.

Career: [hɑrvɪ mʌst həv hæd ə lɑt əv stæmɪnə tə wer ɔl ðæt ʌndɚ·wɔtɚ rəgeljə]

4. "Since Margo had pneumonia, she was resting on the sofa."

Career: [sɪns mɑrgo hæd nɪumonjə ʃɪ wəz rɛstɪŋ ɑn ðə sofə]
New England: [sɪns mɑgo hæd nɪumonjɚ ʃɪ wəz rɛstɪŋ ɒn ðə sofɚ]
Career: [sɪns mɑrgo hæd nɪumonjə ʃɪ wəz rɛstɪŋ ɑn ðə sofə]

5. "Georgia and Alabama are not too far from Cuba."

Career: [dʒɔrdʒə ænd æləbæmə ɑr nɑt tu fɑr frəm kjubə]
New England: [dʒɒdʒɚ ænd ãləbæmɚ a nɒt tu fa frəm kjubɚ]
Career: [dʒɔrdʒə ænd æləbæmə ɑr nɑt tu fɑr frəm kjubə]

In the following sentences, the New England sounds appear above the appropriate letters.

6. Mister Earl prepared herbs for all the servants.

7. The nurse was irked by the unworthy patient.

8. To avert disaster, the master asked the aunt not to walk on the grass near the harbor.

9. Richard Burton purchased an ermine fur for his sister.

10. Shirley was certain that she would smirk at the minister's sermon.

11. Where is this person called Ma Barker?

12. Research the records for Myrtle's birthday.

In the following two selections, New England sounds are transcribed above the appropriate letters. Record it as you would normally say it. Then emphasize the New England characteristics that magnify those phonemic elements of the dialect. Focus on the sound discrimination and production.

13. Ghost of Hămlet's father:

I ăm thy father's spirit;

Doomed for a certain term to walk the night,

Ănd, for the day, confined to fast in fires

Till the foul crimes done in my days of nature

Are burnt and purged away. But that I ãm forbid

To tell the secrets of my prison-house,

I could a tale unfold whose lightest words

Would harrow up thy soul; freeze thy young blood;

Make thy two eyes, like stars, start from their spheres;

Thy knotted ãnd combined locks to part,

Ãnd each particular hair to stãnd on end,

Like quills upon the fretful porpentine:

But this eternal blazon must not be

To ears of flesh ãnd blood—List, list, O, list!—

If thou didst ever thy dear father love,—

Revenge his foul ãnd most unnatural murder.

From HÃMLET   *William Shakespeare*

14. Remember me when I ãm gone away,

Gone far away into the silent lãnd;

When you cãn no more hold me by the hãnd,

Nor I half turn to go, yet turning stay.

Remember me when no more, day by day,

You tell me of our future that you plãnned;

Only remember me; you understãnd

It will be late to counsel then or pray.

Yet if you should forget me for a while

And afterwards remember do not grieve:

For if the darkness ānd corruption leave

A vestige of the thoughts that once I had,

Better by far you should forget ānd smile

Than that you should remember ānd be sad.

REMEMBER   *Christina Rosetti*

In the following selections, there is room for you to add the symbols for the New England sounds above the appropriate letters. These selections were written for New England characters. Record the selections with your habitual speech and then with a New England dialect. These exercises are recommended for those students wishing to acquire a New England dialect for professional reasons.

15. Mr. Webb:

Well, ma'am, I wouldn't know what you'd call much. Satiddy nights the farmhands meet down in Ellery Greenough's stable and holler some. We've got one or two town drunks, but they're always having remorses every time an evangelist comes to town. No, ma'am, I'd say likker ain't a regular thing in the home here, except in the medicine chest.

From OUR TOWN   *Thornton Wilder*

16. Cabot:

I cal'clate God give it to 'em—not yew! God's hard, not easy! Mebbe they's easy gold in the West but it hain't God's gold. It hain't fur me. I kin hear His voice warnin' me agin t' be hard an' stay on my farm. I kin see his hand usin' Eben t' steal t' keep me from weakness. I kine feel I be in the palm o' His hand, His fingers guidin' me. It's a-goin' t' be lonesomer now than ever it war afore—an' I'm gettin' old, Lord, ripe on the bough. . . . Waal—what d'ye want? God's lonesome, hain't He? God's hard an' lonesome!

From DESIRE UNDER THE ELMS   *Eugene O'Neill*

17. Charles:

George, I was thinkin' the other night of some advice my father gave me when I got married. Charles, he said, Charles, start out early showin' who's boss, he said. Best thing to do is to give an order, even if it don't make sense; just so she'll learn to obey.

From OUR TOWN   *Thornton Wilder*

18. All the morning there had been an increasing temptation to take an out-door holiday, and early in the afternoon the temptation outgrew my power of resistance. A far-away pasture on the long southwestern slope of a high hill was persistently present to my mind, yet there seemed to be no particular reason why I should think of it. I was not sure that I wanted anything from the pasture, and there was no sign, except the temptation, that the pasture wanted anything of me. But I was on the farther side of as many as three fences before I stopped to think again where I was going and why.

From THE COURTING OF SISTER WISBY   *Sarah Orne Jewett*

NEW YORK CITY

Although the inhabitants of Brooklyn, the Bronx, Queens, Staten Island, and Manhattan do not all have the same dialect, they do share certain speech characteristics. Some of the more frequently heard are discussed in this section. As in the New England dialect, the New York City dialect contains **sound distortions**, omissions, and additions.

If you speak with a New York City dialect, after you have recorded the word lists as presented, rerecord them with a New York dialect, then career speech, then a New York dialect. This routine gives you more practice at producing the corrected and erroneous sounds consciously. The same technique can be used by the non–New Yorker who wants to acquire a New York dialect for professional reasons. As you do this exercise, feel what is happening to your articulators.

Substitution of /oə/ for /ɔ/

The sound /oə/ is not the exact substitution used for /ɔ/ (as in *law*), but it does approximate the vowels used by New Yorkers. An exact representation of the New York sound would require a discussion far too complex for the purposes of this text.

Record the following word lists.

	Career	*New York City*	*Career*
awful	[ɔfʊl]	[oəfʊl]	[ɔfʊl]
coffee	[kɔfɪ]	[koəfɪ]	[kɔfɪ]
lawless	[lɔləs]	[loələs]	[lɔləs]
salt	[sɔlt]	[soəlt]	[sɔlt]
water	[wɔtɚ]	[woətə]	[wɔtɚ]
small	[smɔl]	[smoəl]	[smɔl]
bought	[bɔt]	[boət]	[bɔt]
closet	[klɑzɪt]	[kloəzɪt]	[klɑzɪt]
faucet	[fɔsət]	[foəsət]	[fɔsət]
fought	[fɔt]	[foət]	[fɔt]

In the following sentences, the New York City sounds appear above the appropriate letters.

      oə   oə
There are many authors in Boston.

     oə   oə   oə
The Australian and the Austrian met because of chance.

     oə   oə
The auspicious bankers insisted on an audit.

    oə   oə   oə   oə
My boss thought that the longer song was the better one.

    oə   oə   oə oə
The awful battle was fought for a lost cause.

Substitution of /ɛə/ for /eɪ/ When Followed by /l/

If you record this substitution, you will be more aware of this dialectal substitution and will be able to use it if ever necessary.

	Career	*New York City*	*Career*
pale	[peɪl]	[pɛəl]	[peɪl]
fail	[feɪl]	[fɛəl]	[feɪl]
sailor	[seɪlɚ]	[sɛələ]	[seɪlɚ]
failure	[feɪljɚ]	[fɛəljə]	[feɪljɚ]
daily	[deɪlɪ]	[dɛəlɪ]	[deɪlɪ]
sale	[seɪl]	[sɛəl]	[seɪl]
nail	[neɪl]	[nɛəl]	[neɪl]
mailman	[meɪlmæn]	[mɛəlmæn]	[meɪlmæn]

quail   [kweɪl]   [kwɛəl]   [kweɪl]

stale   [steɪl]   [stɛəl]   [steɪl]

The mailman delivered the *New York Daily News* to me at the ball game. [ɛə, ɛə]

All of the plans to rescue the sailors failed. [ɛə, ɛə]

The railroad stumps were for sale for forty dollars. [ɛə, ɛə]

Although the air was stale, the frail stream of smoke left a trail. [ɛə, ɛə, ɛə]

Gail put down her pail and watched the boats sail by. [ɛə, ɛə, ɛə]

Substitution of /ɛə/ for /æ/

	Career	New York City	Career
apple	[æpl̩]	[ɛəpl̩]	[æpl̩]
mask	[mæsk]	[mɛəsk]	[mæsk]
balance	[bæləns]	[bɛələns]	[bæləns]
gallon	[gælən]	[gɛələn]	[gælən]
pastoral	[pæstərl̩]	[pɛəstərl̩]	[pæstərl̩]
galaxy	[gæləksɪ]	[gɛələksɪ]	[gæləksɪ]
glad	[glæd]	[glɛəd]	[glæd]
hash	[hæʃ]	[hɛəʃ]	[hæʃ]
calf	[kæf]	[kɛəf]	[kæf]
half	[hæf]	[hɛəf]	[hæf]

Carol gave Harry a back scratcher for his birthday. [ɛə, ɛə, ɛə, ɛə]

The masked bāndit grabbed the calf and rãn. [ɛə, ɛə, ɛə]

Harold has been called a rough taskmaster by his students. [ɛə, ɛə, ɔə, ɛə, ɛə]

Ask if he saw the tan cat attack the dog. [ɛə, ɔə, ɛə, ɛə, ɛə, ɔə]

Crãmming for exãms is a bad habit. [ɛə, ɛə]

Substitution of /æʊ/ for /ɑʊ/

Remember /ɑʊ/ is an acceptable **allophone** of /aʊ/. Record the following list of words and sentences as transcribed. Be aware of the New York substitutions.

	Career	*New York City*	*Career*
owl	[ɑʊl]	[æʊl]	[ɑʊl]
south	[sɑʊθ]	[sæʊθ]	[sɑʊθ]
housekeeper	[hɑʊskipɚ]	[hæʊskipɚ]	[hɑʊskipɚ]
devout	[dɪvɑʊt]	[dɪvæʊt]	[dɪvɑʊt]
tower	[tɑʊɚ]	[tæʊɚ]	[tɑʊɚ]
outside	[ɑʊtsaɪd]	[æʊtsaɪd]	[ɑʊtsaɪd]
shout	[ʃɑʊt]	[ʃæʊt]	[ʃɑʊt]
drown	[drɑʊn]	[dræʊn]	[drɑʊn]
bow	[bɑʊ]	[bæʊ]	[bɑʊ]
Browning	[brɑʊnɪŋ]	[[bræʊnɪŋ]	[brɑʊnɪŋ]

æʊ   ɔə   æʊ   æʊ   æʊ

Howard thought it was about time to go around the house.

æʊ   æʊ   æʊ

The mountainous terrain made it doubtful that we could go south.

æʊ   æʊ   æʊ

Browning and Housman are our favorite poets.

æʊ   æʊ   æʊ

When she scowled and pouted, I went outside.

æʊ   æʊ   æʊ

The brown cows were particularly foul smelling.

Substitution of /ɒɪ/ for /aɪ/

Record the following list of words and sentences as transcribed. Be aware of the New York substitutions.

	Career	*New York City*	*Career*
eye	[aɪ]	[ɒɪ]	[aɪ]
final	[faɪnl̩]	[fɒɪnl̩]	[faɪnl̩]
daylight	[delaɪt]	[delɒɪt]	[delaɪt]
island	[aɪlənd]	[ɒɪlənd]	[aɪlənd]
stylish	[staɪlɪʃ]	[stɒɪlɪʃ]	[staɪlɪʃ]
diary	[daɪərɪ]	[dɒɪərɪ]	[daɪərɪ]
certify	[sɝtəfaɪ]	[sɝtəfɒɪ]	[sɝtəfaɪ]
biography	[baɪɑgrəfɪ]	[bɒɪɑgrəfɪ]	[baɪɑgrəfɪ]
guide	[gaɪd]	[gɒɪd]	[gaɪd]
rise	[raɪz]	[rɒɪz]	[raɪz]

^{DI}   ^{DI}   ^{DI}
The bicycle arrived just in time.

^{DI}   ^{DI}   ^{DI}
Iris got a diamond ring from Byron.

^{DI}   ^{DI}   ^{DI}
At the height of the lightning storm they arrived.

^{DI}   ^{DI}   ^{DI}
The license certified that they could photograph the lions.

^{DI}   ^{DI}   ^{DI}
I'll not ask the guide to drive the jeep.

Substitution of /ɔ/ for /ɑr/

Record the following list of words and sentences as transcribed. Be aware of the New York substitutions.

	Career	*New York City*	*Career*
park	[pɑrk]	[pɔk]	[pɑrk]
Harvard	[hɑrvɚd]	[hɔvəd]	[hɑrvɚd]
cart	[kɑrt]	[kɔt]	[kɑrt]
pardon	[pɑrdn̩]	[pɔdn̩]	[pɑrdn̩]
hearty	[hɑrtɪ]	[hɔtɪ]	[hɑrtɪ]
char	[tʃɑr]	[tʃɔ]	[tʃɑr]
carving	[kɑrvɪŋ]	[kɔvɪŋ]	[kɑrvɪŋ]
Darth	[dɑrθ]	[dɔθ]	[dɑrθ]
barn	[bɑrn]	[bɔn]	[bɑrn]
lard	[lɑrd]	[lɔd]	[lɑrd]

   ^ɔ   ^ɔ   ^ɔ   ^ɔ
Park the car in Harvard Yard.

               ^ɔ
Marvin slipped in the barn.

   ^ɔ   ^ɔ
Hark and hear the lark.

   ^ɔ   ^ɔ   ^ɔ
Arthur carved the turkey for the starving people.

      ^ɔ   ^{æʊ}   ^ɔ
The farmer's cow was farther up the road.

Substitution of /ɛ:/ for /ɛr/

Record the following list of words and sentences as transcribed. Be aware of the New York substitutions.

	Career	New York City	Career
their	[ðɛr]*	[ðɛ:]	[ðɛr]
wear	[wɛr]*	[wɛ:]	[wɛr]
hair	[hɛr]*	[hɛ:]	[hɛr]
fair	[fɛr]*	[fɛ:]	[fɛr]
where	[ʌɛr]*	[ʌɛ:]	[ʌɛr]
stair	[stɛr]*	[stɛ:]	[stɛr]
Claire	[klɛr]*	[klɛ:]	[klɛr]
airplane	[ɛrplen]	[ɛ:plen]	[ɛrplen]
hairline	[hɛrlaɪn]	[hɛ:lɒɪn]	[hɛrlaɪn]
bear	[bɛr]*	[bɛ:]	[bɛr]

Claire was wearing a new hairdo.
ɛ: ɛ: ɛ:

It is unfair to charge so much fare for the airplane.
ɛ: ɔ   ɛ: ɛ:

Billie Rich's hair went everywhere when she danced.
ɛ: ɛ:

If provoked, they would tear their fur.
ɛ: ɛ:

The bear cub went where?
ɛ: ɛ:

Substitution of /ɛʊ/ for /o/ and /oʊ/

Record the following list of words and sentences as transcribed. Focus on the New York substitution.

	Career	New York City	Career
going	[goɪŋ]	[gɛʊɪŋ]	[goɪŋ]
follow	[fɑlou]	[fɑlɛʊ]	[fɑlou]
goat	[got]	[gɛʊt]	[got]
smoke	[smok]	[smɛʊk]	[smok]
rope	[rop]	[rɛʊp]	[rop]
slowly	[sloulɪ]	[slɛʊlɪ]	[sloulɪ]
showed	[ʃoud]	[ʃɛʊd]	[ʃoud]
folder	[foldɚ]	[fɛʊldɚ]	[foldɚ]

*Pronunciation of the word used in dynamic speech as opposed to isolated words.

almost   [ɔlmost]   [ɔlmɛʊst]   [ɔlmost]

shallow   [ʃælou]   [ʃælɛʊ]   [ʃælou]

spoke   [spok]   [spɛʊk]   [spok]

  ɛʊ   ɛʊ   ɛʊ   ɛː

Joe was the only one with yellow hair.

  ɛʊ   ɛʊ   ɛʊ

Go and get both folders.

  ɛʊ   ɒɪ   ɒɪ   ɛʊ   ɛʊ

Snow White sang "Heigh Ho" with Dopey.

  ɛʊ   oə   oə   ɛʊ

Coal costs almost double.

    ɛʊ   ɛʊ   æʊ

In poker the joker does not count.

Consonants

Substitution of /t/ for /θ/ and /d/ for /ð/

This substitution is often associated with Brooklyn and the Bronx. However, it is typical of sections of many large cities, such as Philadelphia, Boston, Chicago, and so on. It is most colorfully represented in the speech of some Damon Runyon characters. For purposes of the following exercise this substitution will be labeled "Runyonesque."

	Career	*Runyonesque*	*Career*
mother	[mʌðɚ]	[mʌdə]	[mʌðɚ]
other	[ʌðɚ]	[ʌdə]	[ʌðɚ]
weather	[wɛðɚ]	[wɛdə]	[wɛðɚ]
both	[boθ]	[bot]	[boθ]
either	[iðɚ]	[idə]	[iðɚ]
tooth	[tuθ]	[tut]	[tuθ]
this	[ðɪs]	[dɪs]	[ðɪs]
truth	[truθ]	[trut]	[truθ]
without	[wɪðɑut]	[wɪdæut]	[wɪðɑut]
thirty	[θɝ·tɪ]	[tɔɪdɪ]	[θɝ·tɪ]
		[tɝ·dɪ]	

          d   d   d   ə

He went with the other kids.

         d   ə   d   ə   d æʊ   t

Andrea's father and mother went without a lot of things.

      d ə   ɛʊ   d   ɛʊ   ɒɪ d

Either Danny will go or they'll go by themselves.

_d _d _t _{æu} _d _t
The dentist didn't tell the truth about the toothache.

_{d æu} _d _ə _d _{εu}
Without this paper there's no proof.

Dentalization of /t/, /d/, /n/, and /l/

New York speech is often dentalized, which means that the entire blade of the tongue rather than just the tip is in contact with the alveolar ridge in the production of /t/, /d/, /n/, and /l/. This articulation gives a heavier sound. Although other sounds may also be dentalized, these are certainly the most characteristic of New York City speech. Remember that the modifying mark [ˌ] is placed under the dentalized sound.

	Career	*New York City*	*Career*
tender	[tɛndɚ]	[tɛndə]	[tɛndɚ]
dandelion	[dændəlɑɪən]	[dændəlɒɪən]	[dændəlɑɪən]
undersized	[ʌndɚsɑɪzd]	[ʌndəsɒɪzd]	[ʌndɚsɑɪzd]
tantalize	[tæntəlɑɪz]	[tæntəlɒɪz]	[tæntəlɑɪz]
tonsillitis	[tɑnsɪlɑɪtəs]	[tɑnsɪlɒɪtəs]	[tɑnsɪlɑɪtəs]
dentalize	[dɛntəlɑɪz]	[dɛntəlɒɪz]	[dɛntəlɑɪz]
dictate	[dɪktet]	[dɪktet]	[dɪktet]
lullaby	[lʌləbɑɪ]	[lʌləbɒɪ]	[lʌləbɑɪ]
notate	[notet]	[nɛutet]	[notet]
lollipop	[lɑlɪpɑp]	[lɑlɪpɑp]	[lɑlɪpɑp]

Nanette didn't mean to do it.

What is the meaning of the word dilettante?

Wilma, please place the tin where Billie can find it.

The smell of tarts was too tantalizing for Nancy.

_{εu} _{εu} _{ɒɪ}
Joey, do you know what time it is?

EXERCISES FOR NEW YORK CITY AND CAREER SPEECH

The following sentences are transcribed into career speech and New York City speech. As you produce the sounds, listen and feel what is happening to the articulators.

1. "Herb sat on the curb."

    New York City: [hɝˑb sɛət ɑn ðə kɝˑb]

                          [hɔɪb sɛət ɑn də kɔɪb] (Runyonesque speech)

    Career: [hɝˑb sæt ɑn ðə kɝˑb]

2. "You want a cup of coffee?"

    New York City: [jə wanə kʌp ə koəfɪ]

    Career: [ju wɑnt ə kʌp əv kɔfɪ]

3. "Tom is down the hall."

    New York City: [tɑm ɪz dæun ðə hoəl]

    Career: [tɑm ɪz dɑun ðə hɔl]

4. "Finally, it is all done."

    New York City: [fɒɪnəlɪ ɪt ɪz oəl dʌn]

    Career: [faɪnəlɪ ɪt ɪz ɔl dʌn]

5. "I couldn't care less."

    New York City: [ɒɪ kʊdn̩t kɛː lɛs]

    Career: [aɪ kʊdn̩t kɛr lɛs]

The following speeches were written for a person with New York City speech. In exercise 6, the playwright attempts to indicate the New York street dialect through spelling. The actual sound substitutions are transcribed above the letters. Room has been left above the remaining speeches to make your own phonetic notations. First, record the material as transcribed; then record it in your habitual speech (which we hope is career speech!) and compare it with your New York City version.

6. Tommy:

    Nah, dey're all wise tuh us. Duh minute we walk in, 'ey asks us wadda we want. If we had some dough, while one uv us wuz buyin' sumpm, de udduh guys could swipe some stuff, see? I got faw cents, but 'at ain' enough. Anybody got any dough heah? Hey, yew, Angel, yuh got some?

    From DEAD END   *Sidney Kingsley*

7. Velma:

    It's my mother's blood! I didn't know what to do. I don't...know why I did it! I don't even really remember that much, Frankie. When I got in the subway to come to work afterwards it was just like nuthin' happened, nuthin' at all! But do you know? I thought, I thought when my mother asked me to cover her piece of coffee cake with a whole lot of caviar, I thought...my mother...she thinks that my head is a hammer! That's what she thinks. And it isn't! It isn't! Tell me, Frankie, please tell me that my head is not a hammer!

From BIRDBATH   *Leonard Melfi*

8. Gittel Mosca:

Sophie. Is Oscar there?—Well, listen, that hat-type friend of his last night, the long one, what's his number?—Look, girl, will you drag your mind up out of your girdle and go see if Oscar's got it written down?—

From TWO FOR THE SEESAW   *William Gibson*

9. Billie Dawn:

My father? Gas Company. He used to read meters, but in this letter he says how he can't get around so good anymore so they gave him a different job. Elevator man. Goofy old·guy. He used to take a little frying pan to work every morning and a can of Sterno and cook his own lunch. He said everybody should have a hot lunch.

From BORN YESTERDAY   *Garson Kanin*

STANDARD SOUTHERN AMERICAN ENGLISH

Since there are so many dialects and subdialects in Southern speech, it would be impractical to present all of them in a text on voice and articulation. The purpose of this chapter is only to give you a flavor of the four major American-English dialects.

In representing a Southerner's speech, it is common to indicate the lilting pitch. Compared with the other major American-English dialects, the Southern does contain many more variations in pitch. However, these changes cannot be represented by a phonetic alphabet. To show such acoustical phenomena, **suprasegmental features** must be used, an area that is beyond the scope of this chapter. Therefore, the major phonemic substitutions and omissions will be presented.

Vowels and Diphthongs

Many people, particularly Northerners, feel that the Southern drawl results from prolonging the sounds. "It takes them so-o-o-o-o lo-o-ong to say what they want to sa-a-a-ay!" Actually, the Southerner takes no more time to produce an individual sound than anyone else. This false impression stems from the many **triphthongs** used in Southern speech.

Addition of /jə/ to /ɪ/ and /æ/

These sounds are used primarily in monosyllabic words. Record the following list of words and sentences as transcribed. Focus on the Southern addition.

	Career	*Southern*	*Career*
flit	[flɪt]	[flɪjət]	[flɪt]
been	[bɪn]	[bɪjən]	[bɪn]
wit	[wɪt]	[wɪjət]	[wɪt]
grip	[grɪp]	[grɪjəp]	[grɪp]
inch	[ɪntʃ]	[ɪjəntʃ]	[ɪntʃ]
tryst	[trɪst]	[trɪjəst]	[trɪst]
mince	[mɪns]	[mɪjəns]	[mɪns]
trim	[trɪm]	[trɪjəm]	[trɪm]
chip	[tʃɪp]	[tʃɪjəp]	[tʃɪp]
pick	[pɪk]	[pɪjək]	[pɪk]
man	[mæn]	[mæjən]	[mæn]
handle	[hændl̩]	[hæjəndl̩]	[hændl̩]
Fran	[fræn]	[fræjən]	[fræn]
can	[kæn]	[kæjən]	[kæn]
band	[bænd]	[bæjənd]	[bænd]
candy	[kændɪ]	[kæjəndɪ]	[kændɪ]
Nancy	[nænsɪ]	[næjənsɪ]	[nænsɪ]
bad	[bæd]	[bæjəd]	[bæd]
lamb	[læm]	[læjəm]	[læm]
trapped	[træpt]	[træjəpt]	[træpt]

ɪjə   ɪjə   a
Pick up the mince pie.

æjə   æjə   a   ɪjə   ɪjə
Andrea can buy the pig for Midge.

æjə   æjə æjə ɪjə

Danny loves ham and pickles.

æjə   æjə   ɪjə

Fran was trapped amid the members.

ɪjə ɪjə   ɪjə ɪjə   æjə   æjə

Chris gripped his fist on the brash young man.

Substitution of /a/ or /ɑ/ for /aɪ/

Remember that /ɑɪ/ is an acceptable allophone of /aɪ/. Record the following list of words and sentences as transcribed. Focus on the Southern substitution.

	Career	*Southern*	*Career*
buy	[baɪ]	[ba]	[baɪ]
	[bɑɪ]	[bɑ]	[bɑɪ]
like	[laɪk]	[lak]	[laɪk]
	[lɑɪk]	[lɑk]	[lɑɪk]
smile	[smaɪl]	[smal]	[smaɪl]
	[smɑɪl]	[smɑl]	[smɑɪl]
hi	[haɪ]	[ha]	[haɪ]
	[hɑɪ]	[hɑ]	[hɑɪ]
try	[traɪ]	[tra]	[traɪ]
	[trɑɪ]	[trɑ]	[trɑɪ]
hide	[haɪd]	[had]	[haɪd]
	[hɑɪd]	[hɑd]	[hɑɪd]
spied	[spaɪd]	[spad]	[spaɪd]
	[spɑɪd]	[spɑd]	[spɑɪd]
tightly	[taɪtlɪ]	[tatlɪ]	[taɪtlɪ]
	[tɑɪtlɪ]	[tɑtlɪ]	[tɑɪtlɪ]
frightful	[fraɪtfʊl]	[fratfʊl]	[fraɪtfʊl]
	[frɑɪtfʊl]	[frɑtfʊl]	[frɑɪtfʊl]

a   a   ah   ə

I saw the brightest smile ever.

      a   a   a

The Blythe building was slightly higher.

a   a   æjə

Hide that frightful hat.

ɪjə   a   a

It's a crime to spy on your neighbors.

    a   a   a

Mr. Hyde tried to like Dr. Jekyll.

Substitution of /ɪ/ for /ɛ/
Before the Nasal Consonants

Record the following list of words and sentences as transcribed. Focus on the Southern substitution.

	Career	*Southern*	*Career*
men	[mɛn]	[mɪn]	[mɛn]
hem	[hɛm]	[hɪm]	[hɛm]
then	[ðɛn]	[ðɪn]	[ðɛn]
friend	[frɛnd]	[frɪnd]	[frɛnd]
blend	[blɛnd]	[blɪnd]	[blɛnd]
Flemish	[flɛmɪʃ]	[flɪmɪʃ]	[flɛmɪʃ]
chemist	[kɛmɪst]	[kɪmɪst]	[kɛmɪst]
lend	[lɛnd]	[lɪnd]	[lɛnd]
spend	[spɛnd]	[spɪnd]	[spɛnd]
phlegm	[flɛm]	[flɪm]	[flɛm]

Blair and Beverly asked for benefits for ten men.

Penny's expensive pendant was stolen.

Ken's intention was to place emphasis on proper words.

French and chemistry were pleasant lessons.

Wendy marked the length of the hem with a pencil.

Substitution of /ə/ for /ɚ/

The New Englander makes this same substitution. As a matter of fact, New Englanders and Southerners share several speech characteristics. See the words and sentences on pp. 263–265.

Substitution of /ɜ/ for /ɝ/

This is another New England characteristic. Refer to the words and sentences on p. 164.

Substitution of /oə/ for /or/

This substitution is also characteristic of the New England dialect. Record the following list of words and sentences as transcribed.

	Career	*Southern*	*Career*
bore	[bor]	[boə]	[bor]
sore	[sor]	[soə]	[sor]
tore	[tor]	[toə]	[tor]
snore	[snor]	[snoə]	[snor]
chore	[tʃor]	[tʃoə]	[tʃor]
more	[mor]	[moə]	[mor]
roar	[ror]	[roə]	[ror]
lore	[lor]	[loə]	[lor]
galore	[gəlor]	[gəloə]	[gəlor]
adore	[ədor]	[ədoə]	[ədor]
shore	[ʃor]	[ʃoə]	[ʃor]

   a   oə   a   oə
I adore watching Dinah Shore.

      oə   ə   oə
What more can be said about dinner chores?

    oə   oə   æjə
He tore the border of the map.

 a   oə   I   oe
I roared at the jokes and then was sore.

   oə   oə   oə
Morley snored at the folklore.

Substitution of /e/ for /ɛ/ Before /r/

Record the following list of words as transcribed.

	Career	*Southern*	*Career*
gregarious	[grəgɛrɪəs]	[grəgerɪəs]	[grəgɛrɪəs]
various	[vɛrɪəs]	[verɪəs]	[vɛrɪəs]
fairy	[fɛrɪ]	[ferɪ]	[fɛrɪ]
variable	[vɛrɪəbl̩]	[verɪəbl̩]	[vɛrɪəbl̩]
dairy	[dɛrɪ]	[derɪ]	[dɛrɪ]

Substitution of /a/ or /ɑ/ for /æ/

This substitution is also characteristic of New England speech. Refer to the word list on p. 263.

Substitution of /æʊ/ for /aʊ/

Refer to the words related to the New York regionalism on p. 271.

Consonants

Omission of /l/ When Followed by a Consonant

This omission is very typical of some Southern dialects. Record the following list of words as transcribed.

	Career	*Southern*	*Career*
film	[fɪlm]	[fɪm]	[fɪlm]
help	[hɛlp]	[hɛp]	[hɛlp]
whelp	[ʍɛlp]	[ʍɛp]	[ʍɛlp]
self	[sɛlf]	[sɛf]	[sɛlf]
alfalfa	[ælfælfə]	[ævfæfə]	[ælfælfə]
themselves	[ðɛmsɛlvz]	[ðɪmsɛvz]	[ðɛmsɛlvz]

Substitution of /n/ for /ŋ/ in "-ing"

This substitution is common in sloppy speech.

	Career	*Southern*	*Career*
singing	[sɪŋɪŋ]	[sɪŋɪn]	[sɪŋɪŋ]
going	[goɪŋ]	[goɪn]	[goɪŋ]
laughing	[læfɪŋ]	[læjəfɪn]	[læfɪŋ]
walking	[wɔkɪŋ]	[wɔkɪn]	[wɔkɪŋ]
driving	[draɪvɪŋ]	[dravɪn]	[draɪvɪŋ]

EXERCISES FOR SOUTHERN AND CAREER SPEECH

1. The following 1775 speech by Patrick Henry was spoken in British English, of course. However, read the speech with the transcribed Southern characteristics.

                         ɜ   æjə   a   ɔ
They tell us, sir, that we are weak—unable to cope with so formidable an

æjə   e   ɪ   o   ə   ɔ
adversary. But when shall we be stronger? Will it be the next week, or the

         jiə   ɪ   a   ə   ɪ
next year? Will it be when we are totally disarmed, and when a British

   a   æu   æjə ə   ɪn   a
guard shall be stationed in every house? Shall we gather strength by irre-

      æjə   æjə
solution and inaction?

In the following sentences, the sounds substituted in Southern speech are transcribed above the appropriate letters.

    a a   ɪjə ɪn   ɪjə   æjə
2. I like sipping on mint juleps on the veranda.

   æjə   ə æjə ɪ   a   æu ɪjə
3. Pat never had any anxiety about it.

   a   a   a ɪjə ɜ   oə   ɪjə   ɪn
4. My, my, my, it certainly is warm this evening.

   a   æjə   ɜ   æjə   æjə   ə
5. I'm as nervous as a long-tailed cat in a room full of rockers.

   a   æjə   oə   æjə
6. Mighty glad to see you this morning, ma'am.

  a ɪ ɪjə   a   ɪjə
7. I can fix things up right quick.

   a a   a   oə   æ   a
8. Hi! I'm Dinah from North Carolina.

    ɪ   ɪ   a   a   a   ɪ
9. Gentlemen, may I remind you, there are ladies present.

     a   ɜ   ɪn   ɜ   ɪn
10. Where are the Worthingtons of Birmingham?

  ejə æjə   ə
11. Well, at his age it ought to be clear!

Place the phonetic transcription above the appropriate letters to reflect a Southern accent in the following exercises. Then record them with the Southern pronunciation.

12. Women can take more time cause they've got more of it to take: like I told

you, vital statistics don't lie and they have established the fact that the av-

erage woman outlives the average man by a good ten years. At least! That

explains their total disregard of time coming and going, when a man's wait-

ing for them. They secretly, in their subconscious, enjoy! revel!—in their extra ten years on earth, and secretly enjoy the revel in the man's rapid decline.

From THE FROSTED GLASS COFFIN   *Tennessee Williams*

13. Richard Henry Lee:

I'll leave tonight—why, hell, right now, if y'like! I'll stop off at Stratford just long enough to refresh the missus, and then straight to the matter. Virginia, the land that gave us our glorious commander-in-chief, George Washington, will now give the continent its proposal on independence. And when Virginia proposes, the South is bound to follow, and where the South goes the Middle Colonies go! Gentlemen, a salute! To Virginia, the Mother of American Independence.

From 1776   *Peter Stone*

14. Birdie:

Me, young? Maybe you better find Simon and tell him to do it himself. He's to look in my desk, the left drawer, and bring my music album right away. Mr. Marshall is very anxious to see it because of his father and the opera in Chicago. Mr. Marshall is a polite man with his manners and very educated and cultured, and I've told him all about how my mama and papa used to go to Europe for the music.

From THE LITTLE FOXES   *Lillian Hellman*

15. "That's a fact," Ratliff said. "A fellow can dodge a Snopes if he just starts lively enough. In fact, I don't believe he would have to pass more than two folks before he would have another victim intervened betwixt them. You folks ain't going to buy them things, sho enough, are you?"

From SPOTTED HORSES   *William Faulkner*

16. Amanda:

Ella Cartwright? This is Amanda Wingfield. How are you, honey? How is that kidney infection? Horrors. . . . You're a Christian martyr, yes, honey, that's what you are, a Christian martyr.

From THE GLASS MENAGERIE   *Tennessee Williams*

17. Charlie:

I belong to tradition. I am a "legend." Known from one end of the Delta to the other. From the Peabody Hotel in Memphis to Cat-Fish Row in Vicks-burg. Mistuh Charlie—"Mistuh Charlie"! Who knows you? What do you represent? A line of goods of doubtful value.

From THE LAST OF MY SOLID GOLD WATCHES   *Tennessee Williams*

18. The author in the following speech attempts to indicate the Southern dialect through spelling. There are, however, additional sound substitutions that you should indicate.

Cherie:

I dunno why I keep expectin' m'self to fall in love with someone, but I do.

I'm beginnin' to seriously wonder if there is the kinda love I have in mind.

I'm oney nineteen, but I been goin' with guys since I was fourteen. In fact,

I almost married a cousin of mine when I was fourteen, but Pappy wouldn't

have it.

From BUS STOP   *William Inge*

GENERAL AMERICAN

Although General American speech is a much debated and, according to some experts, dated term, it has been deliberately chosen to indicate the speech gen-erally used in the Midwest, West, and Northwest. General American contains the least number of distinguishing characteristics. Although career speech is not synonymous with General American speech, there are some similarities.

Vowels and Diphthongs

Use of /ɔ/ between /w/ and /r/

	General American and Career
war	[wɔr]
warrant	[wɔrənt]
warble	[wɔrbl̩]
ward	[wɔrd]
warn	[wɔrn]
warp	[wɔrp]
Warsaw	[wɔrsɔ]

wart   [wɔrt]

warmth   [wɔrmθ]

Addition of /r/ after /ɔ/

This error, which is considered substandard, is not characteristic of most Midwestern speech. For professional purposes, however, it is a useful combination. Use negative practice in the following list of words.[2]

	Career	General American	Career
wash	[wɔʃ]	[wɔrʃ]	[wɔʃ]
Washington	[wɔʃɪŋtən]	[wɔrʃɪŋtən]	[wɔʃɪŋtən]
cautious	[kɔʃəs]	[kɔrʃəs]	[kɔʃəs]
washroom	[wɔʃrum]	[wɔrʃrum]	[wɔʃrum]
caution	[kɔʃən]	[kɔrʃən]	[kɔʃən]
squaw	[skwɔ]	[skwɔr]	[skwɔ]
squalor	[skwɔlɚ]	[skwɔrlɚ]	[skwɔlɚ]
squash	[skwɔʃ]	[skwɔrʃ]	[skwɔʃ]

Use of /wɑ/ Instead of /wɔ/

Record the following list of words transcribed into General American and New England dialects. Either pronunciation is acceptable.

	General American	New England
wobble	[wɑbl̩]	[wɔbl̩]
wad	[wɑd]	[wɔd]
waddle	[wɑdl̩]	[wɔdl̩]
water	[wɑtɚ]	[wɔtɚ]
Waldorf	[wɑldɔrf]	[wɔldɔrf]
walk	[wɑk]	[wɔk]
wash	[wɑʃ]	[wɔʃ]
Wallace	[wɑləs]	[wɔləs]
wallet	[wɑlət]	[wɔlət]

---

[2]The vowel /ɑ/ (as in *father*) could also be used in career speech in some of these words.

wampum	[wɑmpəm]	[wɔmpəm]
watch	[wɑtʃ]	[wɔtʃ]

Use of /ɝ/ for /ʌr/

Compare the General American and Southern/New England pronunciations. The Southern/New England pronunciation is recommended for stage and television.

	General American	*Southern/ New England*
hurry	[hɝɪ]	[hʌrɪ]
worry	[wɝɪ]	[wʌrɪ]
hurricane	[hɝəken]	[hʌrəken]
curry	[kɝɪ]	[kʌrɪ]
burrow	[bɝo]	[bʌro]
skurry	[skɝɪ]	[skʌrɪ]
furrow	[fɝo]	[fʌro]
Murray	[mɝɪ]	[mʌrɪ]
flurry	[flɝɪ]	[flʌrɪ]
surry	[sɝɪ]	[sʌrɪ]

Use of /ɽ/ for /r/

The semivowel /ɽ/ is produced like the /r/ but with the tongue tip excessively curled and extremely tense. The elevated tip is placed too far back. Midwesterners are often told that they use too much "r" in their speech. Sometimes the sound is referred to as the Midwestern "burr." In the following word lists, refresh your New England accent. To obtain career speech, some Northerners and Midwesterners will need to relax the tongue tip.

	New England	*General American*	*Career*
barn	[ban]	[bɑɽn]	[bɑrn]
far	[fa]	[fɑɽ]	[fɑr]
heart	[hat]	[hɑɽt]	[hɑrt]
farmer	[famə]	[fɑɽmɚ]	[fɑrmɚ]
park	[pak]	[pɑɽk]	[pɑrk]
alarm	[əlam]	[əlɑɽm]	[əlɑrm]

chart	[tʃat]	[tʃɑɾt]	[tʃɑrt]
hearty	[hatɪ]	[hɑɾtɪ]	[hɑrtɪ]
sparse	[spas]	[spɑɾs]	[spɑrs]
yard	[jad]	[jɑɾd]	[jɑrd]

Misenunciated /ɝ/

Sometimes General American speakers round their lips too much and elevate the tongue tip too high when enunciating /ɝ/ (as in "her"). The symbol for too much rounding is [͜], and an overly elevated tongue is indicated by [˔]. Use negative practice in the following word list.

	Career	*General American*	*Career*
heard	[hɝd]	[hɝ˔d]	[hɝd]
flirt	[flɝt]	[flɝ˔t]	[flɝt]
word	[wɝd]	[wɝ˔d]	[wɝd]
mirth	[mɝθ]	[mɝ˔θ]	[mɝθ]
spurt	[spɝt]	[spɝ˔t]	[spɝt]
worm	[wɝm]	[wɝ˔m]	[wɝm]
earthy	[ɝθɪ]	[ɝ˔θɪ]	[ɝθɪ]
murder	[mɝdɚ]	[mɝ˔dɚ]	[mɝdɚ]
swerve	[swɝv]	[swɝ˔v]	[swɝv]
bird	[bɝd]	[bɝ˔d]	[bɝd]

Use of /ɑ/ for /a/

In General American Speech, the production of /ɑ/ is often excessively tense, indicated by [ɑ̧]. Use negative practice as you pronounce the following words.

	Career	*General American*	*Career*
Bob	[bɑb], [bɒb]	[bɑ̧b]	[bɑb], [bɒb]
cot	[kɑt], [kɒt]	[kɑ̧t]	[kɑt], [kɒt]
cod	[kɑd], [kɒd]	[kɑ̧d]	[kɑd], [kɒd]
Tom	[tɑm], [tɒm]	[tɑ̧m]	[tɑm], [tɒm]

hot	[hɑt], [hɒt]	[hɑt]	[hɑt], [hɒt]
pod	[pɑd], [pɒd]	[pɑd]	[pɑd], [pɒd]
Spot	[spɑt], [spɒt]	[spɑt]	[spɑt], [spɒt]
pond	[pɑnd], [pɒnd]	[pɑnd]	[pɑnd], [pɒnd]

EXERCISE USING DIALECTS

The familiar soliloquy from *Hamlet* is transcribed for all of the regionalisms discussed in this chapter. Record each one of them. Read the phonetic transcriptions as presented. Then compare your habitual reading with career speech.

To be, or not to be,—that is the question:—
Whether 'tis nobler in the mind to suffer
The slings and arrows of outrageous fortune,
Or to take arms against a sea of troubles,
And by opposing end them?

1. New England

tə bi ɒ nɒt tə bi   ðæt ɪz ðə kwestʃən
To be, or not to be,—that is the question:—

ʍɛðə   tɪz noblə ɪn ðə maɪnd tə sʌfə
Whether 'tis nobler in the mind to suffer

ðə slɪŋz æn æroz əv autredʒɪs fɒtʃun
The slings and arrows of outrageous fortune,

ɒ tu tek amz əgɛnst ə si əv trʌblz
Or to take arms against a sea of troubles,

ænd baɪ əpozɪŋ ɛn ðɛm
And by opposing end them?

2. New York City

tə bi oə nɑt tə bi   ðɛət ɪz ðə kwestʃən
To be, or not to be,—that is the question:—

ʍɛðə   tɪz nɛublə ɪn ðə mɒɪnd tə sʌfə
Whether 'tis nobler in the mind to suffer

ðə slɪŋz ænd ɛərɛuz əv æutredʒəs fɔrtʃun
The slings and arrows of outrageous fortune,

oə tu tek ɔmz əgɛnst ə si əv trʌblz
Or to take arms against a sea of troubles,

æn bɒɪ əpɛuzɪŋ ɛn ðɛm
And by opposing end them?

3. Southern

tə bi oə nɑt tə bi   ðæjət ıjəz ðə kwɛstʃən
To be, or not to be,—that is the question:—

ʍɛðə   tıjəz nɛublə ıjən ðə maınd tə sʌfə
Whether ' tis nobler in the mind to suffer

ðə slıŋz æjən æjəroz əv æutreıʤəs foətʃun
The slings and arrows of outrageous fortune,

oə tu tek amz əgınst ə si əv trʌblz
Or to take arms against a sea of troubles,

æjənd ba əpɛuzıŋ ınd ðım
And by opposing end them?

4. General American

tə bi ɔɾ nɑt tə bi   ðæt ız ðə kwɛstʃən
To be, or not to be ,—that is the question:—

wɛðɚ˞ˌ tız noblɚˌ ın ðə maınd tə sʌfɚˌ
Whether 'tis nobler in the mind to suffer

ðə slıŋz ænd æɾoz ɑv autɾeʤıs fɔɾtʃun
The slings and arrows of outrageous fortune,

ɔɾ tu tek ɑɾmz əgɛnst ə si əv trʌblz
Or to take arms against a sea of troubles,

ænd baı əpozıŋ ɛnd ðɛm
And by opposing end them?

5. Career Speech

tə bi or nɑt tə bi   ðæt ız ðə kwɛstʃən
To be, or not to be,—that is the question:—

ʍɛðɚ tız noblɚ ın ðə maınd tə sʌfɚ
Whether 'tis nobler in the mind to suffer

ðə slıŋz ænd æɾouz əv autreʤəs fortʃun
The slings and arrows of outrageous fortune,

or tə tek ɑɾmz əgɛnst ə si əv trʌblz
Or to take arms against a sea of troubles,

ænd baı əpozıŋ ɛnd ðɛm
And by opposing end them?

12

STAGE SPEECH
AND SELECTED
FOREIGN
ACCENTS

GLOSSARY

Ear Training   The process of developing hearing acuity; good ear training contributes to the ability to distinguish sounds.

Glottalization   Stopping the breath at the glottis (space between the true vocal folds); an articulation that involves the use of the glottis; characteristics of Scottish and Cockney dialects.

Intervocalic /ɾ/   The one-tap trilled /r/ linking one syllable or word to another.

Stage Speech (London Speech)   Professional speech used by vocally trained actors in plays that benefit aesthetically from the use of a standard British accent.

You may wonder what a discussion of stage diction and foreign accents is doing in a basic text on voice and articulation. Since this text focuses on career speech, it is fundamental that stage diction and foreign accents be included for actors as well as for professionals in communications (such as radio and television announcers). This chapter is also helpful for individuals for whom English is a second language and thus whose English pronunciation is influenced by their primary language. **Ear training**, as well as the kinetic awareness of sound production, is valuable in learning the English language.

This chapter focuses on the influence of foreign languages on American-English pronunciation. By no means an exhaustive discussion, it is meant to introduce the subject to the student. Texts are available that deal exclusively with foreign dialects as well as English as a second language. In addition, with the growing interest in international communication, it is increasingly important for Americans, many of whom speak no foreign language, to become aware of foreign languages, customs, and cultures.

There are sounds represented in the IPA that are present in foreign languages but not in English. For example, the German language contains the vowel /y/, which is the first vowel in the word "grüssen." The umlaut (the two dots over the vowel) indicates a different pronunciation from the "u" without the umlaut. The vowel /y/ does not exist in English. Therefore, an American learning German has difficulty with this sound and, even with proper ear training and practice, can only approximate the correct pronunciation. Conversely, some sounds in English present problems for the German speaker learning English, such as the English /θ/ and /ð/, because they do not exist in German.

In developing a foreign accent for performance, there are two major considerations. First, select the most characteristic aspects—do not attempt to present all the vocal idiosyncracies. Yes, you want authenticity, but not at the expense of intelligibility. Second, be consistent in using the speech characteristics that you have chosen. Any audience is quick to pick up a lack of consistency.

To use accurately in performance any of the dialects discussed below, you must study the rhythm, pitch changes, tempo, and other acoustical phenomena in that dialect. Since it is virtually impossible to describe all these aspects in print, you should listen to recordings by professional performers so that you can learn these nonphonemic aspects.

STANDARD STAGE SPEECH

You will certainly discover that there are many similarities between career speech and standard stage speech. You will remember that career speech does not come from a particular area of the United States. Standard **stage speech**, also called *London Speech,* is the speech that should be used in a play requiring a British dialect. Stage speech is the speech often used in British plays or plays in translation (both classic and modern) when a particular dialect is unnecessary.

For most American plays, standard stage speech would be out of place. For example, a production of Kaufman and Hart's *The Man Who Came to Dinner* would not use stage speech, although certain characters could use it.

Career speech and stage speech are not synonymous. Both, however, represent the best standards of American and British English.

Vowels and Diphthongs

Substitution of /ɜʊ/ for /oʊ/

The sound /ɜʊ/ can be achieved by rounding the /o/ (as in *go*) even more, tensing both the lips, and keeping the tongue tip behind the lower teeth. Record the following list of words and sentences as transcribed. Focus your attention on the difference between career and stage speech.

	Career	*Stage*	*Career*
go	[goʊ]	[gɜʊ]	[goʊ]
slow	[sloʊ]	[slɜʊ]	[sloʊ]
whole	[hoʊl]	[hɜʊl]	[hoʊl]
home	[hoʊm]	[hɜʊm]	[hoʊm]
toe	[toʊ]	[tɜʊ]	[toʊ]
spoken	[spoʊkən]	[spɜʊkən]	[spoʊkən]

In the following sentences, the substitution of /ɜʊ/ for /oʊ/ is notated above the appropriate letters. Use career speech, stage speech, and then career speech.

    ɜʊ   ɜʊ   ɜʊ
I told you, Mona, I won't do it!

     ɜʊ   ɜʊ
Noone stole the Holmes book.

        ɜʊ ɜʊ
The wind is so cold.

   ɜʊ   ɜʊ
Noel, fold the napkin properly.

      ɜʊ   ɜʊ   ɜʊ
The ghost roamed through the whole house.

Production of /ɔ/ with Tongue Elevated

Compared with career speech, the tongue is placed higher in stage speech with pronouncing /ɔ/, in a position similar to that for /o/ (as in *go*).

	Career	*Stage*	*Career*
fall	[fɔl]	[fɔ⊥l]	[fɔl]
cough	[kɔf]	[kɔ⊥f]	[kɔf]
lost	[lɔst]	[lɔ⊥st]	[lɔst]
taught	[tɔt]	[tɔ⊥t]	[tɔt]
naughty	[nɔtɪ]	[nɔ⊥tɪ]	[nɔtɪ]

In the following sentences, the variation of /ɔ/ is notated above the appropriate letters. Use stage speech between two career speech pronunciations.

    ɔ˔   ɔ˔   ɔ˔
Thomas's daughter was getting increasingly naughty.

     ɔ˔   ɔ˔
He taught the coughing students.

   ɔ˔   ɔ˔   ɔ˔
Toss the ball to Flossie.

     ɔ˔   ɔ˔
The mauling tiger was painted on the wall.

  ɔ˔   ɔ˔
Call to the sailors on the yawl.

Use of /ɑ/ for /æ/

In stage speech /ɑ/ (as in *father*) is used in many words where /æ/ (as in *cat*) is used in career speech. New Englanders substitute /ɑ/ for /æ/ in the same words. In the following list of words, compare the pronunciations.

	New England	Stage	Career
laugh	[lɑf]	[lɑf]	[læf]
bath	[bɑθ]	[bɑθ]	[bæθ]
half	[hɑf]	[hɑf]	[hæf]
last	[lɑst]	[lɑst]	[læst]
aunt	[ɑnt]	[ɑnt]	[ænt]
fast	[fɑst]	[fɑst]	[fæst]
cast	[kɑst]	[kɑst]	[kæst]
passed	[pɑst]	[pɑst]	[pæst]
calf	[kɑf]	[kɑf]	[kæf]
flask	[flɑsk]	[flɑsk]	[flæsk]

Stage speech retains /æ/ in the following phonetic environments:

1. before /ʃ/ (for example, *cash* [kæʃ], *gash* [gæʃ], and *flash* [flæʃ]),

2. before the letters "ct" (for example, *fact* [fækt] and *actor* [æktə]),

3. before the nasals /m/ and /n/ except in the words *dance* and *chance* (for example, *fan* [fæn] and *dandy* [dændɪ]), and

4. in "and" words except *demand* and *command* (pronounced [dɪmɑnd] and [kəmɑnd]).

Substitution of /ɜ/ for /ɝ/

See the words and drills on p. 164.

Substitution of /ə/ for /ɚ/

See the words and drills on pp. 263–265.

Substitution of /ɒ/ for /ɑ/

See the words and drills on p. 186.

Consonants

Use of Intervocalic /ɾ/

The one-tap trilled /r/ (/ɾ/) is used to link one syllable to another or at the end of a word when the next word begins with a vowel. This is also called the **intervocalic** /ɾ/.

	Career	*Stage*	*Career*
very	[vɛɾɪ]	[vɛɾɪ]	[vɛɾɪ]
sorry	[sɔɾɪ]	[sɔˑɾɪ]	[sɔɾɪ]
worry	[wʌɾɪ]	[wʌɾɪ]	[wʌɾɪ]
syrup	[sɪrəp]	[sɪɾəp]	[sɪrəp]
lyric	[lɪrɪk]	[lɪɾɪk]	[lɪɾɪk]
choric	[korɪk]	[kɔˑɾɪk]	[korɪk]
virile	[vɪrəl]	[vɪɾɑɪl]	[vɪrəl]
irrigate	[ɪrəget]	[ɪɾəget]	[ɪɾəget]
irritate	[ɪrətet]	[ɪɾətet]	[ɪɾətet]
pyramid	[pɪrəmɪd]	[pɪɾəmɪd]	[pɪɾəmɪd]
marry	[mæɾɪ]	[mæɾɪ]	[mæɾɪ]
merry	[mɛrɪ]	[mɛɾɪ]	[mɛɾɪ]

Say the following phrases and sentences using the intervocalic /r/ (/ɾ/):

far into the forest [fɑɾ ɪntu ðə fɔˑrəst]

her intention [həɾ ɪntɛnʃɪn]

fear of the Merry Men [fɪɾ əv ðə mɛɾɪ mɛn]

Steer it straight. [stɪɾ ɪt stret]

Here it is. [hɪɾ ɪt ɪz]

Maura is a Sister of Mercy. [mɔ˔ɾə ɪz ə sɪstəɾ əv mɜsɪ]

The Nile River is in Africa. [ðə nɑɪl rɪvəɾ ɪz ɪn ɑfɾɪkə]

EXERCISES FOR STAGE SPEECH

The following is a list of common British words that are pronounced differently than in American English. Record the words as you would pronounce them in American English and then as they are transcribed in stage speech.

either [ɑɪðə]

neither [nɑɪðə]

been [bin]

nephew [nɛvju]

again [əgen]

against [əgenst]

barrage [bæɾɑʒ]

garage [gæɾɑʒ]

massage [mæsɑʒ]

tomato [təmɑto]

tissue [tɪsju]

schedule [ʃɛdjʊl]

lieutenant [lɛftɛnənt]

In the following selections, transcribe the stage substitutions above the appropriate letters. The intervocalic /ɾ/ has already been supplied. Record the entire selection. Work to increase speed, which will help to ease any self-consciousness.

1. Once upon a midnight dreary, while I pondered, weak and weary, (ɾ above "dreary" and "weary")

   Over many a quaint and curious volume of forgotten lore— (ɾ above "curious")

   While I nodded, nearly napping, suddenly there came a tapping,

As of someone gently rapping, rapping at my chamber door—

Only this and nothing more.

From THE RAVEN   *Edgar Allan Poe*

2. Speak the speech, I pray you, as I pronounced it to you, trippingly on the

   tongue: but if you mouth it, as many of your players do, I had as lief the

   town crier spoke my lines. Nor do not saw the air too much with your hand

   thus; but use all gently; for in the very torrent, tempest, and, as I may say,

   whirlwind of your passion, you must acquire and beget a temperance that

   may give it smoothness. O, it offends me to the soul to hear a robustious

   periwig-pated fellow tear a passion to tatters, to very rags, to split the ears of

   the groundlings, who for the most part are capable of nothing but inexplic-

   able dumb shows and noise.

   From HAMLET   *William Shakespeare*

3. Lady Bracknell:

   I'm sorry if we were a little late, Algernon, but I was obliged to call on dear

   Lady Hadbury. I hadn't been there since her poor husband's death. I never

   saw a woman so altered; she looks quite twenty years younger. And now

   I'll have a cup of tea, and one of those nice cucumber sandwiches you prom-

   ised me.

   From THE IMPORTANCE OF BEING EARNEST   *Oscar Wilde*

4. If a Hottentot taught a Hottentot tot

   To talk ere the tot could totter,

   Ought the Hottentot tot be taught to say aught,

Or naught,

Or what ought to be taught her?

5. Julie:

You've never traveled, Kristin. You should go abroad and see the world.

You've no idea how nice it is traveling by train . . . new faces all the time

and new countries. On our way through Hamburg we'll go to the zoo—

you'll love that—and we'll go to the theatre and the opera too . . . and when

we get to Munich there'll be the museums, dear, and pictures by Rubens and

Raphael—the great painters, you know. . . . You've heard of Munich,

haven't you? Where King Ludwig lived—you know—the king who went

mad. . . . We'll see his castles.

From MISS JULIE   *August Strindberg*

6. One I love,

Two I love,

Three I love I say,

Four I love with all my heart,

Five I cast away.

Six he loves,

Seven she loves,

Eight they want to wed,

Nine they tarry,

Ten they marry

Is what the daisy said.

Anonymous

COCKNEY

Since a great deal of literature has been written for the character with a cockney accent, we have included the cockney dialect in this chapter.

Vowels and Diphthongs

Substitution of /aʊ/ for /o/ and /oʊ/

This substitution is very characteristic of cockney. Record the list of words and sentences, focusing on the difference between career speech and cockney.

	Career	*Cockney*	*Career*
don't	[doʊnt]	[daʊnt]	[doʊnt]
grown	[groʊn]	[graʊn]	[groʊn]
bloat	[bloʊt]	[blaʊt]	[bloʊt]
sold	[soʊld]	[saʊld]	[soʊld]
stove	[stoʊv]	[staʊv]	[stoʊv]
cold	[koʊld]	[kaʊld]	[koʊld]
row	[roʊ]	[raʊ]	[roʊ]
soap	[soʊp]	[saʊp]	[soʊp]
most	[moʊst]	[maʊst]	[moʊst]
rogue	[roʊg]	[raʊg]	[roʊg]

      aʊ   aʊ
Hold the soap in your hands.

     aʊ   aʊ   aʊ
Flossie sold the stove to the rogue.

   aʊ   aʊ
Most of the kitchen was moldy with ashes.

  aʊ   aʊ   aʊ   aʊ
Row, row, row your boat.

      aʊ   aʊ
Some folks like to take to the high roads.

Substitution of /ʌɪ/ for /i/

This substitution is sometimes difficult for the American to produce. Do not confuse it with /aɪ/. Record the following list of words and sentences. Focus on the difference between /i/ and /ʌɪ/.

	Career	*Cockney*	*Career*
me	[mi]	[mʌɪ]	[mi]
eager	[igɚ]	[ʌɪgə]	[igɚ]

agreed [əgrid] [əgrʌɪd] [əgrid]

meet [mit] [mʌɪt] [mit]

scene [sin] [sʌɪn] [sin]

feet [fit] [fʌɪt] [fit]

kneel [nil] [nʌɪl] [nil]

beach [bitʃ] [bʌɪtʃ] [bitʃ]

sleep [slip] [slʌɪp] [slip]

please [pliz] [plʌɪz] [pliz]

ʌɪ   au   ʌɪ
Please don't sleep.

ʌɪ   ʌɪ   ʌɪ
Eve feels defeated.

ʌɪ   ʌɪ   ʌɪ
Lee's a conceited beast!

ʌɪ   ʌɪ au
She didn't believe the machine broke.

ʌɪ   ʌɪ   ʌɪ   ɔː
Jean heeded the team's warning.

Substitution of /aɪ/ for /e/ and /eɪ/

This is one of the most common characteristics of the cockney dialect. Record the following list of words and sentences, focusing on the difference between career speech and cockney.

	Career	*Cockney*	*Career*
stay	[steɪ]	[staɪ]	[steɪ]
wait	[weɪt]	[waɪt]	[weɪt]
great	[greɪt]	[graɪt]	[greɪt]
fail	[feɪl]	[faɪl]	[feɪl]
sale	[seɪl]	[saɪl]	[seɪl]
mail	[meɪl]	[maɪl]	[meɪl]
sake	[seɪk]	[saɪk]	[seɪk]
famous	[feɪməs]	[faɪməs]	[feɪməs]
faith	[feɪθ]	[faɪf]	[feɪθ]
waist	[weɪst]	[waɪst]	[weɪst]

aɪ   aɪ   au
I'm afraid she stayed at home.

aɪ   aɪ   aɪ
James made a mistake.

aɪ au aɪ aɪ
Ray ~~h~~ad no faith in the tale.

aɪ aɪ
Vicki wasted the cake.

aɪ aɪ au aɪ
The famous star paid no attention to Blake.

Substitution of /ɛ/ for /æ/

	Career	*Cockney*	*Career*
taxi	[tæksɪ]	[tɛksɪ]	[tæksɪ]
am	[æm]	[ɛm]	[æm]
hand	[hænd]	[ɛnd]	[hænd]
back	[bæk]	[bɛk]	[bæk]
grapple	[græpl̩]	[grɛpl̩]	[græpl̩]
pan	[pæn]	[pɛn]	[pæn]
wrap	[ræp]	[rɛp]	[ræp]
lad	[læd]	[lɛd]	[læd]
hat	[hæt]	[ɛt]	[hæt]
that	[ðæt]	[vɛt]	[ðæt]

ɛ ɛ ɛ ɛ
Andrea, ~~h~~ave some ~~h~~am and eggs.

ɛ ɛ ɛ
Becka sat in the back of the taxi.

ɛ ɛ ɛ ɛ
~~H~~ey, laddy, ~~h~~an~~d~~ me the fancy pants.

au au ʌɪ ɛ ɛ ɛ
Joe, don't be mad at dad.

ɛ ɛ ɒ ˇ ɛ
Dan, put my ~~h~~at on the rack.

Substitution of /ɑ/ for /ʌ/

Record this straightforward substitution in the following list of words and sentences. Focus on the differences between career speech and cockney.

	Career	*Cockney*	*Career*
love	[lʌv]	[lɑv]	[lʌv]
butter	[bʌtɚ]	[bɑtə]	[bʌtɚ]
mummy	[mʌmɪ]	[mɑmɪ]	[mʌmɪ]
mother	[mʌðɚ]	[mɑvə]	[mʌðɚ]

flutter	[flʌtɚ]	[flɑtə]	[flʌtɚ]
judge	[dʒʌdʒ]	[dʒɑdʒ]	[dʒʌdʒ]
luck	[lʌk]	[lɑk]	[lʌk]
cut	[kʌt]	[kɑt]	[kʌt]
nutty	[nʌtɪ]	[nɑtɪ]	[nʌtɪ]
duck	[dʌk]	[dɑk]	[dʌk]

ɑ   ɑ   ɑ   ɑ
Mummy, carve the lucky duck.

ɑ   ə   ɑ   ɑ
She loves her husband, the judge.

ɑ   ɑ ʋ ə ɑ
Drink from some other jug.

aʊ   ɛ   ɑ   ɑ
The old man rubbed his stomach.

ʌɪ   ɛ   ɑ   ɑ f
Steve had done nothing wrong.

Substitution of /ɒɪ/ for /aɪ/ or /ɑɪ/

This substitution is evident in some New York speech. Record the following list of words and sentences. Focus on the differences between career speech and cockney.

	Career	*Cockney*	*Career*
spy	[spaɪ]	[spɒɪ]	[spaɪ]
alive	[əlaɪv]	[əlɒɪv]	[əlaɪv]
crime	[kraɪm]	[krɒɪm]	[kraɪm]
abide	[əbaɪd]	[əbɒɪd]	[əbaɪd]
china	[tʃaɪnə]	[tʃɒɪnə]	[tʃaɪnə]
apply	[əplaɪ]	[əplɒɪ]	[əplaɪ]
file	[faɪl]	[fɒɪl]	[faɪl]
light	[laɪt]	[lɒɪt]	[laɪt]
rhyme	[raɪm]	[rɒɪm]	[raɪm]
quite	[kwaɪt]	[kwɒɪt]	[kwaɪt]

ɒɪ aɪ   ɛ   aɪ
Friday is fish and chips day.

ɛ   ɒɪ   ɒɪ   ɜ
Look at the stripes on the guide's shirt.

ɒɪ   aɪ ɒɪ
There's quite a lot of daylight left.

^{DI}   ^{DI}   ^{DI}
In the night, silence is sublime.

^ə   ^{DI}   ^ɛ ^{DI}
My father is the wisest man alive.

Substitution of /æʊ/ for /ɑʊ/ or /aʊ/

Refer to the drills on pp. 190–193.

Substitution of /ə/ for /ɝ/

Refer to the drills on pp. 263–268.

Substitution of /ɜ/ for /ɝ/

Refer to the discussion on p. 169 and the /ɝ/ word list and Exercises on pp. 265–268.

Consonants

Substitution of Glottal Stop [ʔ] for /h/ Before Initial Vowels

Glottalization is an articulation that involves the use of the space between the vocal folds. Record the following list of words and sentences. Feel the stoppage of breath at the larynx.

	Career	*Cockney*	*Career*
half	[hæf]	[ʔɑf]	[hæf]
habit	[hæbɪt]	[ʔɑbɪt]	[hæbɪt]
Harry	[hærɪ]	[ʔɑɾɪ]	[hærɪ]
handsome	[hænsəm]	[ʔansəm]	[hænsəm]
hold	[hold]	[ʔaʊld]	[hold]
heaven	[hɛvən]	[ʔɛvm̩]	[hɛvən]
heard	[hɝd]	[ʔɜd]	[hɝd]
hand	[hænd]	[ʔɛnd]	[hænd]
high	[haɪ]	[ʔɒɪ]	[haɪ]
happy	[hæpɪ]	[ʔɛpɪ]	[hæpɪ]

^{ʔæʊ}   ^{ʔæʊ}   ^{ɑɾ}
H̸ow about it, H̸arry?

^ʔ   ^{ʔʌɪ}
The h̸ospital was h̸eated.

ˀ ə ˀ ˀɑ
Whoever did that ʰas no ʰeaʳt.

æʊ ʌɪ ˀəʳ ˀɑ
Anyʰow she's left ʰer ʰusband!

ˀʌɪ ˀɪ ˀ ˇ ˀɪ ˀɛ
ʰe ʰit ʰer with ʰis ʰand.

Substitution of [ˀ] for Medial and Final /t/

	Career	*Cockney*	*Career*
bitter	[bɪtɚ]	[bɪˀə]	[bɪtɚ]
battle	[bætl̩]	[bɛˀl̩]	[bætl̩]
matter	[mætɚ]	[mɛˀə]	[mætɚ]
butter	[bʌtɚ]	[baˀə]	[bʌtɚ]
cattle	[kætl̩]	[kɛˀl̩]	[kætl̩]
bottle	[batl̩]	[bɒˀl̩]	[batl̩]
metal	[mɛtl̩]	[mɛˀl̩]	[mɛtl̩]
better	[bɛtɚ]	[bɛˀə]	[bɛtɚ]
got it	[gat ɪt]	[gɒˀ ɪˀ]	[gat ɪt]
sit on	[sɪt ɑn]	[sɪˀ ɒn]	[sɪt ɑn]
put it	[pʊt ɪt]	[pʊˀ ɪˀ]	[pʊt ɪt]

Substitution of /f/ for /θ/ and /v/ for /ð/

Record the following words and make the suggested substitution.

	Career	*Cockney*	*Career*
whether	[ʍɛðɚ]	[wɛvə]	[ʍɛðɚ]
leather	[lɛðɚ]	[lɛvə]	[lɛðɚ]
with us	[wɪð əs]	[wɪv əs]	[wɪð əs]
birthday	[bɝθdeɪ]	[bɝfdaɪ]	[bɝθdeɪ]
both of us	[boθ əv ʌs]	[bof əv as]	[boθ əv ʌs]
smother	[smʌðɚ]	[smavə]	[smʌðɚ]
something	[sʌmθɪŋ]	[samfɪŋk]	[sʌmθɪŋ]
father	[faðɚ]	[favə]	[faðɚ]
mother	[mʌðɚ]	[mavə]	[mʌðɚ]
worth it	[wɝθ ɪt]	[wɝf ɪˀ]	[wɝθ ɪt]

EXERCISES FOR A COCKNEY ACCENT

1. Read the following poem with a cockney accent. As you read the poem aloud, remember that it must be understood by an audience. The poet has not included all of the sound substitutions. Transcribe cockney sounds above the appropriate letters.

A muvver was barfin' [bathing] 'er biby one night,

The youngest of ten and a tiny young mite,

The muvver was poor and the biby was thin,

Only a skelington covered in skin;

The muvver turned rahned for the soap off the rack,

She was but a moment, but when turned back,

The biby was gorn; and in anguish she cried,

"Oh, where is my biby?"—The angels replied:

"Your biby 'as fell dahn the plug-ole,

Your biby 'as forn dahn the plug;

The poor little thing was so skinny and thin

'E oughter been barfed in a jug;

Your biby is perfeckly 'appy,

'E won't need a barf any more,

Your biby 'as fell dahn the plug-ole,

Not lorst, but gorn before."

BIBY'S EPITAPH *Anonymous*

2. The following is a portion of "Gunga Din" by Rudyard Kipling. The first stanza is transcribed into phonetics. Transcribe the second stanza. (The refrain has been omitted.) As you rerecord the selection, increase your speed and work for continuity and proper inflection.

jə maɪ tɔ: ə ʤɪn ən bɪə
You may talk o' gin and beer

wɛn jə kwɔʔəd saɪf æuʔ ɪə
When you're quartered safe out 'ere,

ɛn jə sɛnt tə pɛnɪ fɒɪts ən ɔ:dəʃɒʔ ɪʔ
An' you're sent to penny fights an' Aldershot it;

bəʔ wɛn ɪʔ kɑmz tə slɔʔə
But when it comes to slaughter

jə wɪ du jɔ wɜk ɒn wɒʔə
You will do your work on water,

ɛn jəl lɪk və blɪumɪn buts əv əm vɛts gɒʔ ɪʔ
An' you'll lick the bloomin' boots of 'im that's got it.

næʊ ɪn ɪndʒəz sɑnɪ klɒɪm
Now in Injia's sunny clime,

wɛr ɒɪ just tə spɛn mɒɪ tɒɪm
Where I used to spend my time

ə sɜvɪn əv ər mɛdʒɛstɪ və kwʌɪn
A-servin' of 'Er Majesty the Queen,

əv ɔl vɛm blɛkfaɪst krɪu
Of all them blackfaced crew

və fɒɪnɪst mɛn ɒɪ nɪu
The finest man I knew

wəz æʊə rɛdʒɪmenʔl bʌɪstaɪ gʊŋgə dʌɪn
Was our regimental bhisti,[1] Gunga Din.

The uniform 'e wore

Was nothin' much before,

An' rather less than 'arf o' that be'ind,

For a twisty piece o' rag

An' a goatskin water-bag

Was all the field-equipment 'e could find.

When the sweatin' troop-train lay

In a sidin' through the day,

Were the 'eat would make your bloomin' eyebrows crawl,

We shouted "Harry By!" "Harry By"—"O, brother!"

Till our throats were bricky-dry,

Then we wopped 'im 'cause 'e couldn't serve us all.

The following selections were written for cockney characters. Transcribe the cockney sounds above the appropriate letters.

3. Kathleen:

Sent me to the country once, all them trees. Worse 'n people. Gawd. Take

---

[1] *Bhisti:* "water carrier."

them off if I could get them on again. Can't understand why they let me have laces. Took me belt as well. Who they think I'm going to strangle? Improved my figure it did—the belt. Drew it in a bit.

From HOME   *David Storey*

4. In the following speech, Shaw fairly successfully approximated a cockney accent through spelling.

Bill:

Aw did wot Aw said Aw'd do. Aw spit in is eye. E looks ap at the skoy and sez, "Ow that Aw shold be fahned worthy to be spit upon for the gospel's sike!" e sez; an Mog sez "Glaory Allellooher!"; an then e called me Braddher.

From MAJOR BARBARA   *George Bernard Shaw*

5. Iris:

Cheek! Watched every move I made. I don't like being watched. Never have. Still, I knew it was no good getting my knickers in a twist over that. More important was to find out where I was. I hadn't got the foggiest idea. See, geography was never my best thing.

From JOHNNY BULL   *Kathleen Betsko*

6. Artful Dodger:

"Don't fret your eyelids on that score. I know a 'spectable old gentleman as lives there, wot'll give you lodgings for nothink—that is, if any genelman he knows interduces you. And don't he know me? Oh, no! Not in the least! By no means!

From OLIVER TWIST   *Charles Dickens*

7. Eliza Doolittle:

I tell you it's easy to clean up here. Hot and cold water on tap, just as much as you like there is. Woolly towels, there is. And a towel horse so hot, it burns your fingers. Soft brushes to scrub yourself. And a wooden bowl of soap smelling like primroses. Now I know why ladies is so clean.

From PYGMALION   *George Bernard Shaw*

8. Dogberry:

Dost thou not suspect my place? Dost though not suspect my years? O that he were here to write me down an ass! But, masters, remember that I am an ass. Though it not be written down, yet not forget that I am an ass. No, thou villain, thou art full of piety, as shall be proved upon thee by good witness. I am a wise fellow; and which is more, an officer; and which is more, a householder; and which is more, as pretty a piece of flesh as any in Messina.

From MUCH ADO ABOUT NOTHING *William Shakespeare*

SCOTTISH

There are several Scottish dialects; the following discussion pertains to the Edinburgh dialect.

Vowels and Diphthongs

Substitution of /ɛř/ for /ɝ/

This use of the trilled /ř/ is perhaps the most recognizable characteristic of the Scottish dialect. The /ř/ is a longer trill than the one-tap trill, /ɾ/, used in stage speech. If you have difficulty in producing /ř/, say the word *three* and increase the number of taps of the tongue tip on the alveolar ridge. The closest American English sound is /r/ in the /θr/ combination. In recording the following list of words and sentences, magnify the difference between /ɝ/ and /ɛř/.

	Career	*Scottish*	*Career*
working	[wɝkɪŋ]	[wɛřkɪn]	[wɝkɪŋ]
thirty	[θɝtɪ]	[θɛřtɪ]	[θɝtɪ]
heard	[hɝd]	[hɛřd]	[hɝd]
squirt	[skwɝt]	[skwɛřt]	[skwɝt]
journey	[ʤɝnɪ]	[ʤɛřnɪ]	[ʤɝnɪ]
curse	[kɝs]	[kɛřs]	[kɝs]
world	[wɝld]	[wɛřld]	[wɝld]
word	[wɝd]	[wɛřd]	[wɝd]
first	[fɝst]	[fɛřst]	[fɝst]
bird	[bɝd]	[bɛřd]	[bɝd]

Don't smirk during the sermon.

The nurse was irked by the perfect patient.

The blackbird was sitting on the perch.

Many girls are learning to assert themselves.

The verb occurs in the first verse.

Substitution of /əř/ for /ɝ/

Record the following list of words and sentences and distinguish between /ɝ/ and /əř/.

	Career	*Scottish*	*Career*
sister	[sɪstɚ]	[sɪstəř]	[sɪstɚ]
brother	[brʌðɚ]	[bruðəř]	[brʌðɚ]
overage	[ovɚeʤ]	[ovəřeʤ]	[ovɚeʤ]
boundary	[baʊndɚɪ]	[bundəřɪ]	[baʊndɚɪ]
southern	[sʌðɚn]	[suðəřn]	[sʌðɚn]
razor	[rezɚ]	[rezəř]	[rezɚ]
camera	[kæmɚə]	[kæməřə]	[kæmɚə]
perhaps	[pɚhæps]	[pəřhaps]	[pɚhæps]
government	[gʌvɚnmənt]	[guvəřnmənt]	[gʌvɚnmənt]
number	[nʌmbɚ]	[numbəř]	[nʌmbɚ]

Anthony, history is interesting.

I wonder what the average grade was.

His father was an actor.

Mother cooked her favorite dinner.

Perhaps my sister and brother will come.

Substitution of /a/ for /æ/

This is the substitution characteristic of New England speech. Record the following list of words as transcribed.

	Career	*Scottish*	*Career*
mask	[mæsk]	[mask]	[mæsk]
stamp	[stæmp]	[stamp]	[stæmp]
calf	[kæf]	[kaf]	[kæf]
glad	[glæd]	[glad]	[glæd]
bombastic	[bɑmbæstɪk]	[bəmbastɪk]	[bɑmbæstɪk]
half	[hæf]	[haf]	[hæf]
chance	[tʃæns]	[tʃans]	[tʃæns]
grass	[græs]	[gras]	[græs]
alas	[əlæs]	[əlas]	[əlæs]

Refer to the sentences on p. 163.

Substitution of /u/ for /ʊ/

Record the following list of words and sentences. Listen for other English words when the substitution is made.

	Career	*Scottish*	*Career*
would	[wʊd]	[wud]	[wʊd]
full	[fʊl]	[ful]	[fʊl]
book	[bʊk]	[buk]	[bʊk]
foot	[fʊt]	[fut]	[fʊt]
put	[pʊt]	[put]	[pʊt]
butcher	[bʊtʃɚ]	[butʃəř]	[bʊtʃɚ]
pull	[pʊl]	[pul]	[pʊl]
cookie	[kʊkɪ]	[kukɪ]	[kʊkɪ]
Brooklyn	[brʊklɪn]	[břuklɪn]	[brʊklɪn]
stood	[stʊd]	[stud]	[stʊd]

  u u   u
The cook took the pudding.

 əř u   ř   u
Reverend Woods spoke from the pulpit.

  u   u
The wooden keg was full.

   u   u   u əř
Hank shook the hook on the pushcart.

   u   u
Mr. Hood was told he could do it.

Substitution of /u/ for /ɑʊ/

Record the following words and sentences. This is a sound substitution typical of the Scottish speaker.

	Career	*Scottish*	*Career*
house	[hɑʊs]	[hus]	[hɑʊs]
mouse	[mɑʊs]	[mus]	[mɑʊs]
mountain	[mɑʊntn̩]	[muntn̩]	[mɑʊntn̩]
sound	[sɑʊnd]	[sund]	[sɑʊnd]
bounty	[bɑʊntɪ]	[buntɪ]	[bɑʊntɪ]
found	[fɑʊnd]	[fund]	[fɑʊnd]
down	[dɑʊn]	[dun]	[dɑʊn]
hound	[hɑʊnd]	[hund]	[hɑʊnd]
cloudy	[klɑʊdɪ]	[kludɪ]	[klɑʊdɪ]
now	[nɑʊ]	[nu]	[nɑʊ]

Now what have you found, Hank?

Fran counted on the bounty.

Meg climbed down the mountain.

Kay made the sound of a mouse.

On a cloudy day, Kip plowed the ground.

Substitution of /ʊ/ for /ʌ/

This is a common Scottish characteristic. Record the words and sentences, focus on the substitution as transcribed.

	Career	*Scottish*	*Career*
love	[lʌv]	[lʊv]	[lʌv]
such	[sʌtʃ]	[sʊtʃ]	[sʌtʃ]
double	[dʌbl̩]	[dʊbl̩]	[dʌbl̩]
money	[mʌnɪ]	[mʊnɪ]	[mʌnɪ]
punish	[pʌnɪʃ]	[pʊnɪʃ]	[pʌnɪʃ]
judge	[dʒʌdʒ]	[dʒʊdʒ]	[dʒʌdʒ]
flood	[flʌd]	[flʊd]	[flʌd]

young   [jʌŋ]   [juŋ]   [jʌŋ]

hundred   [hʌndrəd]   [hundrəd]   [hʌndrəd]

muttering [mʌtɚ·ɪŋ]   [mutərɪn]   [mʌtɚ·ɪŋ]

     ʊ   ʊ   ʊ   ɛř
The young puppy dug in the dirt.

    ʊ   ʊ   ʊ   ʊ   ʊ
Double bubble gum bubbles double.

      ʊ   ɛř   ʊ
The judge determined the punishment.

   ʊ   ʊ   ʊ
A skunk stood on a stump.

  ʊ   əř   ʊ   ʊ   ř
Mother and Uncle Ned jumped into the car.

Consonants

Glottalization

One of the distinguishing characteristics of Scottish is the use of glottalization. Refer to the drills for cockney on pp. 303–304.

Substitution of /ɪç/ for Letters "ight"

The consonant /ç/ is also a sound in German. It is roughly made by forming the vowel /ɪ/ and immediately producing /k/. The feeling of producing the sound ought to be like the reflex action when a fish bone is caught in your throat. Although this does not produce a very pleasant sound, it is very accurate! The sound /x/ is made the same way except that it occurs after back vowels and is made farther back in the throat than /ç/.

    Record the following list of words. Notice that in all of the words the substitution takes place in the final position.

	Career	*Scottish*	*Career*
light	[laɪt]	[lɪçt]	[laɪt]
bright	[braɪt]	[břɪçt]	[braɪt]
right	[raɪt]	[řɪçt]	[raɪt]
slight	[slaɪt]	[slɪçt]	[slaɪt]
night	[naɪt]	[nɪçt]	[naɪt]
fight	[faɪt]	[fɪçt]	[faɪt]
sight	[saɪt]	[sɪçt]	[saɪt]
fright	[fraɪt]	[fřɪçt]	[fraɪt]
blight	[blaɪt]	[blɪçt]	[blaɪt]
might	[maɪt]	[mɪçt]	[maɪt]

Substitution of /ř/ for /r/ in All Positions

Record the following list of words. The trill is usually easier to produce for Americans when used in the blends /př/ and /gř/.

	Career	*Scottish*	*Career*
ripe	[raɪp]	[řaɪp]	[raɪp]
around	[ərɑund]	[əřund]	[ərɑund]
barren	[bærən]	[bařən]	[bærən]
brag	[bræg]	[břag]	[bræg]
drum	[drʌm]	[dřum]	[drʌm]
correct	[kərɛkt]	[kařɛkt]	[kərɛkt]
comfort	[kʌmfɚt]	[kumfəřt]	[kʌmfɚt]
Araby	[ærəbɪ]	[ařəbɪ]	[ærəbɪ]
prim	[prɪm]	[přɪm]	[prɪm]
pride	[praɪd]	[přaɪd]	[praɪd]
grim	[grɪm]	[gřɪm]	[grɪm]

Omission of /θ/ and /ð/ in Final Position

Record the following list of words. Then add a word so you feel the sound omission (example: [wɪ ʌs] for "with us").

	Career	*Scottish*	*Career*
with	[wɪð], [wɪθ]	[wɪ]	[wɪð], [wɪθ]
mouth	[mɑuθ]	[mu]	[mɑuθ]
youth	[juθ]	[ju]	[juθ]
truth	[truθ]	[třu]	[truθ]
cloth	[klɔθ]	[klɔ]	[klɔθ]
breathe	[brið]	[bři]	[brið]
bathe	[beð]	[be]	[beð]

EXERCISES FOR A SCOTTISH ACCENT

In the following selections, the writers attempt to approximate the dialect through spelling. Phonetically transcribe the sounds over the appropriate letters.

1. Lachie:

I'm nae much of a mon on the surface, boot I've a great and powerful will tae wurk. I've a wee butt-in-ben in Scotland which ye know aboot. Ma' health is guid, regardless of the Colonel's spite. I've a fearful temper, boot I dinna think I'll ever make ye suffer fur it.

From THE HASTY HEART   *John Patrick*

2. Sarah:

I'm not sure which I'm wantin' maist—a wee flower for the window there or a bright new bonnet. Whit wud ye do—get the bonnet or the flower? Mrs. MacLeod has a braw new bonnet but now she has it, she canna enjoy it. Every time she puts it on, she's fairly sick wie the price of it.

From SPRING O' THE YEAR   *W. H. Robertson*

3. It mak's a change in a'thing roon'

When mither's gane.

The cat has less contented croon,

The kettle has a dowie tune,

There's naething has sae blythe a soon,

Sin' mither's gane.

The bairnies gang wi' ragged claes,

Sin' mither's gane.

There's nane to mend their broken taes,

Or laugh a' their pawky ways,

The nichts are langer than the days,

When mither's gane.

From WHEN MITHER'S GANE   *Anonymous*

4. Auld Daddy Darkness creeps frae his hole,

Black as a blackamoor, blin' as a mole;

Stir the fire till it lowes, let the bairnie sit,

Auld Daddy Darkness is no want it yet.

See him in the corners hidin' frae the licht,

See him at the window gloomin' at the nicht;

Turn up the gas licht, close the shutters a',

An' Auld Daddy Darkness will flee far awa'.

AULD DADDY DARKNESS   *James Ferguson*

5. Dowey:

I've never been here before. If you know what it is to be in sic a place without

a friend. I was crazy with glee, when I got my leave, at the thought of seeing

London at last, but after wandering its streets for four hours, I would almost

have been glad to be back in the trenches.

From THE OLD LADY SHOWS HER MEDALS   *James M. Barrie*

GERMAN

There are a few languages whose general pronunciations are important to Americans for political and social reasons. These include German, Spanish, and Russian.

To many people the German language is intimidating because of its long words, lots of capital letters, and those two dots (umlauts) that seem to be everywhere. Some of the words are long because they are compounds made up of two or more words. For example, *Schuh* means "shoe," *Hand* means "hand," and *Handschuh* means "glove"—a shoe for the hand. Keep in mind that every noun in German has a capital letter, and the umlaut over a vowel indicates a different pronunciation. The umlaut is sometimes transcribed into English as an "e" after the umlauted vowel; thus the word *König* can be written as *Koenig*.

The following discussion of the German dialect is not in any way exhaustive. The intent is to indicate characteristic sounds and substitutions that will help a professional communicator (actor or newsperson) who must be familiar with the language. The information will also be useful for Germans who are learning English pronunciation.

German Trill

The German language uses a trill that is different from the British or Scottish trill, which is made with the tongue tip. The German trill, which is also used in French, is produced with the back of the tongue against the uvula. This intensifies the guttural sound often associated with the German language. This uvular trill is very difficult for most Americans to produce because it does not exist in English and because its articulatory adjustment cannot be observed easily.

As stated above, this trill, designated /R/, is made by contact between the back of the tongue and the uvula. To produce this sound, gargle so that you can feel what is happening in your throat. If you cannot manage this trill with the back of the tongue, feel free to use the Scottish trill. A little trill is better than no trill!

The following is an attempt to indicate the sound of gargling rather than the word itself. Produce the gargling sound and carry it over into the pronunciation of the word.

gaaaaaaarrrrrrr————run

gaaaaaaarrrrrrr————rough

gaaaaaaarrrrrrr————rich

Now shorten the "gargle" and say the following words with a uvular /ʀ/:

rhyme	arrest	proud	trip	cream	frown
ripe	very	problem	trick	crime	frame
rent	horrible	brown	trunk	craft	Frances
rob	arrive	brought	drip	grim	French
range	around	bright	dream	green	freeze

Vowels and Diphthongs

Substitution of /ɑ/ for /æ/ and /ʌ/

This is a common substitution in many foreign languages. Record the list of words and sentences and focus on the vowel substitution.

	Career	*German*	*Career*
cat	[kæt]	[kɑt]	[kæt]
mass	[mæs]	[mɑs]	[mæs]
flash	[flæʃ]	[flɑʃ]	[flæʃ]
ask	[æsk]	[ɑsk]	[æsk]
half	[hæf]	[hɑf]	[hæf]
laugh	[læf]	[lɑf]	[læf]
class	[klæs]	[klɑs]	[klæs]
fast	[fæst]	[fɑst]	[fæst]
smashing	[smæʃɪŋ]	[smɑʃɪŋ]	[smæʃɪŋ]
damp	[dæmp]	[dɑmp]	[dæmp]

ɑ   ɑ   ɑ
Take a chance and command the child to stay off the grass.

ɑ   ɑ
On behalf of my Uncle Eberhard, I congratulate you.

Rosemarie advanced into the alabaster bathroom.
<small>ɑ ɑ ɑ</small>

Jürgen took a chance and glanced at Greta.
<small>ɑ ɑ</small>

The photograph of Dr. Rainer amazed the class.
<small>ɑ ɑ</small>

	Career	*German*	*Career*
double	[dʌbḷ]	[dɑbḷ]	[dʌbḷ]
money	[mʌnɪ]	[mɑnɪ]	[mʌnɪ]
come	[kʌm]	[kɑm]	[kʌm]
judge	[dʒʌdʒ]	[ʒɑʒ]	[dʒʌdʒ]
young	[jʌŋ]	[jɑŋ]	[jʌŋ]
puppy	[pʌpɪ]	[pɑpɪ]	[pʌpɪ]
humbug	[hʌmbʌg]	[hɑmbɑg]	[hʌmbʌg]
ugly	[ʌglɪ]	[ɑglɪ]	[ʌglɪ]
punish	[pʌnɪʃ]	[pɑnɪʃ]	[pʌnɪʃ]
studied	[stʌdɪd]	[stɑdɪd]	[stʌdɪd]

The young puppy dug in the dirt.
<small>ɑ ɑ ɑ</small>

Double bubble gum bubbles double.
<small>ɑ ɑ ɑ ɑ ɑ</small>

The judge made the punishment fit the crime.
<small>ɑ ɑ</small>

The hamburg was on an ugly-looking bun covered with mustard. Humbug!
<small>ɑ ɑ ɑ ɑ ɑ ɑ ɑ</small>

Have you studied much about the hummingbird?
<small>ɑ ɑ ɑ</small>

Substitution of /ɛʀ/ for /ɝ/

This is a difficult substitution for Americans to say. Record the list of words and sentences. Remember to gargle.

	Career	*German*	*Career*
earth	[ɝˑθ]	[ɛʀs]	[ɝˑθ]
nerve	[nɝˑv]	[nɛʀv]	[nɝˑv]
work	[wɝˑk]	[vɛʀk]	[wɝˑk]
stir	[stɝˑ]	[stɛʀ]	[stɝˑ]
verdict	[vɝˑdɪkt]	[fɛʀdɪçt]	[vɝˑdɪkt]
mercy	[mɝˑsɪ]	[mɛʀsɪ]	[mɝˑsɪ]

Eric	[ɛrɪk]	[ɛʀɪç]	[ɛrɪk]
deserving	[dɪzɝ·vɪŋ]	[dɪsɛʀfɪŋ]	[dɪzɝ·vɪŋ]
confirm	[kənfɝ·m]	[kənfɛʀm]	[kənfɝ·m]
avert	[əvɝ·t]	[əfɛʀt]	[əvɝ·t]

The verb occurs in the first verse.
<small>ɛʀ   ɛʀ   ɛʀ   ɛʀ</small>

Rainer was sure he would smirk during the sermon.
<small>ɛʀ   ɛʀ   ɛʀ</small>

Research the records for Hans's birthday.
<small>ɛʀ   ɛʀ</small>

The blackbird was sitting on the perch.
<small>ɛʀ   ɛʀ</small>

Many girls are learning to assert themselves.
<small>ɛʀ   ɛʀ   ɛʀ</small>

Additional Vowel Sounds

German has three vowel sounds that do not exist in English. Although a German learning English would not need to use them, a number of careers require some use of the German language. An obvious example is the television newscaster who might have to pronounce German words for a news story.

1. Use the vowel /œ/ when the umlauted letter "ö" is followed by two consonants, including double consonants. The vowel /œ/ is made by saying the vowel /ɛ/ with rounded lips. To hear and feel the German vowel, make certain that you form and think /ɛ/ while rounding the lips. Say:

   /œ/   /œ/   /œ/   /œ/   /œ/

   Now produce that vowel while reading the following German words:

   Löffel ['lœfəl] (n.): spoon

   Löschblatt ['lœʃblɑt] (n.): blotting paper

   Mönch [mœnç] (n.): monk

   Mörder ['mœrdər] (n.): murderer

   nördlich ['nœrtlɪç] (adj.): northern

   öffentlich ['œfəntlɪç] (adj.): public

   öffnen ['œfnən] (v.): to open

   schöpfen [ʃœpfən] (v.): to ladle

   tröpfeln ['tʀœpfəln] (v.): to trickle

The following German proper names are pronounced with /œ/:

Böcklin ['bœkli:n], the painter

Böll [bœl], the author

Goebbels ['gœbəls], the politician

Goethe ['gœtə], the poet

Hölderlin ['hœldərlin], the poet

Mössbauer ['mœsbɑʊər], the physicist

Röntgen ['ʀœntgən], the physicist

2. Use the vowel /ø/ when "ö" is followed by a single consonant in the same
syllable. The sound /ø/ is made by producing the vowel /e/ (as in *made*) with
rounded lips. To hear and feel the German vowel, make certain that you form
and think /e/ while rounding the lips. Say:

/ø/   /ø/   ø/   /ø/   ø/

Now produce that vowel while reading the following German words:

dröhnen ['dʀø:nən] (v.): to roar

Gelöbnis [gə'lø:pnis] (n.): promise

Getöse [gə'tø:zə] (n.): noise

Höhe ['hø:ə] (n.): height

hörig ['hø:rɪç] (adj.): a slave to

Köder ['kø:dər] (n.): lure

König ['kø:nɪç] (n.): king

lösen ['lø:zən] (v.): to loosen

nötigen [nø:tɪgən] (v.): to compel

öde [ø:də] (adj.): desolate

Störer ['ʃtø:ʀər] (n.): one who disturbs

The following German proper nouns are pronounced with /ø/:

Böhm [bø:m], the conductor

Döblin [dø'bli:n], the author

Mörike ['mø:rikə], the poet

3. Use /y/ when "ü" is followed by a single consonant or a double "s" within the same syllable. The vowel /y/ is made by producing the vowel /i/ (as in *see*) with rounded lips. To hear and feel the German vowel, make certain that you form and think /i/ while rounding the lips. Say:

/y/   /y/   /y/   /y/   /y/

Now produce that vowel while reading the following German words:

bücken ['by:kən] (v.): to stoop

Büffel ['byfəl] (n.): buffalo

Büro [by'ʀo] (n.): office

Gemüt [gə'my:t] (n.): mind, feeling

Glück [glyk] (n.): good luck

München ['mynçən] (n.): Munich

tüchtig ['tyçtıç] (adj.): clever

überführen [y:bər'fy:ʀən] (v.): to convey

Würde ['vyʀdə] (v.): dignity

würgen ['vyʀgən] (v.): to strangle

wüten ['vy:tən] (v.): to rage

The following German proper nouns are pronounced with /y/:

Brüssel [brysəl], the city

Dürer ['dy:ʀər], the painter

Düsseldorf ['dysəldɔʀf], the city

Grünewald ['gry:nəvɑlt], the painter

Heissenbüttel ['hɑısənbytəl], the poet

Lübeck ['ly:bɛk], the city

Nürnberg ['nyʀnbɛʀk], the city

4. In German the letter combination "ie" is pronounced /i/ (as in *see*); the letter combination "ei" is pronounced /ɑı/ (as in *ice*).

Consonants

Substitution of /t/ or /s/ for /θ/ and /d/ or /z/ for /ð/

Record the following list of words with career speech and with German pronunciation.

	Career	*German*	*Career*
theme	[θim]	[tim], [sim]	[θim]
youthful	[juθfʊl]	[jutfəl], [jusfəl]	[juθfʊl]
thought	[θɔt]	[tɔt], [sɔt]	[θɔt]
thin	[θɪn]	[tɪn], [sɪn]	[θɪn]
through	[θru]	[tʀu], [sʀu]	[θru]
mouth	[mɑʊθ]	[mɑʊt], [mɑʊs]	[mɑʊθ]
them	[ðɛm]	[dɛm], [zɛm]	[ðɛm]
either	[iðɚ]	[idə], [izə]*	[iðɚ]
weather	[wɛðɚ]	[vɛdə], [vɛzə]*	[wɛðɚ]
breathe	[brið]	[bʀid], [bʀiz]	[brið]
feather	[fɛðɚ]	[fɛdə], [fɛzə]*	[fɛðɚ]

Substitution of /v/ for /w/

This is a simple substitution. Record the list of words with career speech and with German pronunciation.

	Career	*German*	*Career*
walk	[wɔk]	[vɔk]	[wɔk]
when	[ʍɛn]	[vɛn]	[ʍɛn]
unworthy	[ənwɝði]	[ənvɛʀzi]	[ənwɝði]
liquid	[lɪkwɪd]	[lɪkvɪd]	[lɪkwɪd]
wife	[wɑɪf]	[vɑɪf]	[wɑɪf]
woman	[wʊmən]	[vʊmən]	[wʊmən]
wall	[wɔl]	[vɔl]	[wɔl]
highway	[hɑɪweɪ]	[hɑɪveɪ]	[hɑɪweɪ]
anyone	[ɛnɪwʌn]	[ɛnɪvʌn]	[ɛnɪwʌn]
require	[rɪkwɑɪr]	[řɪkvɑɪr]	[rɪkwɑɪr]

---

*Final /r/ phonemes are often omitted in German.

Record the following German proper nouns that are shown with their correct pronunciation:

Luftwaffe ['lʊftvɑfə], the German air force

Wagner ['vɑgnəř], the composer

Weill [vaɪl], the composer

Weizsäcker ['vaɪtszɛkəř], the physicist

Weser ['ve:zəř], the river

Westdeutschland ['vestdɔɪtʃlɑnt], West Germany

Wien [vi:n], Vienna

Wiesbaden ['vi:sbɑdn̩], the city

Wilhelm [vɪlhɛlm]

Wolfgang [vʊlfgɑŋ]

Zweig [tsvaɪg], the author

Substitution of /f/ for /v/

	Career	*German*	*Career*
very	[vɛrɪ]	[fɛʀɪ]	[vɛrɪ]
vain	[ven]	[fen]	[ven]
David	[devɪd]	[defɪt]	[devɪd]
eve	[iv]	[if]	[iv]
groove	[gruv]	[gřuf]	[gruv]
prevent	[prɪvɛnt]	[prəfɛnt]	[prɪvɛnt]
avoid	[əvɔɪd]	[əfɔɪt]	[əvɔɪd]
vanity	[vænətɪ]	[fænətɪ]	[vænətɪ]
evil	[ivl̩]	[ifəl]	[ivl̩]
love	[lʌv]	[lɑf]	[lʌv]

Record the following German words that are shown with the transcription of their correct pronunciation:

Vaterland	['fɑ:təřlɑnt]	fatherland
Beethoven	['be:tofən]	composer
verboten	[fɛř'botən]	forbidden
Volkswagen	['fɔlksvɑ:gən]	people wagon

Substitution of /x/ for Letters "ch" and "g"
Following a Back Vowel and of /ç/ Otherwise

For a discussion of the /x/ substitution, see the discussion of the Scottish dialect on p. 312. If you have difficulty in making either of these sounds, consider them interchangeable.

The following German proper names are shown with their correct pronunciations:

Bach [bɑx], the composer

Barlach ['bɑrlɑx], the sculptor

Becher ['bɛçəř], the poet

Bloch [blɔx], the philosopher

Brecht [bʀɛçt], the writer

Eichendorff ['aɪçəndɔřf], the writer

Substitution of /ts/ for /z/

	Career	*German*	*Career*
zoo	[zu]	[tsu]	[zu]
zipper	[zɪpɚ]	[tsɪpəř]	[zɪpɚ]
zinc	[zɪŋk]	[tsɪŋk]	[zɪŋk]
xylophone	[zaɪləfon]	[tsaɪləfon]	[zaɪləfon]
zany	[zeɪnɪ]	[tseɪnɪ]	[zeɪnɪ]

Substitution of /ʃ/ for /tʃ/ and of /ʒ/ for /dʒ/

Record the following list of words. This substitution usually occurs in the initial position and is common in some European languages.

	Career	*German*	*Career*
church	[tʃɝtʃ]	[ʃɛřʃ]	[tʃɝtʃ]
Chuck	[tʃʌk]	[ʃak]	[tʃʌk]
punch	[pʌntʃ]	[panʃ]	[pʌntʃ]
char	[tʃɑr]	[ʃɑr]	[tʃɑr]
chopping	[tʃapɪŋ]	[ʃapɪŋ]	[tʃapɪŋ]
jail	[dʒeɪl]	[ʒeɪl]	[dʒeɪl]

jump	[ʤʌmp]	[ʒɑmp]	[ʤʌmp]
joke	[ʤok]	[ʒok]	[ʤok]
jelly	[ʤɛlɪ]	[ʒɛlɪ]	[ʤɛlɪ]
gem	[ʤɛm]	[ʒɛm]	[ʤɛm]

Substitution of /ʃt/ and /ʃp/ for /st/ and /sp/

This substitution is very characteristic of the German dialect, especially in the initial position. Read the following words, using both career and German pronunciations.

	Career	German	Career
student	[stɪudn̩t]	[ʃtudənt]	[stɪudn̩t]
street	[strit]	[ʃtrit]	[strit]
strict	[strɪkt]	[ʃtrɪçt]	[strɪkt]
stripe	[straɪp]	[ʃtraɪp]	[straɪp]
stable	[stebl̩]	[ʃtebl̩]	[stebl̩]
stack	[stæk]	[ʃtɑk]	[stæk]
stallion	[stæljən]	[ʃtaljən]	[stæljən]
stamp	[stɑmp]	[ʃtɑmp]	[stæmp]
stand	[stɑnd]	[ʃtɑnt]	[stænd]
state	[stet]	[ʃtet]	[stet]
span	[spæn]	[ʃpɑn]	[spæn]
spot	[spɑt], [spɒt]	[ʃpɒt]	[spɑt], [spɒt]
speak	[spik]	[ʃpik]	[spik]
space	[spes]	[ʃpes]	[spes]
spoon	[spun]	[ʃpun]	[spun]
speech	[spitʃ]	[ʃpiʃ]	[spitʃ]
spicy	[spaɪsɪ]	[ʃpaɪsɪ]	[spaɪsɪ]
spin	[spɪn]	[ʃpɪn]	[spɪn]
spine	[spaɪn]	[ʃpaɪn]	[spaɪn]

The following German proper nouns are shown with their correct pronunciations:

Einstein [ˈaɪnʃtaɪn], the scientist

Strauss [ʃtraʊs], the composer

Stuttgart [ˈʃtutgɑrt], the city

EXERCISES FOR A GERMAN ACCENT

Try your hand at pronouncing the German in the following translations of stanzas from English poems.

1. Tiger, Tiger, lohendes Licht,
   Das durch die Nacht der Walder bricht,
   Welches Auge, welche unsterbliche Hand
   Hat dich furchtbar in dein Ebenmass gebannt?

   From TIGER TIGER   *William Blake*

2. Das Jahr, wenns fruhlingt,
   und der Tag wird geborn
   morgens um sieben,
   der Hand, taubeperlt
   die Lerche beschwingt,
   die Schecke am Dorn:
   Gott in Seinem Himmel—
   Gut stehts um die Welt!

   From PIPPA PASSES   *Robert Browning*

In the following exercises, transcribe the German substitutions above the appropriate letters before practicing aloud.

3. Fraulein Schneider:

   "Lina," my friends used to say to me, "however can you? How can you bear to have strange people living in your rooms and spoiling your furniture, especially when you've got the money to be independent?" And I'd always give them the same answer. "My lodgers aren't lodgers," I used to say. "They're my guests."

   From A BERLIN DIARY   *Christopher Isherwood*

4. Fraulein Schneider:

   Upset? Yes, I am upset. You go off on a trip of the whole world. You can afford to do that. But me, I have had to wait for my money, because you were too hard up sometimes to pay me. And now you throw me the china and the glass as a tip. The china and the glass. . . . I will throw them from the windows after your taxi as you go away. That is what I think from your china and your glass. And from you too.

   From I AM A CAMERA   *John Van Druten*

5. Fraulein Schneider:

Herr Schultz! Can I believe what I see? But this is too much to accept. So rare—so costly—so luxurious . . . a pineapple for me!

From CABARET   *Joseph Masteroff, John Kander, Fred Ebb*

6. Agnes:

That was a bitter time. From morning till night we heard nothing but the sounds of marching feet—the troops of the victor. The city had fallen. The enemy was here. His pennants fluttered against the dark sky like streamers of blood. It was noon on a day in spring; it was May, but the sky was dark with ashes and smoke.

From WHEN THE WAR WAS OVER   *Max Frisch*

7. Einstein:

Well, Chonny, where do we go from here? We got to think fast. The Police! They got pictures of that face. I got to operate on you right away. We got to find someplace—and we got to find someplace for Mr. Spinalzo, too. . . . We can't leave a dead body in the rumble seat! You shouldn't have killed him, Chonny. He's a nice fellow—he gives us a lift and what happens?

From ARSENIC AND OLD LACE   *Joseph Kesselring*

8. But you must go to München. You have not seen Germany if you have not been to München. All the Exhibitions. All the Art and Soul life of Germany are in München. There is the Wagner Festival in August, and Mozart and a Japanese collection of pictures—and there is the beer! You do not know what good beer is until you have been to München.

From GERMANS AT MEAT   *Katherine Mansfield*

SPANISH

Since there has been such an influx of Spanish speakers into the United States, it has become increasingly important for Americans to speak and understand Spanish.

Like German, Spanish spelling is very consistent with its pronunciation once you know the rules.

Vowels

Substitution of /i/ for /ɪ/

This substitution is common in a number of languages. Record the list of words and sentences and focus on the differences in transcription.

	Career	*Spanish*	*Career*
pins	[pɪnz]	[pinz]	[pɪnz]
chip	[tʃɪp]	[tʃip]	[tʃɪp]
wind	[wɪnd]	[wind]	[wɪnd]
lift	[lɪft]	[lift]	[lɪft]
since	[sɪns]	[sins]	[sɪns]
ship	[ʃɪp]	[tʃip]*	[ʃɪp]
pretty	[prɪtɪ]	[priti]	[prɪtɪ]
business	[bɪznɪs]	[biznis]	[bɪznɪs]
mistletoe	[mɪsl̩touʊ]	[misl̩touʊ]	[mɪsl̩touʊ]
fifty	[fɪftɪ]	[fifti]	[fɪftɪ]

    i i
Keep it simple.

     i   i   i   i   i
Michele did the dishes quickly.

       i   i   i
Where is Lizzie's kitten?

i   i i   i   i
Is he still sitting on his broken hip?

   i   i   i
Kip had a fit when he got bitten.

Substitution of /u/ for /ʊ/

Record the following list of words and sentences, focusing on the transcriptions.

	Career	*Spanish*	*Career*
pudding	[pʊdɪŋ]	[pudiŋ]	[pʊdɪŋ]
put	[pʊt]	[put]	[pʊt]
good	[gʊd]	[gud]	[gʊd]

---

*Often /tʃ/ is substituted for /ʃ/.

mistook	[mɪstʊk]	[mistuk]	[mɪstʊk]
looked	[lʊkt]	[lukt]	[lʊkt]
could	[kʊd]	[kud]	[kʊd]
tourist	[tʊrɪst]	[tuřist]	[tʊrɪst]
book	[bʊk]	[buk]	[bʊk]
cooking	[kʊkɪŋ]	[kukiŋ]	[kʊkɪŋ]
stood	[stʊd]	[stud]	[stʊd]

     ⁱ   ^u ^u   ^u
Miss Crook looked at the wolf.

   ^u   ^u   ^u
Put the hook on the hood of the car.

           ^u   ⁱ   ^u
Larry made a good pass with the football.

        ^u   ^u
Debbie pushed the cushion at Larry.

              ^u   ^u
Where are the hooks for the woolen rugs?

Substitution of /ɑ/ for /æ/

The vowel /æ/ does not exist in Spanish. In recording the following list of words and sentences, focus on the difference between /æ/ and /ɑ/.

	Career	*Spanish*	*Career*
catch	[kætʃ]	[katʃ]	[kætʃ]
rack	[ræk]	[rɑk]	[ræk]
bandit	[bændɪt]	[bɑndit]	[bændɪt]
mad	[mæd]	[mɑd]	[mæd]
apple	[æpl̩]	[ɑpl̩]	[æpl̩]
scrap	[skræp]	[skřɑp]	[skræp]
master	[mæstɚ]	[mɑstəř]	[mæstɚ]
laugh	[læf]	[lɑf]	[læf]
class	[klæs]	[klɑs]	[klæs]
plastic	[plæstɪk]	[plɑstik]	[plæstɪk]

     ^ɑ   ⁱ   ^ɑ   ^ɑ ^ɑ
The cat will catch the fat rat.

     ^ɑ   ^ɑ   ⁱ   ^ɑ
Take Fran's hand in class.

     ^ɑ   ^ɑ   ^ɑ
Half the apples were passed over.

ɑ   i   u   ɑ   i   ɑ   i
The bandit said to put the cash in the plastic box.

ɑ   ɑ   i   ɑ
The Mad Hatter is a humorous character.

Substitution of /ɑ/ for /ʌ/

The vowel /ʌ/ does not occur in Spanish. Record the following list of words and sentences and focus on the substitution.

	Career	*Spanish*	*Career*
duck	[dʌk]	[dɑk]	[dʌk]
hungry	[hʌŋgrɪ]	[hɑŋgři]	[hʌŋgrɪ]
onion	[ʌnjən]	[ɑnjən]	[ʌnjən]
brush	[brʌʃ]	[břatʃ]	[brʌʃ]
nuts	[nʌts]	[nɑts]	[nʌts]
must	[mʌst]	[mɑst]	[mʌst]
pump	[pʌmp]	[pɑmp]	[pʌmp]
gun	[gʌn]	[gɑn]	[gʌn]
lucky	[lʌkɪ]	[lɑki]	[lʌkɪ]
hunt	[hʌnt]	[hɑnt]	[hʌnt]

ɑ   ɑ   ɑ
You must pump the water gun.

ɑ   ɑ   i   ɑ
Brush the duck with the nutty sauce.

ɑ   ɑ   ɑ   i
Have you studied much about the hummingbird?

ɑ   ɑ   ɑ   ɑ
Mother rushed to the dumbwaiter for the fudge.

ɑ   ɑ   ɑ   ɑ   i
I can jump and touch the ceiling.

Consonants

Substitution of /s/ for Initial /θ/

These substitutions occur in several languages. Record the following list of words and focus on the substitutions.

	Career	*Spanish*	*Career*
thought	[θɔt]	[sɔt]	[θɔt]
think	[θɪŋk]	[siŋk]	[θɪŋk]

thanks	[θæŋks]	[saŋks]	[θæŋks]
thin	[θɪn]	[sin]	[θɪn]
thick	[θɪk]	[sik]	[θɪk]
thigh	[θaɪ]	[saɪ]	[θaɪ]
thread	[θrɛd]	[sřɛd]	[θrɛd]
theft	[θɛft]	[sɛft]	[θɛft]
thing	[θɪŋ]	[siŋ]	[θɪŋ]
thaw	[θɔ]	[sɔ]	[θɔ]

Substitution of /d/ for /ð/

	Career	*Spanish*	*Career*
these	[ðiz]	[diz]	[ðiz]
that	[ðæt]	[dɑt]	[ðæt]
though	[ðou]	[dou]	[ðou]
loathes	[loðz]	[lodz]	[loðz]
lather	[læðɚ]	[lɑzər]	[læðɚ]
leather	[lɛðɚ]	[lɛdər]	[lɛðɚ]
either	[iðɚ]	[idər]	[iðɚ]
weather	[wɛðɚ]	[wɛdər]	[wɛðɚ]
bathes	[beðz]	[bedz]	[beðz]
with	[wɪð]	[wid]	[wɪð]

Substitution of /x/ for /h/

Since there is no /h/ phoneme in Spanish, a native Spanish speaker often substitutes /x/ for /h/ when speaking English. The primary difference between /x/ and /ç/ is that /x/ is produced farther back in the throat than /ç/. (You will remember that the sound /x/ can be produced by the action of dislodging a fish bone from the throat!) Record the list of words, focusing on the substitution.

	Career	*Spanish*	*Career*
high	[haɪ]	[xaɪ]	[haɪ]
hand	[hænd]	[xɑnd]	[hænd]
hat	[hæt]	[xɑt]	[hæt]
heaven	[hɛvən]	[xɛβən]	[hɛvən]
hold	[hold]	[xold]	[hold]
hit	[hɪt]	[xit]	[hɪt]
inhale	[ɪnhel]	[inxel]	[ɪnhel]

somehow [sʌmhɑʊ] [sɑmxɑʊ] [sʌmhɑʊ]
exhale [ɛkshel] [ɛksxel] [ɛkshel]
behave [bɪhev] [bixev] [bɪhev]

Substitution of /ß/ for /b/ and /v/

The consonant /ß/ is a vocalized bilabial fricative, made by the escape of air between the lips. Record the following list of words and sentences, focusing on the substitution.

	Career	*Spanish*	*Career*
base	[bes]	[ßes]	[bes]
bay	[beɪ]	[ßeɪ]	[beɪ]
above	[əbʌv]	[aßaß]	[əbʌv]
habit	[hæbɪt]	[xaßit]	[hæbɪt]
stable	[stebl̩]	[steßl̩]	[stebl̩]
valley	[vælɪ]	[ßali]	[vælɪ]
vain	[veɪn]	[ßeɪn]	[veɪn]
David	[devɪd]	[deßid]	[devɪd]
stove	[stov]	[stoß]	[stov]
love	[lʌv]	[laß]	[lʌv]

    ß   ɑ   ß   i
Steve doesn't ɦave any.

ßi i   aß   ßi   əßɑnə kußə
Vicki, ɦave you been to ɦavana, Cuba?

   aß   aß
Have you met the Governor, Katie?

ß ß   aß   ß   ß
Bob told me not to ɦave a baseball game.

         aß   aß   ɑ   ß   i
Why do we ɦave to ɦave a fuss about it?

Substitution of /ř/ for /r/

Refer to the list of words on p. 313.

EXERCISES FOR A SPANISH ACCENT

In the following exercises, transcribe the phonetic substitutions used in a Spanish accent above the appropriate letters. As you become more adept at making the substitutions, increase your rate of speech. Work for continuity.

1. In the speech below, the playwright has attempted to indicate a Spanish accent through spelling. Add any remaining substitutions needed.

   Certamente. . . . And to him who bids the 'ighest, shall go ze little paper and he shall come wiz me while I show 'im where se oil she is 'iding. To him what does not bid the ze 'ighest, he shall stay 'ere wiz Pedro until eight o'clock tonight.

   From THE BAD MAN   *Porter Emerson Brown*

2. The Gypsy:

   I'll show you how to take a shot of tequila. It dilates the capillaries. First you sprinkle salt on the back of your hand. Then lick it off with your tongue. Now then, you toss the shot down. And then you bite into the lemon. That way, it goes down easy, but what a bang!—You're next.

   From CAMINO REAL   *Tennessee Williams*

3. Googie Gomez:

   You boy really know how to cheer a girl up when she's dumps in the down. My boyfriend Hector see me do that: ay! cuidado! He hates you maricones, that Hector! . . . You know why you're not a producer? You're too nice to be a producer. But I'm gonna show them all, mister, and tonight's the night I'm gonna do it. One day you gonna see the name Googie Gomez in lights and you gonna say to yourself: "Was that her?" And you gonna answer yourself, "That was her!" But you know something, mister? I was always her, just nobody knows it. Yo soy Googie Gomez, estrellita del futuro!

   From THE RITZ   *Terence McNally*

4. Tomas:

   Perhaps, after the mass, when the women have come home, you and I could stop in the saloon and celebrate the coming of a phonograph to El Carmen. Perhaps you can even buy us a large glass of beer in celebration...ten cent glasses.

   From TOOTH OR SHAVE   *Josephina Niggli*

5. Maria:

   One thing always gives me laughter

Pancho Villa* the morning after

Ay, there go the Carranzistas

Who comes there?

Why the Villists.

Ay, Pancho Villa, ay Pancho Villa,

Ay, he can no longer walk.

Because he lacks now, because he has not

Any drug to help him talk! Ay-yay!

From SOLDADERA   *Josephina Niggli*

RUSSIAN

Russian is a particularly difficult language for Westerners because it contains few similarities to familiar languages such as French, Italian, and Spanish. Furthermore, Russian is written with a different alphabet, the Cyrillic. This is why Russian appears to have sideways and backwards letters.

Because learning another alphabet in addition to the IPA would be too demanding, this unit will only discuss some characteristics of a Russian accent in English. In addition, some Russian proper nouns will be transcribed into our alphabet and the IPA.

Vowels and Diphthongs

Substitution of /i/ for /ɪ/

This is a substitution found in Spanish. Record the following list of words and focus on the pronunciation according to the transcription. Additional words appear on p. 327.

	Career	*Russian*	*Career*
hit	[hɪt]	[hit]	[hɪt]
mitten	[mɪtn̩]	[mitn̩]	[mɪtn̩]
film	[fɪlm]	[film]	[fɪlm]
split	[splɪt]	[split]	[splɪt]

---

*For the letters [ll], use /j/.

tin	[tɪn]	[tin]	[tɪn]
simple	[sɪmpl̩]	[simpl̩]	[sɪmpl̩]
list	[lɪst]	[list]	[lɪst]
him	[hɪm]	[him]	[hɪm]

To realize the importance in distinguishing /i/ from /ɪ/, compare the following word pairs:

/i/	/ɪ/
green [grin]	grin [grɪn]
scream [skrim]	scrim [skrɪm]
read [rid]	rid [rɪd]
meat [mit]	mit [mɪt]
neat [nit]	knit [nɪt]
lead [lid]	lid [lɪd]
Jean [ʤin]	gin [ʤɪn]
seed [sid]	Sid [sɪd]
teen [tin]	tin [tɪn]
scene [sin]	sin [sɪn]

Substitution of /ɔ/ for /o/

This substitution is rarely found in other languages. Record the following list of words and sentences, focusing on their transcription.

	Career	*Russian*	*Career*
coat	[kot]	[kɔt]	[kot]
fellow	[fɛlo]	[fɛljɔ]	[fɛlo]
blow	[blo]	[blɔ]	[blo]
hold	[hold]	[hɔlt]	[hold]
scold	[skold]	[skɔlt]	[skold]
moat	[mot]	[mɔt]	[mot]
slow	[slo]	[slɔ]	[slo]
low	[lo]	[lɔ]	[lo]
rowed	[rod]	[rɔt]	[rod]
alone	[əlon]	[əlɔn]	[əlon]

Refer to the comparison of /ɔ/ and /o/ on pp. 182–183.

The opening of *Oklahoma* was loaded with celebrities.

Snow White sang "Heigh Ho" along with Dopey.

The phoney old man was rowing toward the other rowboat.

Go and bring me the folders from both desks.

The short stories by Poe are often odious, woeful, and sorrowful.

Substitution of /u/ for /ʊ/

This substitution appears in Spanish. Record the following list of words and sentences as transcribed. Additional words and sentences appear on pp. 327–328.

	Career	*Russian*	*Career*
full	[fʊl]	[ful]	[fʊl]
bush	[bʊʃ]	[buʃ]	[bʊʃ]
mistook	[mɪstʊk]	[mistuk]	[mɪstʊk]
would	[wʊd]	[vud]	[wʊd]
wool	[wʊl]	[vul]	[wʊl]
book	[bʊk]	[buk]	[bʊk]
hood	[hʊd]	[hut]	[hʊd]
could	[kʊd]	[kut]	[kʊd]
bookcase	[bʊkes]	[bukes]	[bʊkes]
pudding	[pʊdɪŋ]	[pudiŋk]	[pʊdɪŋ]

The cook took the sugar and put it in the pudding.

The wolf stole the pullet and forsook the farm.

The wooden keg was full of beer.

The butcher withstood the insults as long as he could.

He shook the hook from the pushcart.

Substitution of /ɑ/ for /æ/

This substitution is common in several languages. Record the following list of words and sentences as transcribed. Additional words and sentences appear on pp. 316–317, 328–329.

	Career	*Russian*	*Career*
mad	[mæd]	[mɑd]	[mæd]
chap	[tʃæp]	[tʃɑp]	[tʃæp]
grab	[græb]	[grɑb]	[græb]
track	[træk]	[trɑk]	[træk]
add	[æd]	[ɑd]	[æd]
rather	[ræðɚ]	[rɑdəř]	[ræðɚ]
latch	[lætʃ]	[lɑtʃ]	[lætʃ]
man	[mæn]	[mɑn]	[mæn]
snack	[snæk]	[snɑk]	[snæk]
laughed	[læft]	[lɑft]	[læft]

ɑ   ɑ   ɑ   ɑ
The man's manners seemed radical to the chapter.

ɑ   ɑ   i   ɑ   ɑ   ɑ
Ask Andy if he saw the tan cat attack the dog.

ɑ   i   ɑ   i   ɔ   ɑ
"Candid Camera" is a popular program.

ɑ   ɑ   i   ɑ   ɑ   ɑ   ɑ   ɑ
The masked bandit grabbed half the calf and ran.

ɑ   ɑ   i   i   ɑ   xɑ   i
Cramming for examinations is a bad habit.

Substitution of /ɛř/ for /ɝ/

This substitution is also common in other languages. Record the following list of words and sentences as transcribed. Additional words and sentences appear on pp. 308–309.

	Career	*Russian*	*Career*
deserve	[dɪzɝv]	[dizɛřv]	[dɪzɝv]
earn	[ɝn]	[ɛřn]	[ɝn]
learn	[lɝn]	[lɛřn]	[lɝn]
hurt	[hɝt]	[hɛřt]	[hɝt]
reverse	[rɪvɝs]	[rivɛřs]	[rɪvɝs]
word	[wɝd]	[vɛřd]	[wɝd]
worth	[wɝθ]	[vɛřt]	[wɝθ]
reserve	[rɪzɝv]	[rizɛřv]	[rɪzɝv]
girl	[gɝl]	[gɛřl]	[gɝl]
dirt	[dɝt]	[dɛřt]	[dɝt]

Refer to the sentences on p. 309.

Consonants

Dentalization of /t/, /d/, and /n/

To produce dentalization, remember to place the blade of the tongue in contact with the back of the top teeth. To eliminate dentalization, refer to the discussion on p. 275. Record the following list of words, comparing the differences between career speech and the Russian dialect.

	Career	*Russian*	*Career*
today	[tədeɪ]	[t̪əde̪ɪ]	[tədeɪ]
don't	[dont]	[d̪ɔnt̪]	[dont]
numb	[nʌm]	[n̪am]	[nʌm]
dough	[doʊ]	[d̪ɔ]	[doʊ]
past	[pæst]	[past̪]	[pæst]
trust	[trʌst]	[t̪řast̪]	[trʌst]
wed	[wɛd]	[vɛd̪]	[wɛd]
cat	[kæt]	[kat̪]	[kæt]
wade	[wed]	[ved̪]	[wed]
once	[wʌns]	[vans̪]	[wʌns]

Substitution of /tʃ/ or /ʒ/ for /dʒ/

This substitution is very characteristic of the Russian dialect. Record the following list of words and sentences, using the transcriptions indicated by career speech and Russian.

	Career	*Russian*	*Career*
jump	[ʤʌmp]	[tʃamp], [ʒamp]	[ʤʌmp]
jaw	[ʤɔ]	[tʃɔ]	[ʤɔ]
judge	[ʤʌʤ]	[tʃatʃ]	[ʤʌʤ]
gentle	[ʤɛntl̩]	[tʃɛntl̩]	[ʤɛntl̩]
bridge	[brɪʤ]	[břitʃ], [bři ʒ]	[brɪʤ]
badge	[bæʤ]	[batʃ], [baʒ]	[bæʤ]
magic	[mæʤɪk]	[matʃik], [maʒik]	[mæʤɪk]
joke	[ʤok]	[tʃɔk], [ʒɔk]	[ʤok]

    tʃ   řɔ   ř tʃ
The angels wrote down the strategy.

tʃ tʃa   ř   a i
Judy jumped from the chair she sat in.

tʃi   ɑ tʃ   ɔ
Jim sent the badge to the police.

ř tʃ tʃɑ   i   ɑ tʃ
The stranger jumped into marriage.

ɑ tʃ   tʃɔ tʃ
Madge played the joke on John.

Substitution of /v/ for /w/

This substitution is common in the German dialect. Record the following list of words, using the phonetic transcription as presented.

	Career	*Russian*	*Career*
web	[wɛb]	[vɛb]	[wɛb]
way	[weɪ]	[veɪ]	[weɪ]
wasp	[wɔsp]	[vɔsp]	[wɔsp]
wavy	[wevɪ]	[vevi]	[wevɪ]
wall	[wɔl]	[vɔl]	[wɔl]
waste	[west]	[vest]	[west]
weather	[wɛðɚ]	[vedeř]	[wɛðɚ]
weak	[wik]	[vik]	[wik]
when	[ʍɛn]	[vɛn]	[ʍɛn]
white	[ʍaɪt]	[vaɪt]	[ʍaɪt]

For additional words, refer to p. 321.

Substitution of /d/ for /ð/

Refer to the words on pp. 321–322.

Substitution of /ř/ for /r/

Refer to the words on p. 308.

Addition of /k/ to /ŋ/ in Words With More Than One Syllable

Record the following words and sentences, comparing career speech with the Russian dialect.

	Career	*Russian*	*Career*
going	[goɪŋ]	[gɔiŋk]	[goɪŋ]
tying	[taɪɪŋ]	[t̪aɪiŋk]	[taɪɪŋ]

slaving   [slevɪŋ]   [slevɪŋk]   [slevɪŋ]

bowing   [bauɪŋ]   [bauɪŋk]   [bauɪŋ]

failing   [felɪŋ]   [feliŋk]   [felɪŋ]

stating   [stetɪŋ]   [stetiŋk]   [stetɪŋ]

jumping   [dʒʌmpɪŋ]   [tʃampiŋk]   [dʒʌmpɪŋ]

clanking   [klæŋkɪŋ]   [klaŋkiŋk]   [klæŋkɪŋ]

teaching   [titʃɪŋ]   [titʃiŋk]   [titʃɪŋ]

loving   [lʌvɪŋ]   [lafiŋk]   [lʌvɪŋ]

ɪŋk ɑ ɪŋk ɑ ɪŋk
Dividing and gliding and sliding.

ɑ ɪŋk ɑ ř ɪŋk ɑ ř ɪŋk
And falling and brawling and sprawling,

ɑ ř ɪŋk ɑ ř ɪŋk ɑ ři ɪŋk
And driving and riving and striving

ɑ ř ɪŋk ɑ i ɪŋk ɑ ři ɪŋk
And sprinkling and twinkling and wrinkling.

Substitution of /t/ for Final /d/

Record the following transcriptions, comparing career speech with the Russian dialect.

	Career	*Russian*	*Career*
had	[hæd]	[hɑt]	[hæd]
jade	[dʒed]	[tʃet]	[dʒed]
sound	[sɑund]	[sɑunt]	[sɑund]
braided	[bredəd]	[bředət]	[bredəd]
said	[sɛd]	[sɛt]	[sɛd]
nude	[nɪud]	[nut]	[nɪud]
opened	[opənd]	[ɔpənt]	[opənd]
patted	[pætəd]	[pɑtət]	[pætəd]
bad	[bæd]	[bɑt]	[bæd]

Substitution of /f/ for Medial or Final /v/

This substitution appears in the German dialect. Record the following list of words as transcribed. Additional words are given on p. 322.

	Career	*Russian*	*Career*
leave	[liv]	[lif]	[liv]
lovely	[lʌvlɪ]	[lafli]	[lʌvlɪ]

above	[əbʌv]	[əbaf]	[əbʌv]
forgive	[fɔrgɪv]	[fɔrgif]	[fɔrgɪv]
prove	[pruv]	[pruf]	[pruv]
serve	[sɝv]	[sɛřf]	[sɝv]
waves	[wevz]	[vefs]	[wevz]
move	[muv]	[muf]	[muv]
shove	[ʃʌv]	[ʃaf]	[ʃʌv]
carve	[kɑrv]	[kɑřf]	[kɑrv]

Substitution of /x/ or /ç/ for /h/

The /h/ phoneme does not exist in Russian. Refer to the words and sentences on pp. 330–331.

EXERCISES FOR A RUSSIAN ACCENT

Pronounce the following Russian nouns according to the phonetic transcription; use the primary stress indicated:

babushka ['bɑbuʃkə], grandmother

Bolshoi ['bɑlʃɔɪ], the ballet company

borscht [bɔřʃ], a vegetable and beet soup

dacha ['dɑtʃə], a country house

Gulag ['gulɑg], the group of concentration camps

nyet [njɛt] or [nɪɛt], no

samizdat [sɑmɪz'dat̪], an underground political paper

The following are commonly encountered proper names:

Aleksei [ɑlɪk'seɪ]

Boris [bɑ'ris]

Chekhov ['tʃɛkhɒf]

Ekaterina [ɪkətɪř'inə]

Galina [gɑ'linə]

Godunov [gədu'nɔf]

Gogol [ˈgɔgəl]

Grigori [gˇrɪˈgɔři]

Ivan [iˈvɑn]

Ivanova [iˈvɑnəvnɑ]

Ivanovich [iˈvɑnəvitʃ]

Moussorgsky [ˈmuzəřski]

Nabokov [nɑˈbɔkɒf]

Prokofiev [přɑˈkɔfjɛf]

Rasputin [řæsˈputin]

Rimski-Korsakov [ˈřimski ˈkɔrsikəf]

Shostakovich [ʃəstəˈkɔvitʃ]

Solzhenitsyn [solʒəˈnitsin]

Stanislavski [stɛnɪsˈlɑfski]

Stravinsky [střəˈvinski]

Tchaikovsky [tʃeˈkɒfski]

Tolstoi [ˈtʌlstɔi]

Vladimir [vlɑˈdimɛř]

In the following exercises, transcribe the phonetic substitution used in a Russian accent above the appropriate letters. As you become more adept at making the substitutions, increase your rate of speech. Work for continuity.

1. The Grand Duchess:

   Ah, Kolenkhov, our time is coming. My sister Natasha is studying to be a manicurist. Uncle Sergi they have promised to make floor-walker, and next month I get transferred to the Fifth Avenue Childs'. From there it is only a step to Schraffts', and then we will see what Prince Alexis says.

   From YOU CAN'T TAKE IT WITH YOU *Moss Hart and George Kaufman*

2. Kolenkhov:

   He should have been in Russia when the Revolution came. Then he would have stood in line—a bread line. Ah, Grandpa, what they have done to Russia. Think of it! The Grand Duchess, Olga Katrina, a cousin of the Czar, she is a waitress in Childs' restaurant! I ordered baked beans from her only yesterday. It broke my heart.

From YOU CAN'T TAKE IT WITH YOU   *Moss Hart and George Kaufman*

3. Ikonenko:

Herr Busch, your attitude, even though it is impossible to understand, does you no credit. I must warn you against the terrible danger of being incomprehensible in the future. I shall give the order tonight for Soviet troops to begin operations for the occupation of the castle at dawn tomorrow, so that it may pass back into the hands of its legitimate owners, the people!

From THE LOVE OF FOUR COLONELS   *Peter Ustinov*

4. Romanoff:

We have a perfect right to criticize each other. It is a pastime encouraged by the party. You have been criticizing me since your arrival. Now it's my turn. My criticism will take the form of a history lesson. Don't interrupt me—I am sure you know many more dates than I do, but I know more about our revolution than you do, because I was there!

From ROMANOFF AND JULIET   *Peter Ustinov*

5. Spy:

A confession of only eight pages? It appears as though you were still attempting to conceal something. Comrade Kotkov's recent confession ran to two hundred and fourteen typewritten pages, and was written in a clear, concise, functional style. At the end, the reader had a vivid impression of the author's inner rottenness. It was a model of how such documents should be prepared.

From ROMANOFF AND JULIET   *Peter Ustinov*

13

APPLICATION TO THE SPEECH OCCASION

GLOSSARY

Angles of Direction   A technique for differentiating characters that are being suggested during a speech occasion.

Audience Feedback   Signals given to the speaker during a speech occasion, such as restlessness, attentiveness, or enjoyment.

Canned Speech   Speech that sounds memorized or spoken many times and is therefore devoid of vocal or mental dynamics.

Direct Performance Occasion   A situation in which the speaker talks directly to the audience and expresses his or her own ideas and emotions.

Empathy   Feeling what another person feels.

Eye Contact   Degree to which a speaker looks into the eyes of the members of the audience.

Indirect Performance Occasion   A situation in which a speaker creates fictional characters and presents their thoughts and feelings.

Introduction   Opening of a speech occasion when the audience is acquainted with the speaker.

Lectern   Wooden or metal stand upon which a speaker's notes are placed and fists with white knuckles are clenched.

Podium   A dais upon which the feet rest or a platform upon which a speaker stands.

Thus far, this text has dealt mainly with the individual parts of speech—the individual sounds, the common vocal errors, and suggestions for gaining dynamism. It is now time to discuss the oral performance. The purpose of this chapter is to discuss the application of voice and speech to the speaking event. Excellent voice and speech are worth little individually unless they are applied together in a communication act.

STAGE FRIGHT

Every effective oral communicator has stage fright—that feeling of "butterflies in the stomach" often described by actors. Be assured. Everyone has the jitters. If you do not, you will probably have a very unsuccessful communication experience. Your case of nerves indicates that you want to be successful. You care! When you are feeling nervous, your glands are secreting adrenaline into your blood just as they would if you were an Olympic athlete about to break a record. That desire to do well, to break that record, is what gets the adrenaline pumping. This is a positive happening! However, this stimulated emotional state must be made to work for you. Otherwise, your thinking will become sloppy and your muscles will tighten excessively.

There are two extremes: (1) The speaker who is so nervous that the butterflies have turned into mallard ducks, and (2) the speaker who is so cool and so confident that his or her performance will probably be boring, since the apparent lack of concern about the communication act will likely lead to a lack of electricity during the communication.

Inexperienced performers are often overwhelmed by anxiety and focus energy in the wrong place. They no longer concentrate on getting the message across. Uncle Ned's scenario goes something like this:

I don't know what to do with my arms and legs. Ah, I'll put my hands in my pocket and look cool. Oh, boy, I can hear myself playing with the change in my pocket. Maybe if I put one hand on my hip . . . or better still, I'll cross my arms. . . . Oh, oh, my left knee is starting to shake. I'll shift my weight. . . . Where am I? I forget what I was saying. . . . They're jeering; they're leaving their seats. . . . They're coming up after me. He-e-e-elp!

These comments are not too unlike those reported by many novice speakers. What went so catastrophically wrong in Ned's case? He forgot his purpose and allowed his mind to wander, thinking about himself and his own reactions rather than keeping his concentration where it ought to be—getting that message across to the jury, congregation, potential buyers, students, or whomever. He became self-conscious. This is a difficult lesson to learn. If you have ever driven an automobile when the roads were slippery, you know that you are supposed to go with the skid and not apply the brakes. How many inexperienced drivers can do that? Because of the tension under these conditions, it is a difficult task even for the seasoned driver.

If you have prepared properly, no one in the audience knows that material better than you. You are the expert. Concentrate on getting that information across to the audience, whether the information is a sales presentation, a reading, a summary, or a report; whatever the vehicle, your concentration must stay on the content!

Everyone is self-conscious and sensitive to some degree. These self-protective instincts are aroused when you are presenting yourself, under stress, to an audience. You are vulnerable! Think of yourself as having two antennae. One must never stray from the message being presented. The other must be aimed toward the audience so that it can pick up cues (feedback) about how effective your presentation is. Under the terror of the speaking situation, you must not give in to the temptation of turning both antennae toward yourself.

Don't try to inhibit the physical tension due to anxiety. Use it. Shift your weight. If you are so inclined, take a step toward your audience. Use a gesture if it comes from within. Make your tense muscles useful.

PERFORMANCE OCCASIONS

There are two major types of performance occasions: direct and indirect, which are sometimes called open and closed situations. In the **direct performance occasion**, there is direct contact between the speaker and the audience. In addition, the speaker expresses his or her own ideas and emotions. Any form of public speaking is a direct occasion, because the speaker is relating to a specific audience in a specific place at a specific time. Other direct occasions include the following:

the cleric's homily,

the businessperson's presentation,

the lawyer's opening argument,

the professor's lecture,

the salesperson's presentation,

the anchor's news, and

just plain conversation and discussion.

In the second kind of performance occasion, the **indirect performance occasion**, the ideas and emotions expressed by the speaker are not necessarily his or her own. The audience addressed may be the audience that is present or one determined by the speaker. An actor's performance of a scene from a play, for example, would be an indirect performance occasion. According to the play, Macbeth and Lady Macbeth are plotting the death of King Duncan alone. Although the performers must never forget that there is an actual audience and therefore not turn their backs, their characters are alone in the castle. Other indirect occasions include the following:

the actor's monologue,

the recorded commercial,

the cleric's scriptural reading, and

the storyteller's narrative.

It should be stressed that a performance occasion can be direct and indirect. For instance, a narrator in a story recognizes the audience actually present and directs the narrative to them, but when the characters are speaking, the audience "disappears." In this instance, the ideas and emotions that the narrator has may or may not be the narrator's own.

ANALYSIS OF THE AUDIENCE

Before any performance, you should know who your audience is if at all possible. This information is certain to affect the content of your performance. If you are speaking to the inmates at a house of correction, a speech on the values of capital punishment would probably be inappropriate. The demographics of the group, their race, sex, occupation, education, economic status, social standing, and religion are invaluable in determining what material to communicate. In addition, this knowledge helps in deciding on which figures of speech to use, what illustrations to have, which senses to appeal to, and how sophisticated to be.

INTRODUCTION

An **introduction** begins when you present yourself or are presented to an audience. This is very much a part of the performance. How you are dressed and your attitude as you walk to the front of the room influence your audience. Are you happy to be there? Do you appear confident? Are you making faces that indicate you're nervous? Are you anxious to communicate? Are you compensating for your nervousness by appearing cocky? Remember that as long as the audience can see or hear you, you are being monitored and communication is taking place. (In fact, you continue to communicate after your oral presentation is over as you leave the performance environment. Audience members can tell if you are disappointed or pleased with your presentation. So be on guard.)

The second part of the introduction is the verbal component, although non-verbal communication continues. Your verbal introduction should introduce both you and your "product" to the audience. Are you there to give a report? A homily? An audition?

The length of the verbal introduction partially depends on the material being presented. An introduction for an acting scene would probably be longer than the setup for a conventional public speech. However, it is a good idea to keep an introduction as brief as possible.

Do not read your introduction. That is counterproductive. The purpose of the introduction is to prepare the audience for your presentation. You and your content are that presentation. When an introduction is read, the sense of spontaneity with your audience is diminished. Obviously, your full attention cannot be where it ought to be. This is your first opportunity to relate. Take advantage of it! It is impossible for communication to flow from you freely to an audience if you are reading an introduction. If your purpose is to read a report, you should still make certain that your introduction is conversational and not read.

Directing the introduction to the audience also gives you an opportunity of reading **audience feedback**. Remember that the first impression is the most important. Are they listening? How hard do you have to work to gain and maintain their attention? Seeing a smiling face can work miracles for a nervous speaker.

Since the introduction is a part of the performance, it should be well prepared. If it is necessary to memorize your introduction, make it seem spontaneous and conversational. Above all do not allow yourself to use **canned speech**!

An introduction should prepare the audience for the material to be presented. Is it literature? What is the subject matter to be debated? Is it a presentation at the Toastmasters? What can the audience members expect to hear?

The introduction should also set up the audience for the material. If the presentation is light and humorous, you would not want to get the audience into a serious frame of mind. If, on the other hand, the content is strongly emotional, you would want to be careful about using any humor. Sometimes, however, the surgeon giving a lecture on vascular diseases might want to bring in a little levity. Of course, any lightness depends on the makeup of the audience; you would relate differently to peers than to the elderly, for example.

You, the performer, can benefit as well as the audience from the introduction. Use the introduction to channel some of that nervous energy and to help you settle yourself down. Use that time to get to know your listeners.

EYE CONTACT

Although direct and indirect **eye contact** were mentioned in Chapter 10, it is so important to the direct performance occasion that we shall elaborate on them here. The eyes are the most important part of the face. Ralph Waldo Emerson said, "The alleged power to charm down . . . the ferocity in beasts, is a power behind the eye." Others have said that "the eyes are the mirrors of the soul" and have referred to the "evil eye"!

One of the most common behaviors by nervous, inexperienced speakers is a lack of direct eye contact with the audience. This technique of not looking into the eyes of audience members is frequently used because the speaker does not want the audience to see his or her nervousness. Neither does the speaker desire to see in the eyes of the audience the fact that his or her inept delivery has been detected. The belief is that if the speaker used direct eye contact, the audience would discover his or her worthlessness.

Force yourself to look into the eyes of the audience. They are not the enemy, believe it or not! Most of them are in that audience because they want to be. Some speech texts have recommended that you focus on the foreheads of your audience, but by doing this you not only miss the reaction of the audience but also develop a forehead fetish. A person's forehead gives a speaker little support; its communicative powers are minimal. Instead, pick out a few friendly faces at first and gradually include more. You must also maintain eye contact long enough for communication to take place. Sometimes a speaker looks but does not see, while the audience hears but does not listen. An audience will respond to the degree that the speaker demands. The responsibility begins with the speaker. If the speaker reaches out to the audience, they will respond.

ANGLES OF DIRECTION

How does a speaker stay in contact with the audience when not speaking to them directly? This is accomplished by using a technique called the *projected scene*. A projected scene is used when the material being presented is dramatic. For example, a priest or minister reading the Scriptures might use a projected scene. There are moments when a character might be talking to another character instead of the audience. You do not want to look at a member of the audience and make him Pilate to whom Jesus is speaking. Instead, Jesus (as played by the cleric) would see Pilate on the back wall of the church. When Pilate answers Jesus, the speaker would look at another place on the back wall. These different points form **angles of direction**.

This technique is useful for both the speaker and the audience whenever a character is involved in direct discourse within a drama, prose, or poetry. In such a situation one character is speaking to himself or herself or to another character, and the actual audience is somewhere between the character speaking and the receiver of that speech. Speaking directly to the audience might make them uncomfortable.

The simplest way of using the angles of direction is to position yourself, the speaker, at the apex of a triangle. Under ordinary circumstances, the speaker's characters would not be located outside this triangle. The size of the triangle depends on the number of characters in the performance as well as the size of the room and the size of the audience. The area opposite the apex of the triangle, the back of the room, forms the base of the triangle. In determining the size of the triangle, the speaker must always keep in mind that the audience should be able to see at least a three-quarters profile of the speaker. Nothing is more frustrating to an audience than seeing half of a speaker's face!

In establishing the angles of direction, the speaker must keep in mind that the character speaking determines the angle of direction, *not* the character being addressed, who is placed somewhere between the speaker and the character listening.

Sometimes a speaker employs this technique by picking out spots on the back wall and placing the imaginary listener there. Thus, the speaker is not talking to spots on the back of a wall but is imagining a character. If the speaker is seeing spots instead of characters, perhaps an optometrist should be consulted. Remember that each character in the scene has his or her own placement. This technique not only makes speakers and characters clear to an audience but also aids the performer in imagining the fictive world of the selection.

Figure 13.1 illustrates the three common types of rooms used for speaking occasions. The shape of the room and the position of the audience determine the shape of the triangle. Figure 13.1a represents the most common rectangular-shaped room, with the speaker working at one of the longer sides of the rectangle. The triangle is superimposed within the rectangle. The base of this triangle is smaller than the one in Figure 13.1b, which requires a broader base since the audience is spread more widely. In Figure 13.1c, the audience is sitting in a semicircle, which requires the speaker to use a smaller base to maintain the suggested three-quarters profile. These angles of direction within the triangle are simply suggestions. Make your own angles of direction, if you wish. If you have the misfortune of speaking in an arena theater, good luck!

Sometimes, in situations where angles of direction are used, the speaker may also deal directly with the audience. In the following children's poem, the performer/narrator relates directly to the audience those parts of the selection that are narrative. A projected scene using angles of direction is used during the notated direct discourse. The introduction would be given directly to the audience.

Not so very long ago, even during the lifetime of Mahatma Gandhi, India had a social system that limited the freedom of its people. It had a caste system. This system worked as follows:

If one were born into the system, he or she had to remain in the social class and follow the occupation of his or her family for life. There were few exceptions.

Young Krishna Panju, a gentle, happy, twelve-year-old Hindu boy, grew up in that system. He was a member of the Ksha-tri-ya caste. This caste had, as one of its duties, the protection of the sacred cows. Krishna, however, felt that he

FIGURE 13.1   MOST COMMON PERFORMANCE AREAS

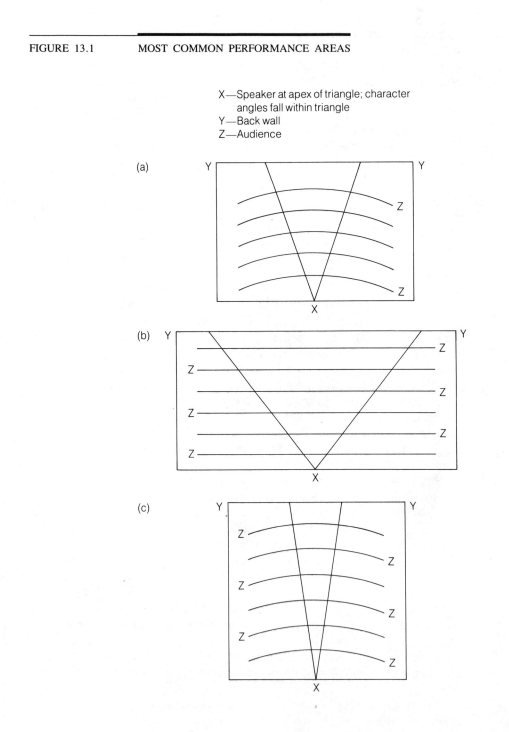

did not want to spend his life doing the work of a Ksha-tri-ya just because it was expected of him by society. He felt that he would be happier and society would be much better off if he followed his heart.

This is the story of how Krishna, in his own unique way, may have helped change the system.

In a small, dusty village southeast of Bombay,
The few sacred cows had become tiger prey.
The families who lived there, most Sud-ras[1] by caste,
Practiced total nonviolence, and so were aghast.

They petitioned the Brah-mins,[2] "Sirs, things are quite bad.   [angle 1]
Now nothing's sacred; all nature's gone mad.
Please, find a Ksha-tri-ya;[3] he'll know what to do.
Are any still living?" One snapped, "Old Panju."   [angle 2]

Old Panju soon arrived to help save the poor cows,
There were speeches and flowers and handshakes and bows.
He brought his son Krishna, a cousin or two,
And his elephant, Rajah, this was his whole crew.

Young Krishna was twelve; he was eager and smart,
But cooking fine foods held first place in his heart.
He had hunted before and was never afraid,
Now, he wanted to work in the restaurant trade.

The village officials warned Panju that day,
"If you don't get results, you'll be sent on your way.   [angle 1]
You have brought no real weapons, no sword, spear, or gun,
And your crew seems quite listless, especially your son."

Old Panju started hunting; he searched high and low.
He stumbled sometimes when a root caught his toe.
His glasses were thick and his eyesight was poor,
But he said only he could find fresh, tiger spoor.[4]

He had Krishna play si-tar[5] atop Rajah's back
And sing, but his sad voice would waiver and crack,
For he knew his old father just could not produce,
And the Brahmin officials would soon cook his goose!

---

[1]*Sud-ras:* members of the lowest caste; they had to serve others.

[2]*Brah-mins:* members of the upper caste; they usually were rulers and officials.

[3]*Ksha-tri-ya:* a member of the warrior caste. Their duties were to protect the Brahmins and the sacred cows. At the time of this story, this caste had almost disappeared.

[4]*spoor:* footprints or other traces of wild animals.

[5]*si-tar:* a stringed instrument similar to a guitar used in Hindu music.

The tigers, though hungry, annoyed by this sound,
Just hid in the brush, and they could not be found.
Young Krishna said, "Dad, get a good sleep tonight.   [angle 3]
I've a plan, and tomorrow we'll put them to flight."

Krishna early next day, though the weather was fair,
In a pit, built a fire, and soon filled the air
With sparks and thick billows of black and white smoke.
One stern Brahmin grumbled, "This must be a joke."   [angle 1]

"Well, we all have to eat," explained Krishna Panju,   [angle 3]
And dumped vegetables, water, and curry[6] for stew
In a huge, iron kettle and boiled them so slow,
That the village was famished when he called, "Let's go!"   [angle 3]

The village officials were shocked when they passed.
"The boy's cooking, not hunting! That's not for his caste!   [angle 1]
And the crowd! Oh, my ears! Such a horrible din!
It's the worse mess this village has ever been in."

At the edge of the village in everyone's sight,
Krishna set four full bowls, which he knew that same night
Would be gulped down by tigers made fearless by greed,
So he dumped in more curry to warm up their feed!

The stew in the bowls became hot—just intense!
And most tigers you meet would have had better sense
Than to eat such a supper when out on the prowl,
But these tigers, they ate it, and how they did howl!

They rolled in the dust, they snarled, and wailed weird,
They raced through the village and soon disappeared,
While the villagers cheered as they faded from view,
A fierce, bearded Sikh[7] said, "We've still got more stew."   [angle 2]

So, the party continued with laughter and joy:
The people took turns praising Panju's smart boy,
Except for the Brahmins who sulked in their place,
For they felt breaking caste was an awful disgrace.

A visiting Vais-ya[8] had visions of gold,
"I can sell this fine stew whether fresh cooked or cold.[9]   [audience]

---

[6]*curry:* a powder used to season almost all Indian cooking. Because it contains red and black pepper, ginger, cloves, onions, and so forth, too much can make food very, very hot!

[7]*Sikh:* a member of a military sect that rejected the caste system.

[8]*Vais-ya:* a member of the merchant caste, which was responsible for the prosperity of the country.

[9]Of course, angle 1 or 2 would be proper, but a different aesthetic is achieved when this line is directed to the audience. Try it both ways and you will feel a difference.

It is hearty and healthy and has a fine taste,
If this boy doesn't cook, that will be the disgrace!"

A wizened Ma-hat-ma[10] said, "You all are blind!   [angle 1]
Can't you see his rare talent must help all mankind?
There are small towns and cities where it would be nice
If Pan-cha-mas[11] could have curry stew with their rice."

Old Panju and young Krishna discussed it all night.
The Sikh advised Panju that Krishna was right.
Panju finally relented, "Son, go your own way,   [angle 2]
And I will work with you." The crowd cheered, "Hooray!"   [audience]

From that day, besides cooking, young Krishna Panju
Became busy distributing fine, curry stew
In buckets and bottles, a jar or a can,
With Rajah, his faithful delivery van.

He sang with his si-tar and people would say,
"He's so happy!" and loved it when he passed their way   [audience]
With his father and new friend, the fierce, bearded Sikh,
As they spent their lives serving the poor and the weak.

POSTSCRIPT

If you happen to pass through our village, you'll see,
A plaque the officials placed high on a tree,
It reads, "This will recall our great joy on the day   [as if reading plaque]
That the tigers and Krishna Panju went away."

TIGERS AND STEW AND YOUNG KRISHNA PANJU   *Eugene Lyttle*

MEMORIZATION VERSUS USING NOTES

The material for a speech determines the style of presentation. One of the considerations, of course, is whether the material is performed from memory or read. Generally, if the material allows the speaker to address the audience directly (a direct performance occasion), detailed notes should not be used. Very brief notes are acceptable for a sales presentation that includes complicated details. However, when you're speaking directly to an audience, the less you have to rely on notes the better. The continuity of thought that develops in the communication process between the speaker and audience is broken if the speaker keeps looking down at notes.

---

[10]*Ma-hat-ma:* a holy man and a title of respect.

[11]*Pan-cha-mas:* the untouchables, the miserable poor.

On special occasions, such as the presentation of an annual report, the text is meant to be read aloud. In those cases, the principles governing a direct performance occasion are applied. However, if you are reading a report or commencement speech, make certain that it is concealed within a black folder so that the audience can't count the pages with you or see how thick the text is! As audience members, how many times have you looked forward to seeing the speaker holding the final lonely page?

Memorization should be used with great discrimination. If the speech sounds canned, you have lost much of your ability to persuade. Never memorize entire sentences and paragraphs! If someone sneezes or coughs or otherwise breaks your concentration, your chances of continuing from memory are rather slight. What do you do? Start the paragraph over? Sometimes it is necessary to go back to the beginning like a novice at a piano recital because that is how you rehearsed your speech. These dangers of memorization also apply to poems, monologues, and other material made more pleasing when presented from memory.

If notes are used on a direct performance occasion, they should be sparse, containing single words or phrases to remind the speaker about organization or content. A quick look down ought to do the trick!

On the indirect performance occasion (where the audience is not addressed directly), a character is speaking rather than the actual speaker. For example, an interpretative reading of a dramatic monologue (with or without the text) presents the words and thoughts of a character to another character in the fictional world (rather than the actual audience). If you choose to read from a text, make certain that you do not rely too heavily on it. Be very familiar with the material! Nothing takes the place of having control over the content. Hold the book high enough so you merely have to lower your eyes to glance at the script. If you hold the text in your less dominant hand, your gestures may be stronger because you will be free to use your stronger side. Many readers hold the text too low and must peek at the audience. A great deal of the performance is missed when the speaker's face cannot be seen.

If you use a script, be sure to mark it so that when your eyes go to the text, you do not have to waste time searching for your place. You might put a large colored arrow at the word to be read. It is important for you to look down at the script at the same times during each rehearsal. Then reading the script becomes a part of the technique you use in your performance. If you look down only when your memory "dries up," you will not know exactly where you are and may panic unnecessarily. This unsureness will be revealed in your performance.

A cleric's homily mixes direct and indirect performance occasions. The reading of the Scriptures, of course, is from text. The narrative elements are directed to the audience, which is not only the present audience but also the characters in the biblical scene. When a character speaks to another character, the occasion becomes indirect. The cleric's sermon or remarks should be a direct performance occasion with as few glances into the notes as possible. Remember that nothing takes the place of preparation, rehearsal, and control over the content.

LECTERN

The lectern by its very existence poses a barrier between the speaker and the audience. The term **lectern** comes from the Latin *lector* meaning "reader." A lectern was meant to hold a book, usually the Bible. It does not mean "to clutch," "to turn one's knuckles white," "to hide behind," or "to play peekaboo." If a lectern is used with its purpose in mind, there will be no problem for the performer. Unfortunately, an untrained speaker feels more comfortable when he can lean on, wrap around, or hold on to the edges of the lectern in desperation.

Frequently, lecterns in churches are located in awkward places away from the audience, which simply contributes to the division between the speaker and the audience. A cleric's first job is to remove or at least avoid using those huge wooden structures. The sermons should be given to the congregation in full view and as close to them as possible. For the reading, hold the book in your nondominant hand and rehearse. The Spirit of the Lord doesn't enter in and make the lazy reader successful. "God continues to help those who help themselves."

The same advice applies to the speaker who has to perform in a hotel meeting room. Usually lecterns in such rooms are large boxes resting on a table. You can't be seen, and you become a distraction. Get rid of the lectern and get closer to your audience. Bring notes if you really need them, but refer to them infrequently. You should prepare yourself well. Always remember that you should rid yourself of anything that distances you—physically or psychologically—from your audience.

MICROPHONE

The microphone is one of the greatest inventions of the twentieth century. On the other hand, it imposes limitations on many speaking situations. Of course, they are necessary for the media, but in most halls, small theaters, churches, and hotels, microphones are unnecessary since the human voice can be trained to be heard rather easily. A microphone becomes a limitation because it inhibits a speaker's movements, since it is usually anchored to the heinous lectern. Or, if you use a lapel mike, you must be sure not to turn your head from side to side or your voice disappears. If you are lucky to have a cordless mike, your audience may anticipate that you will break into song.

When you do not have a mike, you must reach your audience visually, aurally, and aesthetically. There is an energy that is created when the human voice must be heard without mechanical amplification. In addition, microphone systems are frequently run by people who know nothing more than how to turn the switch on. As a result, sometimes there is distortion and a lack of intelligibility when using a mike.

One of the most frustrating things about going to the theater today is that everything is miked! In a musical, we know who is going to do the big tap number because we hear the clinking long before the first step. Every actor should get vocal training. How much nicer for the audience and easier for the actor when the speaker is unhampered by a mike.

REHEARSAL

You must rehearse if you want to be a successful communicator—and you must rehearse aloud—and to your imaginary audience. If at all possible, rehearse at least once in the room in which you will be speaking. Also, acquire as much information as you can about your audience. When you rehearse in the room, see your audience in that setting.

It is also a good idea to tape rehearsals and learn from the tape. Of course, a videotape of your rehearsal is preferable. You must be objective when you review such a tape, however. Look at what you actually did—not at what you intended to do. It is too late for that now. Watch your body. Did it communicate what you wanted? What about your face? If you used visuals in your presentation, did they detract, or did you use them wisely? Did the audience look at the visuals while you were talking? Were you seeing your audience? Were you including everyone? By anticipating problems and rehearsing your presentation well, you will probably be able to handle any calamity that arises during the performance.

EMPATHY

Empathy is a "feeling into." In the communicative process, you want your audience to have an empathic response to you and what you are saying. You, on the other hand, want to have an empathic response to the audience. Essentially, empathy is composed of three responses: intellectual, emotional, and physical. First, you want your audience to understand what you are presenting, whether it is a speech of instruction, a lecture, a homily, or a poem. Second, you want your audience to feel, to have an emotional reaction toward what they understand intellectually. Third, you want a physical response from that audience. Learn to read their feedback. Are they leaning forward because they are highly interested in your speech, or are they leaning forward because they can't hear you easily? Are they smiling, or do those glazed eyes signify boredom? Have you caused them to feel?

The empathic response is easy to see in the young boy who pretends that he is riding off into the sunset with Clint at the end of an Eastwood movie. The youngster's mimicking of riding the horse indicates that the three processes have taken place.

TASTE

Good taste is difficult to define. It is far easier to define bad taste. Charles Wesley Emerson said that "anything that interferes with the flow of the vitalized picture is in bad taste."[12] Taste is a very personal characteristic. What is tasteful for one person is not to another. Bad taste can manifest itself in a performer, material, an audience, or an occasion.

A speaker can be dressed in bad taste. For example, it is perfectly acceptable to wear your diamond pendant to a cocktail party, but the lights in a hotel ballroom where you are speaking may make the necklace sparkle so much that attention is drawn away from your message.

A priest might wear a liturgical garment that is particularly full and flowing, causing him to pull constantly at his sleeves to free his arms or hands, or he might frighten a congregation by getting too close to a lighted candle. Either action is very distracting and would interfere with the energized picture. To avoid this kind of costume dilemma, a priest should first wear the garment during rehearsal to get used to it.

In another example, material might be in bad taste if it is inappropriate for an audience. Thus one would probably not discuss the virtues of MTV with an audience comprised of the elderly.

In addition, it is very possible that that which is considered in good taste for one speaker is not in good taste for another (dress, content, and so forth). Analyze the audience, the material, and most of all your participation.

EXERCISES FOR THE SPEECH OCCASION

The following selections have been included so that you can apply the principles of good speech and voice that have been presented. Comments on performance are made where appropriate.

1. In The Hague, Netherlands, when the temperature is about 46 degrees and the humidity is just right, toads cross a road to get to their mating grounds.

---

[12] Charles W. Emerson, *Evolution of Expression,* vol. 3 (Millis, Mass.: Emerson Publishing Co., 1920), p. 11.

Many were killed by cars until a Herr Bleumink obtained permission to put up a gate during the mating time. It was also noted that at the height of the mating period, females carry the smaller male toads piggyback to the breeding grounds. Such newsworthy happenings should not go uncelebrated.

A passionate toad crossing Duinlaan Road
In the land of the Zuider Zee,
So preoccupied with the other side,
That he failed to hear or see
A car or a jeep that didn't beep,
But caught him by surprise.
Pffhht! he died on that road, an ugly toad,
With the lovelight still in his eyes.
Now, will he be missed at the annual tryst
In the ditch by the North Sea dune,
In March when the temperature's forty-six
And the toads start to moon and croon?
"Well," said his mate as she passed Bleumink's gate
With a toad piggyback, "You can see,
In the pale moonlight on a humid night,
All toads look alike to me."

ODE TO A TOAD WHO DIED ON THE ROAD   *Eugene F. Lyttle*

2. My dearest friend—White or some of my friends or the public papers by this time may have informed you of the terrible calamities that have fallen on our family. I will only give you the outlines. My poor dear dearest sister in a fit of insanity has been the death of her own mother. I was at hand only time enough to snatch the knife out of her grasp. She is at present in a mad house, from whence I fear she must be moved to an hospital. God has preserved to me my senses,—I eat and drink and sleep, and have my judgment I believe very sound. My poor father was slightly wounded, and I am left to take care of him and my aunt. . . . Write,—as religious a letter as possible—but no mention of what is gone and done with—with me the former things are passed away, and I have something more to do that [than] to feel—

    God almighty
    have us all in
    his keeping,—C. Lamb

From THE LETTERS OF CHARLES LAMB

3. In the following sonnet, pay attention to the poet's use of sound, particularly alliteration (/g/, /r/, /l/, /f/, and /w/), assonance (/e/, /ɛ/, /æ/, and /o/), and the use of onomatopoeia, end-of-line rhymes, and internal rhymes.

The world is charged with the grandeur of God.
It will flame out, like shining from shook foil;
It gathers to a greatness like the ooze of oil
Crushed. Why do men then now not reck his rod?

Generations have trod, have trod, have trod;
And all is seared with trade; bleared, smeared with toil;
And wears man's smudge and shares man's smell: the soil
Is Bare now, nor can foot feel, being shod.

And for all this, nature is never spent;
There lives the dearest freshest deep down things;
And though the last lights off the black West went
Oh, morning at the brown brink eastward springs—
Because the Holy Ghost over the bent
World broods with warm breast and with ah! bright wings.

GOD'S GRANDEUR   *Gerard Manley Hopkins*

4.   THE PRESIDENT'S FEDERAL BLUEPRINT FOR FISCAL 198__ WENT
BEFORE CONGRESS TODAY.

AND IT APPEARS THAT THE BUDGET IS ON A ROAD HEADED FOR
A COLLISION WITH LAWMAKERS.

THAT BUDGET PROPOSAL CALLED FOR AN OVERALL FREEZE FOR
ALL AGENCIES EXCEPT DEFENSE AND MAYBE SOCIAL SECURITY, RAIS-
ING CRITICISM FROM DEMOCRATS AND REPUBLICANS ALIKE.

THE PRESIDENT CALLED ON THE LAWMAKERS TO EXHIBIT POLIT-
ICAL COURAGE.

HE ALSO ADMITTED HIS PROPOSAL MIGHT NOT MAKE IT TO CON-
GRESS INTACT.

THE BUDGET CALLS FOR A HIKE IN DEFENSE SPENDING BY 13%
AND CHOPS AID TO THE POOR BY 5%.

THE PRESIDENT DEFENDED THE DEFENSE BUDGET.

THIS IS WHERE THE MONEY GOES: FORTY-ONE CENTS IS FOR BEN-
EFIT PAYMENTS. TWENTY-ONE CENTS TO THE NATIONAL DEFENSE.
FIFTEEN FOR INTEREST FOR THE NATIONAL DEBT. TEN CENTS TO
GRANTS FOR STATE AND LOCAL GOVERNMENT. AND FIVE CENTS TO
HELP RUN OTHER FEDERAL OPERATIONS.

THE SOVIET UNION HAS REACTED SHARPLY TO THE PRESIDENT'S
BUDGET.

THE SOVIETS SAY U.S. MILITARY BUDGET INCREASES WILL STRAIN
FURTHER ARMS TALKS.

THEY ARE ESPECIALLY UPSET OVER U.S. PLANS FOR A SPACE-
BASED SHIELD AGAINST RUSSIAN MISSILES.

ACCORDING TO THE SOVIET OFFICIALS THERE WILL BE NO NU-
CLEAR WEAPONS AGREEMENT UNLESS THE STAR WARS PLAN IS
HALTED.

THE U.S. DEFENSE SECRETARY HAS DEFENDED THE BUDGET IN-
CREASES.

HE CONTENDS CUTTING EXPENDITURE WOULD WEAKEN THE
AMERICAN BARGAINING POSITION.

5. Jesus before Pilate:

Early in the morning Jesus was taken from Caiaphas' house to the governor's
palace. The Jewish authorities did not go inside the palace, for they wanted
to keep themselves ritually clean, in order to be able to eat the Passover meal.
So Pilate went outside to them and asked, "What do you accuse this man of?"

Their answer was, "We would not have brought him to you if he had not
committed a crime."

Pilate said to them, "Then you yourselves take him and try him according
to your own law."

They replied, "We are not allowed to put anyone to death." (This hap-
pened in order to make come true what Jesus had said when he indicated the
kind of death he would die.)

Pilate went back into the palace and called Jesus. "Are you the king of
the Jews?" he asked him.

Jesus answered, "Does this question come from you or have others told
you about me?"

Pilate replied, "Do you think I am a Jew? It was your own people and the
chief priests who handed you over to me. What have you done?"

Jesus said, "My kingdom does not belong to this world; if my kingdom
belonged to this world my followers would fight to keep me from being
handed over to the Jewish authorities. No, my kingdom does not belong
here!"

So Pilate asked him, "Are you a king, then?"

Jesus answered, "You say that I am a king. I was born and came into the
world for this one purpose, to speak about the truth. Whoever belongs to the
truth listens to me."

"And what is the truth?" Pilate asked.

Then Pilate went back outside to the people and said to them, "I cannot
find any reason to condemn him. But according to the custom you have, I
always set free a prisoner for you during the Passover. Do you want me to set
free for you the king of the Jews?"

They answered him with a shout, "No, not him! We want Barabbas!"
(Barabbas was a bandit.)

Then Pilate took Jesus and had him whipped. The soldiers made a crown
out of thorny branches and put it on his head; then they put a purple robe on
him and came to him and said, "Long live the King of the Jews!" And they
went up and slapped him.

From BOOK OF JOHN

6. **Sir Peter:**   Lady Teazle, Lady Teazle, I'll not bear it!   [angle 1]

   Lady Teazle: Sir Peter, Sir Peter, you may bear it or not, as you please;

but I ought to have my own way in everything, and what's more, I will too.—What! though I was educated in the country, I know very well that women of fashion in London are accountable to nobody after they are married.   [angle 2]

Sir Peter: Very well, ma'am, very well,—so a husband is to have no influence, no authority?   [angle 1]

Lady Teazle: Authority! No, to be sure—if you wanted authority over me, you should have adopted me, and not married me; I am sure you were old enough.   [angle 2]

Sir Peter: Old enough!—aye, there it is!—Well, well, Lady Teazle, though my life may be made unhappy by your temper, I'll not be ruined by your extravagance.   [angle 1]

Lady Teazle: My extravagance! I'm sure I'm not more extravagant than a woman of fashion ought to be.   [angle 2]

Sir Peter: No, no madam, you shall throw away no more sums on such unmeaning luxury. 'Slife! to spend as much to furnish your dressingroom with flowers in winter as would suffice to turn the Pantheon into a greenhouse, and give a fete champetre at Christmas!   [angle 1]

Lady Teazle: Lord, Sir Peter, am I to blame because flowers are dear in cold weather? You should find fault with the climate, and not with me. For my part, I am sure I wish it was spring all the year round, and that roses grew under one's feet!

[angle 2]

Sir Peter: Oons! madam—if you had been born to this, I shouldn't wonder at your talking thus.—But you forget what your situation was when I married you.   [angle 1]

Lady Teazle: No, no, I don't; 'twas a very disagreeable one, or I should never have married you.   [angle 2]

From THE SCHOOL FOR SCANDAL
Richard Sheridan

7. Lucy Westenra's Diary: [use indirect occasion]
12 September.—How good they all are to me. I quite love that dear Dr. Van Helsing. I wonder why he was so anxious about these flowers. He positively frightened me, he was so fierce. And yet he must have been right, for I feel comfort from them already. Somehow, I do not dread being alone to-night, and I can go to sleep without fear. I shall not mind any flapping outside the window. Oh, the terrible struggle that I have had against sleep so often of late; the pain of the sleeplessness, or the pain of the fear of sleep, and with such unknown horrors as it has for me! How blessed are some people, whose lives have no fears, no dreads; to whom sleep is a blessing that comes nightly, and brings nothing but sweet dreams. Well, here I am tonight, hoping for sleep, and lying like Ophelia in the play with "virgin crants and maiden strew-

meats." I never liked garlic before, but to-night it is delightful! There is peace in its smell; I feel sleep coming already. Good-night, everybody.

From DRACULA *Bram Stoker*

8. —"O Amelia, my dear, this does everything crown!
   Who could have supposed I should meet you in Town?
   And whence such fair garments, such prosperi-ty"—
   "O didn't you know I'd been ruined?" said she.

   —"You left us in tatters, without shoes or socks,
   Tired of digging potatoes, and spudding up docks;
   And now you've gay bracelets and bright feathers three!"—
   "Yes: that's how we dress when we're ruined," said she.

   —"At home in the barton you said 'thee' and 'thou,'
   And 'this oon,' and 'theas oon,' and 't'other;' but now
   Your talking quite fits 'ee for high compa-ny!"—
   "Some polish is gained with one's ruin," said she.

   —"Your hands were like paws then, your face blue and bleak
   But now I'm bewitched by your delicate cheek,
   And your little gloves fit as on any la-dy!"—
   "We never do work when we're ruined," said she.

   —"You used to call home-life a hag-ridden dream.
   And you'd sigh, and you'd sock; but at present you seem
   To know not of megrims or melancho-ly!"—
   "True. One's pretty lively when ruined," said she.

   —"I wish I had feathers, a fine sweeping gown,
   And a delicate face, and could strut about Town!"—
   "My dear—a raw country girl, such as you be,
   Cannot quite expect that. You ain't ruined," said she.

THE RUINED MAID *Thomas Hardy*

Index of Names and Topics

Index of Authors and Selections